# The Sourcebook for
# Clinical Research

# The Sourcebook
# for Clinical Research
## A Practical Guide for Study Conduct

**Natasha Martien**

**Jeff Nelligan**

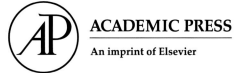

ELSEVIER

ACADEMIC PRESS
An imprint of Elsevier

Academic Press is an imprint of Elsevier
125 London Wall, London EC2Y 5AS, United Kingdom
525 B Street, Suite 1650, San Diego, CA 92101, United States
50 Hampshire Street, 5th Floor, Cambridge, MA 02139, United States
The Boulevard, Langford Lane, Kidlington, Oxford OX5 1GB, United Kingdom

**Notices**
Knowledge and best practice in this field are constantly changing. As new research and experience broaden our understanding, changes in research methods, professional practices, or medical treatment may become necessary.

Practitioners and researchers must always rely on their own experience and knowledge in evaluating and using any information, methods, compounds, or experiments described herein. In using such information or methods they should be mindful of their own safety and the safety of others, including parties for whom they have a professional responsibility.

To the fullest extent of the law, neither the Publisher nor the authors, contributors, or editors, assume any liability for any injury and/or damage to persons or property as a matter of products liability, negligence or otherwise, or from any use or operation of any methods, products, instructions, or ideas contained in the material herein.

**Library of Congress Cataloging-in-Publication Data**
A catalog record for this book is available from the Library of Congress

**British Library Cataloguing-in-Publication Data**
A catalogue record for this book is available from the British Library

ISBN: 978-0-12-816242-2

For information on all Academic Press publications
visit our website at https://www.elsevier.com/books-and-journals

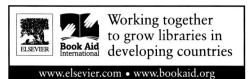

ELSEVIER · Book Aid International
Working together to grow libraries in developing countries
www.elsevier.com · www.bookaid.org

*Publisher:* Andre G. Wolff
*Acquisition Editor:* Erin Hill-Parks
*Editorial Project Manager:* Samuel Young
*Production Project Manager:* Punithavathy Govindaradjane
*Cover Designer:* Mark Rogers

Typeset by SPi Global, India

# Dedication

This book is dedicated to my two beloved children, Dillon and Alexis, and to all of my wonderful friends in Annapolis who bring so much happiness into my life.

**Natasha Martien**

# Contents

**Appendixes Found on Companion Website**
(https://www.elsevier.com/books-and-journals/book-companion/9780128162422)

1. Adverse Events Plus Reporting Table
2. Research Coordinator Work Queue
3. Feasibility Analysis Checklist
4. Contract Content Checklist
5. Consent Form Template
    5.A. New Common Rule Consent Form Template
6. Per Patient Budget Template
7. Cost Reimbursable Budget Template
8. MACs by State List (2016)
9. IDE—JH and JL—Submission Checklist
10. IDE Study Criteria Checklist and Crosswalk Table
11. ClinicalTrials.gov NIH Applicable Clinical Trial Checklist

(Please note that the URL may change over time. For any updates, please see the book's main webpage at the online Elsevier Store.)

# About the Authors

**Natasha Martien**, MBA, CCRP, SSBBP, CRCP, is a Human Subjects Research regulatory expert with 25 years of clinical research and healthcare management experience at institutes including Johns Hopkins Hospital, The Center for Cardiac and Vascular Research, and Scripps Clinic and Research Foundation. Martien has performed every operational role in clinical research at sites, including: training IRB members, Investigators, and Research Coordinators; regulatory management; working for an Office of Human Research Protections supporting an IRB; Research Coordination; writing and negotiating clinical trial agreements and budgets; financial management and billing; Coverage Analysis; CTMS acquisition; data analysis; credentialing; Quality Assurance; writing consent forms and study materials; compliance; advertising and recruiting; and the creation of a Clinical Trials Office. Martien has conducted and managed Investigator-Initiated, Industry- and Grant-funded studies in 24 medical disciplines and for a wide variety of study types, such as INDs, IDEs, biologics, stem cells, behavioral, pilot, observational, chart reviews, and clinical trial Phases I–IV.

**Jeff Nelligan**, J.D., is a Washington, D.C.-based executive with extensive healthcare oversight, regulatory, and finance experience in three Federal Cabinet agencies and in the Legislative branch, including: as a Director at the Centers for Medicare and Medicaid Services (CMS) within the U.S. Department of Health and Human Services; as a Managing Director at the U.S. Government Accountability Office (GAO); and as a senior staffer for three Members of Congress in the U.S. Senate and the U.S. House of Representatives. He is a graduate of Williams College and Georgetown University Law Center.

# Preface

## WHY THIS BOOK?

Despite more than $40 billion in annual funding for clinical trials worldwide, there is no comprehensive book for investigators, institutions, and research organizations which covers beginning, intermediate, and advanced topics in clinical research. And yet, a single study is invariably complex, with numerous federal regulations, administrative processes, medical procedures, time windows, and specific protocol instructions to follow.

This book provides a succinct, useful, and up-to-date roadmap to guide research professionals step-by-step through the clinical trial and clinical research labyrinth. Moreover, *The Sourcebook* is written in such a way as to be understood by a Ph.D., an M.D., nurse, research coordinator, pharmacist, institutional administrator, IRB members, data analysts, and back-office research support personnel.

*The Sourcebook for Clinical Research: A Practical Guide for Study Conduct* has the largest clinical research glossary of any website available today, and has more than 30 Appendix items, including templates, forms, checklists, and diagrams that the reader can customize and download for immediate use. Website can be found at https://www.elsevier.com/books-and-journals/book-companion/9780128162422. Please note that the URL may change over time. For any updates, please see the book's main webpage at the online Elsevier Store. In addition, this book provides knowledge and instruction on how to meet the demands of federal regulations in an urgent clinical situation.

## WHO IS THIS BOOK FOR?

- *Every member of an Investigative Team*
- *Practitioners* who desire to start working in research and have added a clinical trial to their practice but perhaps are not versed in the complexity of clinical trial regulations and project management;
- *Research professionals* who want to have one source they can use in order to stay in compliance with clinical research conduct;
- *The seasoned Principal Investigator* who occasionally needs answers to questions or/and needs guidance in advanced/complex topics;
- *Data Entry Specialists* who need to understand the full scope of trials to better understand the context and importance of their data input;
- *Pharmacists* who need understanding of research protocols and IND regulations;
- *Institutional Administrators/Directors/Managers*, who need to know the myriad of federal and state regulations and to have a sense of certainty the trials conducted under their purview are done so compliantly;
- *Institutional Review Board* members, who need expertise in regulations and ICH GCP to make determinations for the approval, revision or denial of research studies that are submitted;
- *Office of Human Research Protections personnel* within Institutions who must know the federal regulations and ICH GCP at an expert level;

- *Medical students* and other clinical research program students in the health care field;
- *Individuals* working toward a certification in clinical trials; and,
- *Students* pursuing college and graduate degrees in clinical research.

This long-needed book fills a void for the broad range of individuals involved in clinical trials and clinical research. Our hope is that this work serves as a quick, off-the-shelf resource for all research professionals.

**Natasha Martien**
**Jeff Nelligan**

# ICONS for The Sourcebook for Clinical Research: A Practical Guide for Study Conduct

 Take Note

 Warning

 Best Practice

 Consult your IRB

 Consult your Medical Center's Policies and Procedures

 Consult your state law

 ICH GCP reference (E6 R2)

# FOUNDATIONAL ELEMENTS AND REGULATORY REQUIREMENTS

# 1

*Purpose of chapter*:

- Describes the purpose of medical research
- Defines the Types of Research Studies
- Provides the definition of a Clinical Trial
- Explains how a Clinical Trial differs from Clinical Research
- Provides overview of Mandatory Regulations and Ethical Guidelines for Use in Clinical Research: Code of Federal Regulations and ICH GCP (International Council for Harmonisation Good Clinical Practice)
  **a.** Explains FDA versus HHS regulations
- Describes How to Secure a Clinical Trial and Market your Medical Facility to Sponsors
- Explains Principal Investigator Responsibilities
- Explains Research Coordinator Responsibilities
- Describes the Role of HIPAA and PHI in Clinical Research

## 1.1 WHAT IS THE PURPOSE OF MEDICAL RESEARCH?

*Purpose of section*:

- Explains why medical research is conducted

Clinical studies are designed to add to medical knowledge related to the treatment, diagnosis, and prevention of diseases or conditions. Some common reasons for conducting clinical studies include:

- Evaluating one or more interventions (for example, drugs, medical devices, approaches to surgery or radiation therapy) for treating a disease, syndrome, or condition;
- Discovering ways to prevent the initial development or recurrence of a disease or condition;
- Evaluating one or more interventions aimed at identifying or diagnosing a particular disease or condition;
- Examining methods for identifying a condition or the risk factors for that condition, and,
- Exploring and measuring ways to improve the comfort and quality of life through supportive care for people with a chronic illness.[1]

In these textbook-like bullet points, however, the heart and soul of why we conduct studies is not truly conveyed. When you are working in a hospital and see the pain in a patient's eyes, see their family grieving and anxious, or a child in a wheelchair with a shaved head, you want to do anything you can

The Sourcebook for Clinical Research. https://doi.org/10.1016/B978-0-12-816242-2.00001-1

to help. You want to find a cure for what afflicts the people in your care. You want to relieve a family of its burdens. When you see up close this suffering and anxiety, it becomes very easy to understand why medical research is conducted: to find relief or better treatments, so that people can lead a better quality of life or so they can continue to live.

## 1.2  DEFINING THE TYPES OF RESEARCH STUDIES

*Purpose of section*:

- Defines the various types of research studies
- Defines the term "clinical trial"
- Explains the difference between a clinical trial and clinical research

### Types of research studies

1. Adaptive clinical trial

An Adaptive Design Clinical Study is a study that includes a prospectively planned opportunity for modification of one or more specified aspects of the study design and hypotheses based on analysis of data (usually interim data) from subjects in the study. Analyses of the accumulating study data are performed at prospectively planned time points within the study, can be performed in a fully blinded manner or in an unblinded manner (see Chapter 4, Section 4.3 for definitions), and can occur with or without formal statistical hypothesis testing.[2]

An adaptation can be a revision to any part of the protocol. Examples include the eligibility criteria; the treatment duration; the lab tests required; sample size; the data-monitoring schedule; or, statistical analysis.

2. Ascending dose studies

a. Single ascending dose (SAD)

"Single ascending dose" is a part of the clinical trial design for Phase I trials. The SAD tests what the maximum tolerated IND (Investigational New Drug) dose is for subjects. When approximately 1/3 of research subjects experience unacceptable toxicity, the maximum tolerated dose is declared. SAD also serves to identify side effects.

b. Multiple ascending dose (MAD)

After these SAD results are documented, "multiple ascending dose" testing begins. MAD utilizes pharmacokinetics (PK) and pharmacodynamics (PD) to test the safety and tolerability of multiple low doses of an IND. MAD also serves to identify side effects.

3. Blinded study

A study in which the subject, the investigator, or anyone assessing the outcome is unaware of the treatment assignment(s). NOTE: Blinding is used to reduce the potential for bias.[3]

With single blinding, the patient is unaware which treatment he is receiving, while with double blinding, neither the patient nor the investigator knows which treatment is planned… The highest possible degree of blinding should always be selected. The study statistician should also remain blinded until the details of the evaluation have finally been specified.[4]

4. Case-control study

A case-control study is a retrospective observational study conducted to assess the exposure to a risk factor (or risk factors) in two separate cohorts. The cohorts are (comprised of) patients who have a disease or outcome of interest, known as "cases," and patients who do not have the disease or outcome of interest, known as "controls." The case-control study aims to determine the relationship between the risk factor(s) and the disease by comparing how often the patients in each cohort have been exposed to the risk factor(s).

5. Case series study

A case series study (also known as a clinical series study) tracks patients with a known exposure (e.g., to a toxic environmental substance, or to a type of drug, or to second-hand smoke). Patients can be tracked through a collection of reports or through medical chart reviews that compare exposure to health outcomes.

6. Clinical research

Clinical research is medical research that involves people to test new treatments and therapies.[5]

*Types of clinical research*

Clinical studies include both interventional (or experimental) studies and non-interventional (or observational) studies. A clinical drug study is an interventional clinical study, which NIH, in explanatory text on the NIH website, defines according to §4 Paragraph 23 of the Medicines Act [Arzneimittelgesetz; AMG] as "any study performed on man with the purpose of studying or demonstrating the clinical or pharmacological effects of drugs, to establish side effects, or to investigate absorption, distribution, metabolism or elimination, with the aim of providing clear evidence of the efficacy or safety of the drug."

Interventional studies also include studies on medical devices and studies in which surgical, physical, or psychotherapeutic procedures are examined. In contrast to clinical studies, §4 Paragraph 23 of the AMG describes non-interventional studies as follows: "A non-interventional study is a study in the context of which knowledge from the treatment of persons with drugs in accordance with the instructions for use specified in their registration is analyzed using epidemiological methods. The diagnosis, treatment and monitoring are not performed according to a previously specified study protocol, but exclusively according to medical practice."[6]

7. Cohort study

Study of a group of individuals, some of whom are exposed to a variable of interest, in which subjects are followed over time. Cohort studies can be prospective or retrospective.[7]

8. Cross-sectional study

A cross-sectional study is an observational study that takes place at one specific point in time. This is often described as taking a "snapshot." The cross-sectional study is conducted in order to assess the prevailing exposure and disease characteristics in a given population. The subjects are grouped into cohorts whose members share characteristics such as socioeconomic status, educational background, and ethnicity while the subjects vary on one key characteristic such as age.

9. Crossover study

A trial design for which subjects function as their own control and are assigned to receive investigational product and controls in an order determined by randomizations, typically with a washout period between the two products.[8]

The crossover design is, by far, the most common type of repeated measures design. In an experiment with two treatments, the subjects would be randomized into two groups. The first group would be given treatment A followed by treatment B, the second would be given treatment B followed by treatment A. It is also possible to test more than two conditions, if required, and this experiment meets the requirements of randomization, manipulation and control shown in Fig. 1.1.

Like all repeated measures designs, this reduces the chance of variation between individuals.[9]

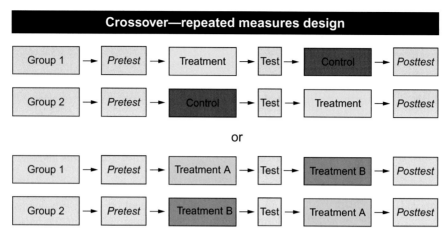

**FIG. 1.1**

Crossover-repeated measures design.

10. Decedent research

Decedent research is medical research conducted with the use of deceased persons' protected health information. (Note, this is different from "cadaver research.") See Chapter 6, Section 6.4.

11. Epidemiology studies

Epidemiology is the method used to find the causes of health outcomes and diseases in populations. In epidemiology, the patient is the community and individuals are viewed collectively. By definition, epidemiology is the study (scientific, systematic, and data-driven) of the distribution (frequency, pattern) and determinants (causes, risk factors) of health-related states and events (not just diseases) in specified populations (neighborhood, school, city, state, country, global). It is also the application of this study to the control of health problems (Source: *Principles of Epidemiology, 3rd Edition* ). Examples of public health problems or events that can elicit an epidemiology study may include environmental exposures, infectious diseases, homicides in a community, increase in a major birth defect or type of cancer, natural disasters, and terrorism (see Fig. 1.2).[10]

12. Field trials

Field trials are experimental studies that are conducted "in the field." This means that study personnel travel to a subject's home, school, or workplace. These trials are often used to study common diseases (such as diabetes and heart disease) and disease prevention.

13. ex vivo/in vitro

These are studies that are conducted outside of a living body or in an artificial environment outside of a living organism, such as a test tube.

14. First-in-man study

A first-in-man study is an exploratory study that occurs after lab testing or/and animal testing. It can also be called a "Phase 0" study. Only a few small doses (This can be known as microdosing.) of a new drug are tested in fewer than 15 people for a very short time, such as 7 days. The purpose is to test how a new drug acts in the human body. FDA Exploratory IND Studies Guidance and the American Cancer Society at www.cancer.org.

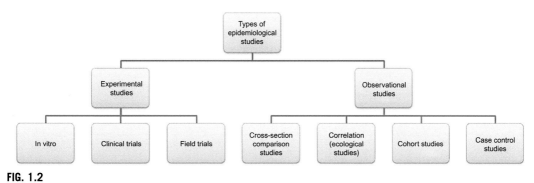

**FIG. 1.2**

Types of epidemiological studies.

15. Investigational device exemption (IDE)

Medical devices researched for human use

A medical device is "an instrument, apparatus, implement, machine, contrivance, implant, in vitro reagent, or other similar or related article, including a component part, or accessory which is:

- recognized in the official National Formulary, or the United States Pharmacopoeia, or any supplement to them,
- intended for use in the diagnosis of disease or other conditions, or in the cure, mitigation, treatment, or prevention of disease, in man or other animals, or
- intended to affect the structure or any function of the body of man or other animals, and which does not achieve any of its primary intended purposes through chemical action within or on the body of man or other animals and which is not dependent upon being metabolized for the achievement of any of its primary intended purposes."[11]

An approved IDE permits a device that otherwise would be required to comply with a performance standard or to have premarket approval to be shipped lawfully for the purpose of conducting investigations of that device. 21 CFR 812.1(a).[12]

An IDE is required for Significant Risk Device Studies. Non-significant risk devices do not require an IDE. A "Significant Risk Device means an investigational device that:

**(1)** Is intended as an implant and presents a potential for serious risk to the health, safety, or welfare of a subject;

**(2)** Is purported or represented to be for a use in supporting or sustaining human life and presents a potential for serious risk to the health, safety, or welfare of a subject;

**(3)** Is for a use of substantial importance in diagnosing, curing, mitigating, or treating disease, or otherwise preventing impairment of human health and presents a potential for serious risk to the health, safety, or welfare of a subject; or

**(4)** Otherwise presents a potential for serious risk to the health, safety, or welfare of a subject." 21 CFR 812.3(m).

16. In vivo

"In vivo" refers to a study that is carried out in a living organism.

17. Longitudinal study

An observational study in which participants are studied over time, with data being collected at multiple intervals.[13] Note: There is no clarity in research definitions regarding the length of time. Longitudinal studies can run from months to decades. The most common usage is a time period of years to decades.

18. Medical device pivotal study

A medical device pivotal study is a definitive study in which evidence is gathered to support the safety and effectiveness evaluation of the medical device for its intended use.

Evidence from one or more pivotal clinical studies generally serves as the primary basis for the determination of reasonable assurance of safety and effectiveness of the medical device of a Premarket Approval Application (PMA) and FDA's overall benefit-risk determination.[14]

19. Meta-analysis study

A Meta-analysis will thoroughly examine a number of valid studies on a topic and mathematically combine the results using accepted statistical methodology to report the results as if it were one large study.[15]

20. Multicenter trial

A clinical trial (one particular protocol) conducted at multiple medical centers

21. N-of-1 study

A trial in which an individual subject is administered a treatment repeatedly over a number of episodes to establish the treatment's effect in that person, often with the order of experimental and control treatments randomized.[16]

22. Nested case-control study (NCC)

A nested case-control study is a type of case-control study that draws its cases and controls from a cohort population that has been followed for a period of time. The investigator compares the exposure frequencies in cases and controls.[17]

23. Non-blinded trial

A clinical trial or other experiment in which the researchers know what treatments are being given to each study subject or experimental group. If human subjects are involved, they know what treatments they are receiving.[18]

24. Non-randomized trial—also known as a quasi-experiment trial

A clinical trial in which the participants are not assigned by chance to different treatment groups. Participants may choose which group they want to be in, or they may be assigned to the groups by the researchers.[19]

25. Open label trial

Describes a clinical trial in which masking is not used. This means that all parties involved in the trial (including participants) know which participants have been assigned to which interventions.[20]

26. Palliative care trials

Palliative Care Trials are also known as Quality-of-Life Trials. They are for subjects with serious illnesses. Their purpose is to provide relief from symptoms, pain, and stress. There is also a holistic focus in these trials that attempt to improve the quality of life of the subjects' families who function as caregivers. Activities such as mental health counseling, support groups, exercise, art therapy, acupuncture, and more can be included in this type of trial.

27. Parallel study

A parallel study is a type of clinical trial in which two or more groups of participants receive different interventions. For example, a "two-arm parallel" design involves two groups of participants. One group receives drug A, and the other group receives drug B. So during the trial, participants in one group receive drug A "in parallel" to participants in the other group, who receive drug B.[21]

28. Non-therapeutic research

This is research that is unlikely to produce a diagnostic, preventive, or therapeutic benefit to current subjects, which might benefit patients with a similar condition in the future.[22]

Non-Therapeutic Research Study examples include:

**Ancillary studies**: These studies are stimulated by, but are not a required part of, a main clinical trial/study that utilizes patients or other resources of the main study to generate relevant information. Ancillary studies must be linked to an active clinical research study and should include only patients accrued to that clinical research study.

**Interventional studies**: Clinical Research Category in which individuals are assigned by an investigator based on a protocol to receive specific interventions. The participant may receive diagnostic, therapeutic, behavioral, or other types of interventions. The assignment of the intervention may or may not be random. The participants are followed and biomedical and/or health outcomes are assessed. Only a subset of non-therapeutic research is designated as interventional. Usually, non-therapeutic interventional studies are biobehavioral in nature.

**Observational studies**: Clinical Research Category in which the studies focus on cancer patients and healthy populations that involve no intervention or alteration in the status of the participants. Biomedical and/or health outcome(s) are assessed in pre-defined groups of participants. The participants in the study may receive diagnostic, therapeutic, or other interventions, but the investigator of the observational study is not responsible for assigning specific interventions to the participants of the study. Epidemiological studies are often included in this research category.

**Prevention studies**: Protocols designed to assess one or more interventions aimed at preventing the development of a specific disease or health condition. The efficacy of smoking cessation groups would be an example of this kind of study.

**Screening studies**: Protocol designed to assess or examine methods of identifying a condition (or risk factor for a condition) in people who are not yet known to have the condition (or risk factor).

**Supportive care studies**: Protocol designed to evaluate one or more interventions where the primary intent is to maximize comfort, minimize side effects, or mitigate against a decline in the participant's health or function. In general, supportive care interventions are not intended to cure a disease. Cognitive behavioral stress management programs designed to reduce stress in cancer patients are usually categorized as supportive care studies.[23]

29. Phase 0 trials

First-in-human trials, in a small number of subjects, which are conducted before Phase 1 trials and are intended to assess new candidate therapeutic and imaging agents. The study agent is administered at a low dose for a limited time, and there is no therapeutic or diagnostic intent. (NOTE: FDA Guidance for Industry, Investigators, and Reviewers: Exploratory IND Studies, January 2006 classifies such studies as (early in) Phase 1. NOTE: A Phase 0 study might not include any drug delivery but may be an exploration of human material from a study (e.g., tissue samples or biomarker determinations).)[24]

30. Phase 1 trials

An experimental drug or treatment in a small group of people (20–80) for the first time. The purpose is to evaluate its safety and identify side effects. The length is several months.[25]

31. Phase 2 trials

The experimental drug or treatment is administered to a larger group of people (100–300) to determine its effectiveness and to further evaluate its safety. The length is several months to 2 years.[26]

32. Phase 2A & 2B trials

- Phase IIA is specifically designed to assess dosing requirements (how much drug should be given).
- Phase IIB is specifically designed to study efficacy (how well the drug works at the prescribed dose(s)).

33. Phase 3 trials

The experimental drug or treatment is administered to large groups of people (1000–3000) to confirm its effectiveness, monitor side effects, and to compare it with standard or equivalent treatments. The length is 1–4 years.[27]

34. Phase 4 trials

After a drug is licensed and approved by the FDA researchers track its safety, seeking more information about its risks, benefits, and optimal use.[28]

35. Pilot study (also known as a Pilot Project or Pilot Experiment)

A pilot study is a small-scale administrative study. The purpose of conducting a pilot study is to examine the feasibility of an approach that is intended to be used in a larger-scale study. For example, a pilot study can be used to evaluate the feasibility of recruitment, randomization, retention, assessment procedures, new methods, and implementation of the novel intervention. A pilot study is not a hypothesis testing study. Safety, efficacy, and effectiveness are not evaluated in a pilot. Pilot results can inform feasibility and identify modifications needed in the design of a larger, ensuing hypothesis testing study.[29]

36. Preclinical studies

Animal studies that support Phase 1 safety and tolerance studies and must comply with good laboratory practice (GLP) NOTE: Data about a drug's activities and effects in animals help establish boundaries for safe use of the drug in subsequent human testing (clinical studies or trials).[30]

37. Prospective

Prospective is an adjective meaning "of or in the future." In clinical research, this means that research activities will occur in the future (and have not occurred yet).

38. Randomized controlled trial (RCT)

A randomized controlled trial is considered the "gold standard" for a clinical trial. Subjects are assigned to one or more interventions through a random process analogous to flipping a coin. One of the interventions is the control, which may be a placebo (e.g., a sugar pill) or the standard of care treatment. The other intervention is the investigational element, such as an investigational new drug or investigational device. Responses to the interventions are compared.

39. Repeated measures design

In a repeated measures design study, all subjects receive all treatments. Each subject is randomly assigned to a sequence of treatments as well as the control.

40. Retrospective

Retrospective means "directed backward" or "directed to the past." In clinical research, this adjective is usually used in conjunction with chart reviews, as in "retrospective chart reviews" meaning that a study is conducted that examines medical chart information from patients visits that have already occurred.

41. Time series study

A time series study is a quasiexperimental research design in which periodic measurements are taken on a defined group of individuals both before and after implementation of an intervention.

42. Uncontrolled study

A clinical study that lacks a comparison (i.e., a control) group. https://www.cancer.gov/.

43. Vaccine trial

A vaccine trial is a clinical trial that purposes to confirm the safety and efficacy of a vaccine prior to it being licensed. A vaccine trial is considered an IND, and therefore, is conducted through Phase I–IV trials.

44. Clinical trial

A research study in which one or more human subjects are prospectively assigned to one or more interventions (which may include placebo or other control) to evaluate the effects of those interventions on health-related biomedical or behavioral outcomes (Fig. 1.3 and Table 1.1).[31]

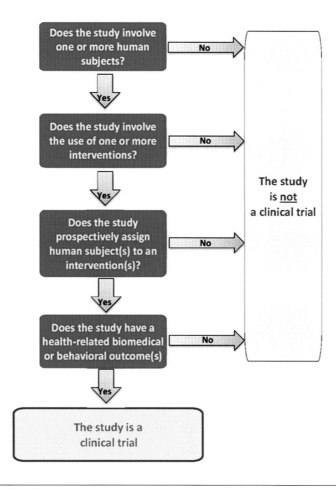

**FIG. 1.3**

Clinical trial determination diagram.

The difference between a clinical trial and clinical research/a clinical study:

**Table 1.1  Clinical Trial vs. Clinical Research**

| Clinical Trial | Clinical Research |
|---|---|
| A **clinical trial** is a research study in which one or more human subjects are prospectively assigned to one or more interventions (which may include placebo or other control) to evaluate the effects of those interventions on health-related biomedical or behavioral outcomes. NIH<br><br>A **clinical trial** is one type of clinical research that follows a predefined plan or protocol. NIH | **Clinical research** is medical research that involves people to test new treatments and therapies. NIH<br><br>**Clinical research** aims to advance medical knowledge by studying people, either through direct interaction or through the collection and analysis of blood, tissues, or other samples. NIH |

As you can see, in the United States, there is a distinct difference between a "clinical trial" and "clinical research," and a "clinical study" is not the same as a "clinical trial." A clinical study takes on the definition of "clinical research." These distinctions are important for the applicability of certain regulations, such as NCD 310.1 (see Chapter 2, Section 2.8).

For the international community, a "clinical trial" and "clinical study" have the same meaning.

꒐ᴵᶜᴴ**1.12 Clinical Trial/Study**

Any investigation in human subjects intended to discover or verify the clinical, pharmacological, and/or other pharmacodynamic effects of an investigational product(s), and/or to identify any adverse reactions to an investigational product(s), and/or to study absorption, distribution, metabolism, and excretion of an investigational product(s) with the object of ascertaining its safety and/or efficacy. The terms clinical trial and clinical study are synonymous.[32]

## 1.3  MANDATORY REGULATIONS AND ICH GCP (INTERNATIONAL COUNCIL FOR HARMONISATION GOOD CLINICAL PRACTICE) ETHICAL GUIDELINES

*Purpose of section*:

- Explains the difference between FDA and HHS regulations
- References ICH GCP ethical guidelines
- Reviews the key regulations for clinical research
- Identifies important Guidance documents for clinical research.

There are two different sets of human subjects protections federal regulations, which govern clinical trials in the United States, those which emanate from the U.S. Department of Health and Human Services (HHS), and those from the U.S. Food and Drug Administration (FDA), which is a division within HHS.

While this can lead to confusion, below is the information you need on what Federal regulation you should follow under what circumstances.

The FDA regulations for human subject protections are found at 21 CFR 50 and the FDA regulations for Institutional Review Boards are found at 21 CFR 56.

**Table 1.2  FDA vs. HHS Regulations**

| FDA Regulations | HHS Regulations |
|---|---|
| 21 CFR 50.1 Scope | 45 CFR 46.101 Scope |
| (a) This part applies to all clinical investigations regulated by the Food and Drug Administration under sections 505(i) and 520(g) of the Federal Food, Drug, and Cosmetic Act, as well as clinical investigations that support applications for research or marketing permits for products regulated by the Food and Drug Administration, including foods, including dietary supplements, that bear a nutrient content claim or a health claim, infant formulas, food and color additives, drugs for human use, medical devices for human use, biological products for human use, and electronic products… Compliance with these parts is intended to protect the rights and safety of subjects involved in investigations filed with the Food and Drug Administration… | All research involving human subjects conducted or supported by HHS or conducted in an institution that agrees to assume responsibility for the research in accordance with 45 CFR 46 regardless of the source of funding |
| 21 CFR 56.101 Scope | |
| IRBs that review clinical investigations regulated by the FDA under sections 505(i), 507(d), and 520(g) of the act, as well as clinical investigations that support applications for research or marketing permits for products regulated by the FDA, including food and color additives, drugs for human use, medical devices for human use, biological products for human use, and electronic products | |

The HHS regulations for human subject protections are found at 45 CFR 46.

The full scopes are in Table 1.2.

HHS is the umbrella or parent institution for 11 Agencies, namely: the Administration for Children and Families (ACF); the Administration for Community Living (ACL); the Agency for Healthcare Research and Quality (AHRQ), the Agency for Toxic Substances and Disease Registry (ATSDR), the Centers for Disease Control and Prevention (CDC), the Centers for Medicare and Medicaid Services (CMS), the Food and Drug Administration (FDA), the Health Resources and Services Administration (HRSA), the Indian Health Service (HIS), the National Institutes of Health (NIH), and the Substance Abuse and Mental Health Services Administration (SAMHA).

*The HHS regulations require assurances and certifications from the grantee institution. FDA regulations generally require assurances of compliance from either or both the sponsor of the research and the clinical investigator.* www.fda.gov.

Your Institution should have a Federal Wide Assurance, otherwise known as an "FWA" through your IRB. The FWA is a written assurance from your institution to the HHS Office of Human Research Protections (OHRP) confirming that your institution will comply with The Common Rule (which is 45 CFR 46 Subpart A). The FWA is legally binding.

Which regulation, **FDA** or **HHS**, do you follow for a particular study?

If you are conducting an IND or IDE clinical trial, you must follow the FDA regulations. Additionally, if the study purposes to support a marketing application, or if the study incorporates a product regulated by the FDA, the FDA regulations must be followed.

If you are conducting a study that is funded by NIH or a division of NIH (including a subaward where NIH is the Primary Sponsor and a university hospital is the Primary Recipient and your Institution is the Secondary Recipient), and there is no IND or IDE in the research, and the research does NOT intend to pursue a marketing application, you will follow 45 CFR 46. In tandem, any research for which there is NO IND or IDE and NO purpose of supporting a marketing application, you will follow 45 CFR 46.

If the study involves an FDA-regulated product and is conducted or supported by HHS (i.e., NIH), both the FDA regulations and HHS human subject protection regulations apply. For example, 21 CFR 50, 54, 56, 312 or 812 … and 45 CFR 46.

In addition, if your study has any of the following types of (vulnerable) subjects, you will ALSO need to follow the 45 CFR 46 regulations beyond the Common Rule in Subparts B through E as applicable:

- Pregnant women
- Human Fetuses
- Neonates
- Prisoners
- Children

> When there is a question as to which regulation should be followed, the strictest regulation is the one that takes precedence.

The 21 CFR 50 and 45 CFR 46 Subpart A regulations mirror each other's language in a lot of ways and differ in others. Of note, 45 CFR 46 Subpart A, "The Common Rule", is a nickname for "The Federal Policy for the Protection of Human Subjects."

Below is the url that delineates the differences between the FDA and HHS regulations, namely, between 21 CFR 56 and 21 CFR 50 in comparison to 45 CFR 46: https://www.fda.gov/ScienceResearch/SpecialTopics/RunningClinicalTrials/EducationalMaterials/ucm112910.htm.

There are more regulations that can apply dependent upon the type of research you are performing. A list is given in Table 1.3.

**Table 1.3  Regulations to Follow**

| Code of Federal Regulations | Title | Most current issue |
|---|---|---|
| 21 CFR 11 | Electronic Records; Electronic Signatures | Revised as of April 1, 2017 |
| 21 CFR 50 | Protection of Human Subjects | Revised as of April 1, 2017 |
| 21 CFR 54 | Financial Disclosure by Clinical Investigators | Revised as of April 1, 2017 |
| 21 CFR 56 | Institutional Review Boards | Revised as of April 1, 2017 |
| 21 CFR 312 | Investigational New Drug Application | Revised as of April 1, 2017 |
| 21 CFR 314 | Applications for FDA Approval to Market a New Drug | Revised as of April 1, 2017 |
| 21 CFR 812 | Investigational Device Exemption | Revised as of April 1, 2017 |
| 21 CFR 814 | Premarket Approval of Medical Devices | Revised as of April 1, 2017 |
| 42 CFR 11 | ClinicalTrials.gov regulations | Revised as of April 1, 2017 |
| 45 CFR 46 | Protection of Human Subjects | Interim Final Rule—January 19, 2018 |
| 45 CFR 164, Subpart A | Security and Privacy, Subpart A—General Provisions, Subpart E—Privacy of Individually Identifiable Health Information | [e-CFR] August 8, 2017 |
| 45 CFR 160 | General Administrative Requirements | [e-CFR] August 8, 2017 |

The Privacy Rule is located at 45 CFR Part 160 and Subparts A and E of Part 164.[33]

## ICH GCP E6 R2

⅄ᴵᶜᴴ INTERNATIONAL COUNCIL FOR HARMONISATION OF TECHNICAL REQUIREMENTS FOR PHARMACEUTICALS FOR HUMAN USE (ICH)
　　INTEGRATED ADDENDUM TO ICH E6(R1):
　　GUIDELINE FOR GOOD CLINICAL PRACTICE E6(R2)
　　Current Step 4 version, Dated 9 November 2016
　　"Good Clinical Practice (GCP) is an international ethical and scientific quality standard for designing, conducting, recording and reporting trials that involve the participation of human subjects. Compliance with this standard provides public assurance that the rights, safety and well-being of trial subjects are protected, consistent with the principles that have their origin in the Declaration of Helsinki, and that the clinical trial data are credible. The objective of this ICH GCP Guideline is to provide a unified standard for the European Union (EU), Japan and the United States to facilitate the mutual acceptance of clinical data by the regulatory authorities in these jurisdictions."
　　ICH GCP E6 R2 references are made throughout the book. The link to the full document is: http://www.ich.org/fileadmin/Public_Web_Site/ICH_Products/Guidelines/Efficacy/E6/E6_R2__Step_4.pdf.

GRANTS
See Tables 1.4 and 1.5.

**Table 1.4　Grant Regulations to Follow**

This regulation took the place of all the Circulars written below and went into effect on 12/26/14.

| Code of Federal Regulations | Title |
|---|---|
| 2 CFR 200 | Uniform Administrative Requirements, Cost Principles, and Audit Requirements for Federal Awards |
| OMB Circular A-21 | Cost Principles for Educational Institutions |
| OMB Circular A-133 | Audits of States, Local Governments, and Non-Profit Organizations |
| OMB Circular A-110 | Uniform Administrative Requirements for Grants and Agreements With Institutions of Higher Education, Hospitals, and Other Non-Profit Organizations |
| OMB Circular A-50 | Audit Follow-up |
| OMB Circular A-102 | Grants and Cooperative Agreements with State and Local Government Organizations |
| OMB Circular A-122 | Cost Principles for Non-Profit Organizations |
| 45 CFR 74, Appendix E | Cost Principles |

**Table 1.5  Guidance Documents List**

*GUIDANCE DOCUMENTS*

**For the online list: http://www.fda.gov/RegulatoryInformation/Guidances/ucm122046.htm**

| | |
|---|---|
| Part 11, Electronic Records: Electronic Signatures—Scope and Application | August 2003 |
| Adverse Event Reporting to IRBs—Improving Human Subject Protection | January 2009 |
| Process for Handling Referrals to FDA Under 21 CFR 50.54—Additional Safeguards for Children in Clinical Investigations | December 2006 |
| Submitting and Reviewing Complete Responses to Clinical Holds | October 2000 |
| The Establishment and Operation of Clinical Trial Data Monitoring Committees for Clinical Trial Sponsors | March 2006 (expires 12/31/18) |
| Data Retention When Subjects Withdraw from FDA-Regulated Clinical Trials | October 2008 |
| Exception from Informed Consent Requirements for Emergency Research | April 2013 |
| Financial Disclosure by Clinical Investigators | February 2013 |
| Oversight of Clinical Investigations—A Risk-Based Approach to Monitoring | August 2013 |
| Patient-Reported Outcome Measures: Use in Medical Product Development to Support Labeling Claims | December 2009 |
| Collection of Race and Ethnicity Data in Clinical Trials | September 2005 |
| Using a Centralized IRB Review Process in Multicenter Clinical Trials | March 2006 |
| Considerations When Transferring Clinical Investigation Oversight to Another IRB | May 2014 |
| IRB Review of Stand-Alone HIPAA Authorizations Under FDA Regulations | October 21, 2003 |
| Questions and Answers on Informed Consent Elements, 21 CFR § 50.25(c) | February 2012 |
| IRB Continuing Review after Clinical Investigation Approval | February 2012 |
| IRB Responsibilities for Reviewing the Qualifications of Investigators, Adequacy of Research Sites, and the Determination of Whether an IND/IDE is Needed | August 2013 |
| The Use of Clinical Holds Following Clinical Investigator Misconduct | September 2004 |
| IND Exemptions for Studies of Lawfully Marketed Drug or Biological Products for the Treatment of Cancer | January 2004 |
| Providing Regulatory Submissions in Electronic Format—Human Pharmaceutical Product Applications and Related Submissions Using the eCTD Specifications | October 2005 |
| Safety Reporting Requirements for INDs and BA/BE Studies | December 2012 |
| Safety Reporting Requirements for INDs and BA/BE Studies—Small Entity Compliance Guide | December 2012 |
| Information Program on Clinical Trials for Serious or Life-Threatening Diseases and Conditions (Clinicaltrials.gov) | March 2002 |
| Guidance for HDE Holders, Institutional Review Boards (IRBs), Clinical Investigators, and FDA Staff—Humanitarian Device Exemption (HDE) Regulation: Questions and Answers | July 8, 2010 (expires 5/31/16) |
| Humanitarian Use Device (HUD) Designations | January 24, 2013 |
| Informed Consent for In Vitro Diagnostic Device Studies Using Leftover Human Specimens that are Not Individually Identifiable | April 25, 2006 |
| Computerized Systems Used in Clinical Investigations | May 2007 |

**Table 1.5    Guidance Documents List—cont'd**

*GUIDANCE DOCUMENTS*

**For the online list: http://www.fda.gov/RegulatoryInformation/Guidances/ucm122046.htm**

| | |
|---|---|
| Electronic Source Data in Clinical Investigations | September 2013 |
| Adaptive Design Clinical Trials for Drugs and Biologics | February 2010 |
| Information Sheet Guidance for IRBs, Clinical Investigators, and Sponsors FDA Inspections of Clinical Investigators | June 2010 |
| Investigator Responsibilities—Protecting the Rights, Safety, and Welfare of Study Subjects | October 2009 |
| Information Sheet Guidance for Sponsors, Clinical Investigators, and IRBs Frequently Asked Questions—Statement of Investigator (Form FDA 1572) Draft Guidance only—not finalized | July 2008 |
| Information Sheet Guidance for Institutional Review Boards, Clinical Investigators, and Sponsors: Clinical Investigator Administrative Actions—Disqualification | May 2010, Updated March 2014 |
| Providing Regulatory Submissions in Electronic Format—Submissions Under Section 745A(a) of the Federal Food, Drug, and Cosmetic Act | December 2014 |
| The Use of Clinical Holds Following Clinical Investigator Misconduct | September 2004 |
| Guidance for Industry Protecting the Rights, Safety, and Welfare of Study Subjects—Supervisory Responsibilities of Investigators | May 2007 |
| Investigational Device Exemptions (IDEs) for Early Feasibility Medical Device Clinical Studies, Including Certain First in Human (FIH) Studies: Guidance for Industry and Food and Drug Administration Staff | October 1, 2013 |
| Guidance on IDE Policies and Procedures | January 1998 |
| Investigators' Responsibilities for Significant Risk Device Investigations | November 1995 |
| Suggested Format for IDE Progress Report (Text Only) | Prior to February 1997 |
| Office of Device Evaluation Final Guidance Documents 2010-2017 (Repository of Device Guidance Documents) | 2010–17 |
| Information Sheet Guidance for IRBs, Clinical Investigators, and Sponsors FDA Inspections of Clinical Investigators | June 2010 |
| Investigator Responsibilities—Protecting the Rights, Safety, and Welfare of Study Subjects | October 2009 |
| Information Sheet Guidance for Sponsors, Clinical Investigators, and IRBs Frequently Asked Questions—Statement of Investigator (Form FDA 1572) Draft Guidance only—not finalized | July 2008 |
| Information Sheet Guidance for Institutional Review Boards, Clinical Investigators, and Sponsors | May 2010, Updated March 2014 |
| Clinical Investigator Administrative Actions—Disqualification | |
| Providing Regulatory Submissions in Electronic Format—Submissions Under Section 745A(a) of the Federal Food, Drug, and Cosmetic Act | December 2014 |
| The Use of Clinical Holds Following Clinical Investigator Misconduct | September 2004 |
| FDA Categorization of Investigational Device Exemption (IDE) Devices to Assist the Centers for Medicare and Medicaid Services (CMS) with Coverage Decisions | December 5, 2017 |

In Appendix 23, there are Quick Reference Pocket Cards that you can download, cut, laminate and carry with you for immediate reference to often-needed regulations, laws, and ICH GCP guidelines.

## 1.4 HOW TO SECURE A CLINICAL TRIAL AND HOW TO MARKET YOUR MEDICAL FACILITY TO SPONSORS

*Purpose of section*:

- How does the Principal Investigator secure a clinical trial?
- Who should he/she contact to secure a trial; who might contact a practitioner to offer a clinical trial?
- How to make your site attractive to Sponsors
- How to reach out to a Sponsor
- What to prepare and what to know when reaching out to a Sponsor

*How to secure a clinical trial*

If you are a physician or PhD and would like to start conducting clinical trials, the authors' first recommendations are that you:

**(1)** Read this book!
**(2)** Read through the complete ICH GCP E6 R2.
**(3)** Take a course and test on clinical trial conduct.
   **IRB** a. Most Institutions have an educational requirement prior to conducting research. Contact your IRB Office or Compliance Department.
**(4)** Volunteer as a sub-investigator on a study with a PI that has performed many clinical trials <u>AND</u> has an established study team (that has also performed many clinical trials).
   **a.** Observe. Ask questions. KNOW THE PROTOCOL EXTREMELY WELL.

If you are a physician or PhD wanting to receive an offer from a CRO or Sponsor to conduct a study as a PI at your site, reach out to CROs and Sponsors.

Do the following:

- Attend clinical research conferences. While at the event, be persistent in seeking out CROs and Sponsors and visit their vendor booths.
  - Leave your business card and an updated Clinical Trial Site Scorecard. See Appendix 34.
    - What is the Clinical Trial Site Scorecard? It's a handy, concise document that highlights the merits of your site and its experience in conducting past trials.
  - SOCRA, ACRP, and MAGI hold conferences. Also, exl events hosts weekly conferences on varying topics in healthcare and clinical research around the United States. Here are their websites:
    - www.socra.org
    - www.acrpnet.org
    - www.magiworld.org/events/
    - http://exlevents.com/event-calendar

- Call a few CROs. Tell them your therapeutic specialty. You will be connected to the division handling that therapeutic specialty. Introduce yourself and let them know of your interest.
  - A list of CRO names can be found here: http://nbscience.com/list-of-contract-research-organizations-cros/
- Publish or/and speak at conferences.
  - Make yourself known in your specialty.
- Ensure the website for your clinical trial site is top notch, kept updated, and telling of the:
  - Quality of care
  - Expertise of the physicians
  - State-of-the-art equipment available
  - Seasoned clinical research support staff

CROs will search their own, internal databases first and will then look to external websites to identify potential clinical trial sites.

**Your web presence should be compelling and inclusive of a research page.**

Reputational marketing

In order to be asked by a CRO or Sponsor to conduct more studies, you will need to provide evidence from studies you previously conducted that:

**(1)** You can recruit participants.
**(2)** You can meet enrollment targets.
**(3)** Your site has a good reputation.
   **a.** This means that:
      **i.** You know and practice "Good Clinical Practice" (ICH GCP).
      **ii.** You are highly skilled in your therapeutic specialty.
      **iii.** You have an efficient study startup process.
         **1.** Coordinated well and timely with the various Departments in your Institution
      **iv.** Your source data and study data match.
         **1.** Your site has been detail oriented and alert.
      **v.** You have a successful Quality Assurance program assuring human subjects protections.
      **vi.** Your data entry is excellent.
      **vii.** You have been ready for monitoring visits, with quickly resolved data queries.
      **viii.** You are vigilant in spotting Adverse Events and have followed proper reporting of AEs and SAEs.
      **ix.** You have sound project management!

How to market your clinical trial site

WEBSITE

As mentioned above, make sure the website for your clinical trial site is top notch, kept updated, and telling of the:

- Quality of care
- Expertise of the physicians
- State-of-the-art equipment available
- Seasoned clinical research support staff

## METRICS

Keep a database from which you can quickly run reports and pull metrics. Keep track of the:

- number of studies you have done
- number of subjects screened in each study
- number of subjects enrolled in each study
- amount of time it took from contract receipt to contract ratification
- amount of time it took from IRB submission to IRB approval
- amount of time it took from template budget receipt to final budget approval
- number of protocol deviations per study
- audits performed and results
- site turnover rate
- types of Electronic Data Capture (EDC) systems your site has used
- equipment available to the study team
- types of research studies performed, i.e., IND, IDE, behavioral, longitudinal, etc.
- Sponsor contacts
- CRO contacts

With the metrics you are tracking, use the Clinical Trial Site Scorecard, found in Appendix 34 to fill in the information and provide a professional report to CROs and Sponsors. This is your marketing tool to demonstrate what a top notch clinical trial site you are!

If your metrics are less than desirable, improve your site's project management and quality assurance programs, and culture, as necessary.

## WHERE TO FIND CROs, SPONSORS, and STUDIES

Begin with www.clinicaltrials.gov, where you can search by Clinical Study "Not yet recruiting" and "By Topic." Refine your search to your therapeutic specialty area and discover what trials are listed. When you click on a study name that is of interest, you can scroll down to the contacts section. The CRO or Sponsor contact information will be available.

Reach out! Ask the CRO or Sponsor contact if they are still looking for sites. If they are, tell them about your site and you and follow up in an e-mail with your Clinical Trial Site Scorecard.

If they already have all of their sites, let them know of your expertise in the designated therapeutic specialty and your interest in conducting other trials with them. Follow up in an e-mail with your Clinical Trial Site Scorecard and great appreciation for their time speaking with you.

## TOURS

Invite a CRO or Sponsor contact to visit you at your site and tour the facility and meet your staff. Offer a working lunch in which your staff are present. Have prepared talking points that each staff member will present to the CRO or Sponsor contact during the lunch speaking to what your site has to offer and what each of them brings to the table. (Make sure the ability to recruit and the recruitment strategy are one of the talking points.) Keep it friendly and relaxed. The CRO and Sponsor will want to know whether they can work with the various personalities while also assessing the facts and facility.

---

## 1.5 PRINCIPAL INVESTIGATOR (PI) RESPONSIBILITIES

*Purpose of section*:

- Outlines the qualifications needed by a Principal Investigator (PI) as noted in FDA and ICH GCP regulations

- Outlines PI responsibilities in the conduct of a trial

*Principal Investigator responsibilities and qualifications*

Principal Investigator responsibilities for PIs in the U.S. as well as abroad are outlined in in the International Council for Harmonisation Good Clinical Practice Guideline E6 R2, dated November 9, 2016.[34]

As determined by ICH GCP, following are the responsibilities and qualifications:

### 4.1. Investigator's Qualifications and Agreements

4.1.1. The investigator(s) should be qualified by education, training, and experience to assume responsibility for the proper conduct of the trial, should meet all the qualifications specified by the applicable regulatory requirement(s), and should provide evidence of such qualifications through up-to-date curriculum vitae and/or other relevant documentation requested by the sponsor, the IRB/IEC, and/or the regulatory authority(ies).

4.1.2. The investigator should be thoroughly familiar with the appropriate use of the investigational product(s), as described in the protocol, in the current Investigator's Brochure, in the product information and in other information sources provided by the sponsor.

4.1.3. The investigator should be aware of, and should comply with, GCP and the applicable regulatory requirements.

4.1.4. The investigator/institution should permit monitoring and auditing by the sponsor, and inspection by the appropriate regulatory authority(ies).

4.1.5. The investigator should maintain a list of appropriately qualified persons to whom the investigator has delegated significant trial-related duties.

### 4.2. Adequate resources

4.2.1. The investigator should be able to demonstrate (e.g., based on retrospective data) a potential for recruiting the required number of suitable subjects within the agreed recruitment period.

4.2.2. The investigator should have sufficient time to properly conduct and complete the trial within the agreed trial period.

4.2.3. The investigator should have available an adequate number of qualified staff and adequate facilities for the foreseen duration of the trial to conduct the trial properly and safely.

4.2.4. The investigator should ensure that all persons assisting with the trial are adequately informed about the protocol, the investigational product(s), and their trial-related duties and functions.

ADDENDUM

4.2.5. The investigator is responsible for supervising any individual or party to whom the investigator delegates trial-related duties and functions conducted at the trial site.

4.2.6. If the investigator/institution retains the services of any individual or party to perform trial-related duties and functions, the investigator/institution should ensure this individual or party is qualified to perform those trial-related duties and functions and should implement procedures to ensure the integrity of the trial-related duties and functions performed and any data generated.

### 4.3. Medical care of trial subjects

4.3.1. A qualified physician (or dentist, when appropriate), who is an investigator or a sub-investigator for the trial, should be responsible for all trial-related medical (or dental) decisions.

4.3.2. During and following a subject's participation in a trial, the investigator/institution should ensure that adequate medical care is provided to a subject for any adverse events, including clinically significant laboratory values, related to the trial. The investigator/institution should inform a subject when medical care is needed for intercurrent illness(es) of which the investigator becomes aware.

4.3.3. It is recommended that the investigator inform the subject's primary physician about the subject's participation in the trial if the subject has a primary physician and if the subject agrees to the primary physician being informed.

4.3.4. Although a subject is not obliged to give his/her reason(s) for withdrawing prematurely from a trial, the investigator should make a reasonable effort to ascertain the reason(s), while fully respecting the subject 's rights.

### 4.4. Communication with IRB/IEC

4.4.1. Before initiating a trial, the investigator/institution should have written and dated approval/favorable opinion from the IRB/IEC for the trial protocol, written informed consent form, consent form updates, subject recruitment procedures (e.g., advertisements), and any other written information to be provided to subjects.

4.4.2. As part of the investigator's/institution's written application to the IRB/IEC, the investigator/institution should provide the IRB/IEC with a current copy of the Investigator's Brochure. If the Investigator's Brochure is updated during the trial, the investigator/institution should supply a copy of the updated Investigator's Brochure to the IRB/IEC.

4.4.3. During the trial, the investigator/institution should provide to the IRB/IEC all documents subject to review.

### 4.5. Compliance with protocol

4.5.1 The investigator/institution should conduct the trial in compliance with the protocol agreed to by the sponsor and, if required, by the regulatory authority(ies) and which was given approval/favorable opinion by the IRB/IEC. The investigator/institution and the sponsor should sign the protocol, or an alternative contract, to confirm agreement.

4.5.2. The investigator should not implement any deviation from, or changes of the protocol without agreement by the sponsor and prior review and documented approval/favorable opinion from the IRB/IEC of an amendment, except where necessary to eliminate an immediate hazard(s) to trial subjects, or when the change(s) involves only logistical or administrative aspects of the trial (e.g., change in monitor(s), change of telephone number(s)).

4.5.3. The investigator, or person designated by the investigator, should document and explain any deviation from the approved protocol.

4.5.4. The investigator may implement a deviation from, or a change of, the protocol to eliminate an immediate hazard(s) to trial subjects without prior IRB/IEC approval/favorable opinion. As soon as possible, the implemented deviation or change, the reasons for it, and, if appropriate, the proposed protocol amendment(s) should be submitted:

**(a)** to the IRB/IEC for review and approval/favorable opinion,
**(b)** to the sponsor for agreement and, if required,
**(c)** to the regulatory authority(ies).

### 4.6. Investigational product(s)

4.6.1. Responsibility for investigational product(s) accountability at the trial site(s) rests with the investigator/institution.

4.6.2. Where allowed/required, the investigator/institution may/should assign some or all of the investigator's/institution's duties for investigational product(s) accountability at the trial site(s) to an appropriate pharmacist or another appropriate individual who is under the supervision of the investigator/institution.

4.6.3. The investigator/institution and/or a pharmacist or other appropriate individual, who is designated by the investigator/institution, should maintain records of the product's delivery to the trial site, the inventory at the site, the use by each subject, and the return to the sponsor or alternative disposition of unused product(s). These records should include dates, quantities, batch/serial numbers, expiration dates (if applicable), and the unique code numbers assigned to the investigational product(s) and trial subjects. Investigators should maintain records that document adequately that the subjects were provided the doses specified by the protocol and reconcile all investigational product(s) received from the sponsor.

4.6.4. The investigational product(s) should be stored as specified by the sponsor (see 5.13.2 and 5.14.3) and in accordance with applicable regulatory requirement(s).

4.6.5. The investigator should ensure that the investigational product(s) are used only in accordance with the approved protocol.

4.6.6. The investigator, or a person designated by the investigator/institution, should explain the correct use of the investigational product(s) to each subject and should check, at intervals appropriate for the trial, that each subject is following the instructions properly.

**4.7. Randomization procedures and unblinding**

The investigator should follow the trial's randomization procedures, if any, and should ensure that the code is broken only in accordance with the protocol. If the trial is blinded, the investigator should promptly document and explain to the sponsor any premature unblinding (e.g., accidental unblinding, unblinding due to a serious adverse event (SAE)) of the investigational product(s).

See the Informed Consent information in Chapter 2, Section 2.5 for the PI's responsibilities regarding consent.

**4.9. Records and Reports**

ADDENDUM

4.9.0. The investigator/institution should maintain adequate and accurate source documents and trial records that include all pertinent observations on each of the site's trial subjects. Source data should be attributable, legible, contemporaneous, original, accurate, and complete. Changes to source data should be traceable, should not obscure the original entry, and should be explained if necessary (e.g., via an audit trail).

4.9.1. The investigator should ensure the accuracy, completeness, legibility, and timeliness of the data reported to the sponsor in the CRFs and in all required reports.

4.9.2. Data reported on the CRF, that are derived from source documents, should be consistent with the source documents or the discrepancies should be explained.

4.9.3. Any change or correction to a CRF should be **dated, initialed, and explained** (if necessary) and should not obscure the original entry (i.e., an audit trail should be maintained); this applies to both written and electronic changes or corrections (see 5.18.4 (n)). Sponsors should provide guidance to investigators and/or the investigators' designated representatives on making such corrections. Sponsors should have written procedures to assure that changes or corrections in CRFs made by sponsor's designated representatives are documented, are necessary, and are endorsed by the investigator. The investigator should retain records of the changes and corrections.

4.9.4. The investigator/institution should maintain the trial documents as specified in Essential Documents for the Conduct of a Clinical Trial (see 8) and as required by the applicable regulatory requirement(s). The investigator/institution should take measures to prevent accidental or premature destruction of these documents.

📝 4.9.5. Essential documents should be retained until at least 2 years after the last approval of a marketing application in an ICH region and until there are no pending or contemplated marketing applications in an ICH region or at least 2 years have elapsed since the formal discontinuation of clinical development of the investigational product. These documents should be retained for a longer period however if required by the applicable regulatory requirements or by an agreement with the sponsor. It is the responsibility of the sponsor to inform the investigator/institution as to when these documents no longer need to be retained (see 5.5.12).

4.9.6. The financial aspects of the trial should be documented in an agreement between the sponsor and the investigator/institution.

4.9.7. Upon request of the monitor, auditor, IRB/IEC, or regulatory authority, the investigator/institution should make available for direct access all requested trial-related records.

**4.10. Progress reports**

4.10.1. The investigator should submit written summaries of the trial status to the IRB/IEC annually, or more frequently, if requested by the IRB/IEC.

4.10.2. The investigator should promptly provide written reports to the sponsor, the IRB/IEC (see 3.3.8) and, where applicable, the institution on any changes significantly affecting the conduct of the trial, and/or increasing the risk to subjects.

**4.11. Safety reporting**

**See the Adverse Event Plus Reporting Table in Appendix 1.**

📝 4.11.1. All SAEs should be reported immediately to the sponsor except for those SAEs that the protocol or other document (e.g., Investigator's Brochure) identifies as not needing immediate reporting. The immediate reports should be followed promptly by detailed, written reports. The immediate and follow-up reports should identify subjects by unique code numbers assigned to the trial subjects rather than by the subjects' names, personal identification numbers, and/or addresses. The investigator should also comply with the applicable regulatory requirement(s) related to the reporting of unexpected serious adverse drug reactions to the regulatory authority(ies) and the IRB/IEC.

4.11.2. Adverse events and/or laboratory abnormalities identified in the protocol as critical to safety evaluations should be reported to the sponsor according to the reporting requirements and within the time periods specified by the sponsor in the protocol.

4.11.3. For reported deaths, the investigator should supply the sponsor and the IRB/IEC with any additional requested information (e.g., autopsy reports and terminal medical reports).

**4.12. Premature termination or suspension of a trial**

If the trial is prematurely terminated or suspended for any reason, the investigator/institution should promptly inform the trial subjects, should assure appropriate therapy and follow-up for the subjects, and, where required by the applicable regulatory requirement(s), should inform the regulatory authority(ies). In addition:

4.12.1. If the investigator terminates or suspends a trial without prior agreement of the sponsor, the investigator should inform the institution where applicable, and the investigator/institution should promptly inform the sponsor and the IRB/IEC, and should provide the sponsor and the IRB/IEC a detailed written explanation of the termination or suspension.

4.12.2. If the sponsor terminates or suspends a trial (see 5.21), the investigator should promptly inform the institution where applicable and the investigator/institution should promptly inform the IRB/IEC and provide the IRB/IEC a detailed written explanation of the termination or suspension.

4.12.3. If the IRB/IEC terminates or suspends its approval/favorable opinion of a trial (see 3.1.2 and 3.3.9), the investigator should inform the institution where applicable and the investigator/institution should promptly notify the sponsor and provide the sponsor with a detailed written explanation of the termination or suspension.

**4.13.  Final report(s) by investigator**

Upon completion of the trial, the investigator, where applicable, should inform the institution; the investigator/institution should provide the IRB/IEC with a summary of the trial's outcome, and the regulatory authority(ies) with any reports required.

The link to all ICH GCP references above can be found here: http://www.ich.org/fileadmin/Public_Web_Site/ICH_Products/Guidelines/Efficacy/E6/E6_R2__Step_4.pdf.

For U.S. Investigators, the FDA has a guidance as well:

It is called the ***Guidance for Industry: Investigator Responsibilities—Protecting the Rights, Safety, and Welfare of Study Subjects***, created by the U.S. Department of Health and Human Services; Food and Drug Administration, the Center for Drug Evaluation and Research (CDER), the Center for Biologics Evaluation and Research (CBER), and the Center for Devices and Radiological Health (CDRH).

Here is the url: https://www.fda.gov/downloads/Drugs/GuidanceComplianceRegulatoryInformation/Guidances/UCM187772.pdf.

A part of the guidance includes the following and is worth special mention:

👍 The Investigator should develop a plan for the supervision and oversight of the clinical trial at the site. Supervision and oversight should be provided even for individuals who are highly qualified and experienced. (Don't assume everyone is doing everything right and is following through.) A plan might include the following elements, to the extent they apply to a particular trial:

- Routine meetings with staff to review trial progress, adverse events, and update staff on any changes to the protocol or other procedures;
- Routine meetings with the sponsor's monitors;
- A procedure for the timely correction and documentation of problems identified by study personnel, outside monitors or auditors, or other parties involved in the conduct of the study;
- A procedure for documenting or reviewing the performance of delegated tasks in a satisfactory and timely manner (e.g., observation of the performance of selected assessments);
- A procedure for ensuring that the consent process is being conducted in accordance with 21 CFR Part 50 and that study subjects understand the nature of their participation and the risks;
- A procedure for ensuring that source data are accurate, contemporaneous, and original;
- A procedure for ensuring that information in source documents is accurately captured on the case report forms (CRFs);
- A procedure for dealing with data queries and discrepancies identified by the study monitor;
- Procedures for ensuring study staff comply with the protocol and adverse event assessment and reporting requirements; and,
- A procedure for addressing medical and ethical issues that arise during the course of the study in a timely manner.

## 1.6 RESEARCH COORDINATOR (RC) RESPONSIBILITIES

*Purpose of section*:

- Provides a detailed overview of Research Coordinator (RC) responsibilities
- Contains a detailed Research Coordinator job description

*Research coordinator responsibilities*

Interestingly, there are neither federal regulations nor ICH GCP guidelines regarding Research Coordinator (RC) responsibilities. Therefore, the RC responsibilities outlined below are from the job descriptions of prominent medical centers, information from clinical trial associations, as well as the authors' experience, which shall suffice to provide us with the necessary understanding.

It cannot be said strongly enough that the Research Coordinator (RC) is an <u>integral member of a study team</u> and must know the federal regulations that apply to human subject protections as well as ICH GCP. The <u>operations</u> of a clinical research study fall predominantly on the shoulders of the RC (so, be very, very kind to your RCs)!

Here is a summary table of RC Responsibilities. These may vary pursuant to your medical center's policies and procedures and delegation of duties among Departments. (See Table 1.6).

| Table 1.6  Table of RC Responsibilities | |
|---|---|
| 1 | Administrative support for the PI for clinical trial conduct |
| 2 | Know the regulations (see regulations and guidance in Section 1.3) |
| 3 | Know ICH GCP (ICH GCP E6 R2) |
| 4 | Regulatory review and editing of consent forms |
| 5 | Completing required study documents, such as screening and enrollment logs, Delegation of Responsibilities forms, 1572, etc. |
| 5 | Perform Activities Preparatory to Research and study start-up tasks. |
| 7 | KNOW YOUR PROTOCOLS IN DETAIL. Create cheat sheets to carry with you |
| 8 | Credentialing of Study Investigators: obtain copies of their current medical licenses (and remind them when their license renewal is coming due) |
| 9 | Obtain Investigator CVs for study startup and every 2 years. Make sure they are signed and dated. |
| 10 | Find out what the Sponsor's and your medical center's requirements are for study team human subjects training. Document that required training for study team members has been completed and when. |
| 11 | Obtain laboratory certification or accreditation for a Sponsor/CRO (CLIA, for example). |
| 12 | Updated normal-range values for each reference laboratory. |
| 13 | Maintain a Regulatory Binder for every study. |
| 14 | Make sure Investigators fill out Financial Disclosure/Conflict of Interest Forms. Retain these in the Regulatory Binder and provide them to the IRB, Sponsor and anyone else required per your Institution's policies and procedures. |
| 15 | Know who reviews budgets in your medical center. Send the budget to the appropriate party. Make sure you receive the final, approved budget for your study records. |
| 16 | Know who reviews contracts and awards in your medical center. Send the contract or award to the appropriate party. Make sure you receive the final, approved contract or award for your study records. |
| 17 | Advertising for study subjects |
| 18 | Coordinate with your Research Pharmacy for the receipt and maintenance of study drugs. Make sure drug dispensation records are completed. |

**Table 1.6    Table of RC Responsibilities—cont'd**

| | |
|---|---|
| 19 | Coordinate with your medical center's Laboratory for lab analyses to be done and for receipt of lab reports/findings. |
| 20 | Inform all medical center staff that will interact with a study subject about the protocol requirements for their part, i.e., technicians performing a radiology procedure, post-op nurses administering medications, etc. The PI, Co-I, or Sub-I may assist with this task. |
| 21 | Arrange for receipt of equipment from a Sponsor or their designee and return of equipment to Sponsor or their designee. |
| 22 | Know the unmasking procedures for blinded trials. |
| 23 | Know your after-hours procedure for subjects experiencing adverse events. |
| 24 | Know your deadlines for reporting. |
| 25 | Recruit study subjects. |
| 26 | Consent study subjects. (The PI has a role in consenting too.) |
| 27 | Retain signed Consent Forms. |
| 28 | Liaison to Sponsors and CROs |
| 29 | Liaison to IRB |
| 30 | Complete all regulatory documentation for IRB/Central IRB review of studies. |
| 31 | Create and maintain a Sponsor/CRO correspondence log for important communications. |
| 32 | Create and maintain an FDA correspondence log. If you are audited or if your PI is a Sponsor-Investigator. |
| 33 | Schedule subject visits. |
| 34 | Register subjects for visits at various Departments in the medical center. |
| 35 | Perform protocol procedures, e.g., taking vital signs, drawing blood, etc. |
| 36 | Collect, label, store, or/and ship specimens. |
| 37 | Dispense drugs or confirm your medical center's policies and procedures for the Research Pharmacy to do so. |
| 38 | Dispense devices or confirm whether an investigator wants to do this. |
| 39 | Fill out Case Report Forms (CRFs) or EDCs to capture study data. |
| 40 | Resolve all Monitors' queries of CRFs and study data. |
| 41 | Enter information into your medical center's CTMS if applicable. |
| 42 | Maintain consent form versions. Replace the previous version with the current version wherever hard copies are. Reconsent subjects if needed per IRB direction. |
| 43 | Process all amendments. |
| 44 | Receive and disseminate Investigator's Brochures and Instructions for Use to Investigators. Maintain these in the Regulatory Binders. |
| 45 | Maintain communication with study subjects to help aid retention. |
| 46 | Dispense subject payments or facilitate the process per your medical center's policies and procedures. |
| 47 | Work with your medical center's financial office to confirm subject visits and medical claim information. |
| 48 | Know your study's budget. Work with your financial office to ensure proper payment for visits completed. See if your PI wants to do this or if he/she is comfortable with assigning this to you. |
| 49 | The PI should keep track of study expenses and make sure they are within budget. The RC may assist in the review of financial statements from your medical center's Finance Department if the PI delegates this. |
| 50 | Fill out and send SAE report forms and Unanticipated Problem Reports. |
| 51 | Receive IND and IDE Safety Reports. Disseminate them to the Investigators and any other stakeholders per your medical center's policies and procedures. |
| 52 | Report protocol deviations and violations. Analyze what caused a protocol deviation or violation. Work with your PI to revise administrative steps in the study to avoid protocol deviations and violations. Document the change in your process as applicable. |

*(Continued)*

**Table 1.6 Table of RC Responsibilities—cont'd**

| 53 | Review CRFs/eCRFs or study databases prior to monitoring visits to assure thorough completion and to correct errors. Be available during monitoring visits to answer questions and provide requested documents. |
|---|---|
| 54 | Prepare for audits. Be available to the auditor during audits. |
| 55 | Prepare progress reports per the Investigator's direction. |
| 56 | Help Investigators prepare presentations for meetings and conferences. |
| 57 | Perform study close out tasks. |
| 58 | Other software-specific and policy- and procedure-specific tasks per your medical center |

See the Research Coordinator Work Queue in Appendix 2. to be used for organizing and tracking the studies your team is managing. There are other tools available for you in the Appendix that are mentioned in separate Chapters and Sections. For example, the Adverse Event Plus Reporting Table, the Study Startup Checklist, and the Study Closeout Checklist.

## 1.7 UNDERSTANDING THE ROLE OF HIPAA AND PHI IN CLINICAL RESEARCH

*Purpose of section*:

- Provides an overview of the Federal law governing the privacy of an individual's health records
- Provides information on how to protect the patient's individually identifiable health information

What is HIPAA and what constitutes Protected Health Information (PHI)?
**HIPAA**

- HIPAA is the Health Insurance Portability and Accountability Act of 1996.
- HIPAA is a FEDERAL LAW. (Many researchers do not realize this, and, therefore, do not give HIPAA the weight it deserves.)
- HIPAA provides rules for protecting health information and the privacy of individuals.[35]

**HIPAA and the privacy rule:**
As stated, HIPAA is a federal law and can be found by looking up "Public Law 104-191".[36]
The Privacy Rule is a regulation. The final modifications were published in final form on August 14, 2002. A text combining the final regulation and the modifications can be found at 45 CFR Part 160 and Part 164, Subparts A and E.[37]
The Privacy Rule protects all *"individually identifiable health information"* held or transmitted by a covered entity or its business associate, in any form or media, whether electronic, paper, or oral. The Privacy Rule calls this information "protected health information (PHI)."[38]

📝 **Protected Health Information (PHI):**

- PHI is information that comes from a health care provider or a health insurance plan.
  - Which includes healthcare claims and billing statements

- PHI identifies an individual or could be used to identify an individual.
- PHI describes the healthcare details/background, condition, or payments of an individual.
- PHI describes the demographics of an individual.

---

Succinctly, Protected Health Information (PHI) is an identifier plus health information that is created by or maintained by a covered entity.

---

**PHI includes:**

(A) Names;

(B) All geographic subdivisions smaller than a State, including street address, city, county, precinct, zip code, and their equivalent geocodes, except for the initial three digits of a zip code if, according to the current publicly available data from the Bureau of the Census:

(1) The geographic unit formed by combining all zip codes with the same three initial digits contains more than 20,000 people; and

(2) The initial three digits of a zip code for all such geographic units containing 20,000 or fewer people is changed to 000.

(C) All elements of dates (except year) for dates directly related to an individual, including birth date, admission date, discharge date, date of death; and all ages over 89 and all elements of dates (including year) indicative of such age, except that such ages and elements may be aggregated into a single category of age 90 or older;

(D) Telephone numbers;

(E) Fax numbers;

(F) Electronic mail addresses;

(G) Social security numbers;

(H) Medical record numbers;

(I) Health plan beneficiary numbers;

(J) Account numbers;

(K) Certificate/license numbers;

(L) Vehicle identifiers and serial numbers, including license plate numbers;

(M) Device identifiers and serial numbers;

(N) Web Universal Resource Locators (URLs);

(O) Internet Protocol (IP) address numbers;

(P) Biometric identifiers, including finger and voice prints;

(Q) Full-face photographic images and any comparable images; and

(R) Any other unique identifying number, characteristic, or code

**PHI Health Conditions include:**

- Information from a health care provider or health plan about an individual's physical or mental condition, including:
  - Past history of a condition
  - Present condition
  - Plans or predictions (prognosis) about the future of a condition

**PHI Health Care includes:**

- Information from a health care provider or health plan about an individual's health care including:
  - Who provided care
  - What type of care was given
  - Where care was given
  - When care was given
  - Why care was given

**Health care employees are required to keep PHI secure.**
PHI must be secured in all forms:

- Written form
  - Reports, charts, X-rays, letters, messages, and so forth.
- Oral communication
  - Phone calls, meetings, and informal conversations; even passing comments in a hospital elevator, corridor, or hospital cafeteria, all of which conversations can be heard by nearby individuals.
- Electronic
  - E-mail, faxes, voicemail, PDA entries, (again) etc.

**HIPAA Fines:**
A Healthcare Institution or an employee of a Healthcare Institution can be fined the following amounts for breaches in PHI:

- $100 fine PER DAY for each violation;
- $50,000 fine and up to 1 year in prison for improperly obtaining or disclosing health information;
- $100,000 fine and up to 5 years in prison for obtaining or disclosing health information under false pretenses; and
- $250,000 fine and up to 10 years in prison for obtaining health information with the intent to sell, transfer or use the information for commercial advantage, personal gain or harm.

# ENDNOTES

[1] Learn About Clinical Studies, https://clinicaltrials.gov/ct2/about-studies/learn [accessed 28.03.18].
[2] Guidance for Industry Adaptive Design Clinical Trials for Drugs and Biologics, U.S. Department of Health and Human Services, Food and Drug Administration, Center for Drug Evaluation and Research (CDER), Center for Biologics Evaluation and Research CBER, February 2010, https://www.fda.gov/downloads/drugs/guidancecomplianceregulatoryinformation/guidances/ucm201790.pdf [accessed 28.03.18].
[3] Clinical Data Interchange Standards Consortium (CDISC), https://www.cdisc.org/standards [accessed 28.03.18].
[4] U.S. National Library of Medicine, National Institutes of Health, https://www.ncbi.nlm.nih.gov/pmc/articles/PMC2689572/ [accessed 28.03.18].
[5] National Institutes of Health, https://search.nih.gov/search?utf8=%E2%9C%93&affiliate=nih&query=what+is+clinical+research&commit=Search [accessed 28.03.18].
[6] U.S. Library of Medicine, National Institutes of Health, https://www.ncbi.nlm.nih.gov/pmc/articles/PMC2689572/ [accessed 28.03.18].
[7] CDISC, https://www.cdisc.org/standards [accessed 28.03.18].

[8]NIH, https://search.nih.gov/search?utf8=%E2%9C%93&affiliate=nih&query=crossover+study&commit=Search [accessed 28.03.18].

[9]NIH, https://www.ncbi.nlm.nih.gov/pmc/articles/PMC3345345/ [accessed 28.03.18].

[10]U.S. Centers for Disease Control, https://www.cdc.gov/careerpaths/k12teacherroadmap/epidemiology.html [accessed 28.03.18].

[11]U.S. Food and Drug Administration, https://www.fda.gov/MedicalDevices/DeviceRegulationandGuidance/Overview/ClassifyYourDevice/ucm051512.htm [accessed 28.03.18].

[12]Following is link to 21 CFR 812 for IDE regulations: https://www.accessdata.fda.gov/scripts/cdrh/cfdocs/cfCFR/CFRSearch.cfm?CFRPart=812 [accessed 28.03.18].

[13]The Free Dictionary, compiled from *The American Heritage Stedman's Medical Dictionary, Second Edition, and Dorland's Medical Dictionary for Health Care Consumers*, http://medical-dictionary.thefreedictionary.com [accessed 28.03.18].

[14]FDA Pre-Market Approval, https://www.fda.gov/medicaldevices/deviceregulationandguidance/howtomarketyourdevice/premarketsubmissions/premarketapprovalpma/default.htm [accessed 28.03.18].

[15]Duke University Medical Center and Archives, http://guides.mclibrary.duke.edu/ebmtutorial [accessed 28.03.18].

[16]NIH, https://search.nih.gov/search?utf8=%E2%9C%93&affiliate=nih&query=N+of+1+study&commit=Search [accessed 28.03.18].

[17]Stanford University School of Medicine, http://cliomods.stanford.edu/trailmaps/design/design/nestedCase-Control/index.html [accessed 28.03.18].

[18]Medical Definition of a Nonblinded Study, http://www.medicinenet.com/script/main/art.asp?articlekey=25411 [accessed 28.03.18].

[19]National Cancer Institute, National Institutes of Health, https://www.cancer.gov/publications/dictionaries/cancer-terms?cdrid=44160 [accessed 28.03.18].

[20]Glossary of Common Site Terms, ClinicalTrials.gov, https://clinicaltrials.gov/ct2/about-studies/glossary#P [accessed 28.03.18].

[21]Ibid (https://clinicaltrials.gov/ct2/about-studies/glossary#P) [accessed 28.03.18].

[22]Nontherapeutic Research, http://medical-dictionary.thefreedictionary.com/nontherapeutic+research [accessed 28.03.18].

[23]All Non-Therapuetic Research studies, https://www.cancer.gov/about-cancer/treatment [accessed 28.03.18].

[24]Improving the Quality of Cancer Clinical Trials: Workshop Summary—Proceedings of the National Cancer Policy Forum Workshop, Improving the Quality of Cancer Clinical Trials (Washington, DC, October 2007), National Academy Press, https://www.nap.edu/read/12146/chapter/1 [accessed 28.03.18].

[25]National Institutes of Health, https://humansubjects.nih.gov/glossary [accessed 28.03.18].

[26]Ibid.

[27]Ibid.

[28]For additional information on Drug Approvals, see: https://www.fda.gov/forpatients/approvals/drugs/ucm405622.htm [accessed 28.03.18].

[29]U.S. National Library of Medicine, National Institutes of Health , https://www.ncbi.nlm.nih.gov/pmc/articles/PMC3081994/ [accessed 28.03.18].

[30]NIH Glossary of Terms, https://search.nih.gov/search?utf8=%E2%9C%93&affiliate=nih&query=preclinical+studies&commit=Search [accessed 28.03.18].

[31]Ibid.

[32]https://www.ich.org/fileadmin/Public_Web_Site/ICH_Products/Guidelines/Efficacy/E6/E6_R1_Guideline.pdf [accessed 28.03.18].

[33]Combined regulation text of Rules, https://www.hhs.gov/hipaa/for-professionals/privacy/laws-regulations/combined-regulation-text/index.html [accessed 28.03.18].

[34]International Council for Harmonisation Good Clinical Practice Guideline E6 R2, https://www.fda.gov/downloads/Drugs/Guidances/UCM464506.pdf [accessed 28.03.18].

[35]Overview, Health Insurance Portability and Accountability Act, U.S. Department of Health and Human Services; https://www.hhs.gov/hipaa/index.html [accessed 28.03.18].

[36]PL 104-191—https://www.gpo.gov/fdsys/pkg/PLAW-104publ191/content-detail.html [accessed 28.03.18].

[37]Summary of HIPPA, U.S. Department of Health and Human Services, https://www.hhs.gov/hipaa/for-professionals/privacy/laws-regulations/index.html [accessed 28.03.18].

[38]Ibid.

# PREPARATION BEFORE A CLINICAL TRIAL BEGINS

*Purpose of chapter*:

- Explains the Clinical Trial Feasibility Analysis
- Describes Conflict of Interest Considerations in a Clinical Trial
- Provides overview of the Confidentiality Disclosure Agreement (also known as the Non-Disclosure Agreement)
- Describes the clinical trial contract (also known as a Clinical Services Agreement or a Clinical Trial Agreement)
- Reviews consent forms and documentation
- Provides overview of the Clinical Trial Budget
- Describes study start-up and sponsor documentation requirements
- Explains the Trial's Medicare Coverage Analysis
- Describes Clinical Trial registration at www.ClinicalTrials.gov
- Provides a flowchart for sequence/timing of all tasks in this chapter

## 2.1  CLINICAL TRIAL FEASIBILITY ANALYSIS

*Purpose of section*:

- Explains the Feasibility Analysis
- Introduces the tool: Feasibility Analysis Checklist (contained in Appendix 3)

An important first step in preparing for a clinical trial or clinical research study is the PI's determination of whether he/she has the required staff, resources, and institutional support to carry a study through from conception to completion. This is called a "Feasibility Analysis," which serves as a recorded assessment of staff, time- eligible study participants, equipment, and financial resources as needed to undertake the trial. A Feasibility Analysis Checklist has been written for your use in Appendix 3, by which to conduct this analysis.

⚠ **DO NOT skip this step. It should not be viewed as additional work, but as an integral part of study preparation.** The authors can attest to the fact, from having seen the outcome time and again, that where Feasibility Analyses are not performed, sites can run short on money to complete studies, or be without the necessary expertise, staffing and time to realistically perform the studies they have contracted to conduct. The PI's relationship with the sponsor, the institution's CFO, direct reports and Clinic Directors will suffer as a result as all are strained to complete the requirements in the protocol. To emphasize again: Do a Feasibility Analysis for EVERY study offered to you.

The Sourcebook for Clinical Research. https://doi.org/10.1016/B978-0-12-816242-2.00002-3
© 2018 Natasha Martien and Jeff Nelligan. Published by Elsevier Inc. All Rights Reserved.

ꙮICH Though ICH GCP does not call it "feasibility analysis," three of the elements of a feasibility analysis are included in its Section 4.2 entitled "Adequate Resources."

4.2.1. The investigator should be able to demonstrate (e.g., based on retrospective data) a potential for recruiting the required number of suitable subjects within the agreed recruitment period.

4.2.2. The investigator should have sufficient time to properly conduct and complete the trial within the agreed trial period.

4.2.3. The investigator should have available an adequate number of qualified staff and adequate facilities for the foreseen duration of the trial to conduct the trial properly and safely.[1]

## 2.2  FINANCIAL CONFLICT OF INTEREST REGULATIONS IN A CLINICAL TRIAL

*Purpose of section*:

- Provides a summary of FDA regulations regarding financial disclosures by clinical investigators
- Provides a summary of conflict-of-interest regulations for clinical investigators funded by the National Institutes of Health

Financial reporting for physicians engaged in clinical research is considered necessary in order to preserve the public's trust that research is conducted in an unbiased manner. To provide clarity for clinical investigators, the relevant information on two federal reporting programs is below. The first are the Federal regulations under which the U.S. Food and Drug Administration monitors clinical trials. The second program regards the reporting requirements for physicians engaged in NIH-funded research.

*Financial Disclosure by Clinical Investigators*

The FDA regulations are located at 21 CFR 54.[2]

As the FDA notes: "Financial Disclosure by Clinical Investigators…requires applicants who submit a marketing application for a drug, biological product, or device to submit certain information concerning the compensation to, and financial interest and arrangements of, any clinical investigator conducting clinical studies covered by the regulation [21 CFR 54]."

"The regulation requires applicants to certify the absence of certain financial interests and arrangements of clinical investigators that could affect the reliability of data submitted to FDA, or to disclose those financial interests and arrangement to the agency and identify steps taken to minimize the potential for bias."

*The Mechanics*

The first scenario: The clinical investigator files with the Sponsor (or CRO) an FDA Form 3454 (see Appendix 35), which documents that there is no financial interest or arrangements between the investigator and the Sponsor.

The second scenario: The clinical investigator files with the Sponsor (or CRO) an FDA Form 3455 (see Appendix 35), which discloses the nature of investigator financial interests and arrangements with the Sponsor and describes any steps taken to minimize the potential for bias resulting from those interests.

*Who is Covered*

The clinical investigator, which per the FDA, means a "listed or identified investigator or subinvestigator who is directly involved in the treatment or evaluation of research subjects, including the spouse and each dependent child of the investigator or subinvestigator."[3]

*What must be disclosed*
From the FDA:

- Any compensation made to the investigator by any sponsor of the covered clinical study in which the value of compensation could be affected by the study outcome.
- A proprietary interest in the tested product including, but not limited to, a patent, trademark, copyright, or licensing agreement.
- Any equity interest in any sponsor of the covered clinical study, i.e., any ownership interest, stock options, or other financial interest whose value cannot be readily determined through reference to public prices. The requirement applies to interests held during the time the clinical investigator is carrying out the study and for one year following completion of the study.
- Any equity interest in any sponsor of the covered study if the sponsor is a publicly held company and the interest exceeds $50,000 in value. The requirement applies to interests held during the time the clinical investigator is carrying out the study and for one year following completion of the study.

Significant payments of other sorts (SPOOS) are payments that have a cumulative monetary value of $25,000 or more (per Guidance: Guidance for Clinical Investigators, Industry, and FDA Staff: Financial Disclosure by Clinical Investigators, February 2013. Note, the regulation at 21 CFR 54.2(f) states, "…a monetary value of more than $25,000…") and are made by any sponsor of a covered study to the investigator or the investigator's institution during the time the clinical investigator is carrying out the study and for one year following completion of the study. This would include payments that support activities of the investigator (e.g., a grant to the investigator or to the institution to fund the investigator's ongoing research or compensation in the form of equipment), exclusive of the costs of conducting the clinical study or other clinical studies, or to provide other reimbursements such as retainers for ongoing consultation or honoraria. See Section IV, Questions C.4, C.5, and C.6 in the Guidance for additional information on SPOOS.[4]

*FDA Enforcement*
The point of the FDA Forms 3454 and 3455 require Sponsors to "certify the absence of certain financial interests and arrangements of clinical investigators that could affect the reliability of data submitted to FDA, or to disclose those financial interests and arrangements to the agency and identify steps taken to minimize the potential for bias (21 CFR § 54.4(a)). If the applicant does not include certification and/or disclosure, or does not certify that he/she was unable to obtain the information despite exercising due diligence, the agency may refuse to file the application (21 CFR § 54.4(c))."

If the FDA determines that the financial interests or arrangements of any clinical investigator raises a serious question about the integrity of the data, FDA will take any action it deems necessary to ensure the reliability of the data (21 CFR § 54.5(c)) including:

- initiating agency audits of the data derived from the clinical investigator in question;
- requesting that the applicant submit further analyses of data, e.g., to evaluate the effect of the clinical investigator's data on the overall study outcome;
- requesting that the applicant conduct additional independent studies to confirm the results of the questioned study; and
- refusing to treat the covered clinical study as providing data that can be the basis for an agency action.[5]

For more information, the Guidance document on Financial Disclosure can be found here: https://www.fda.gov/downloads/regulatoryinformation/guidances/ucm341008.pdf

**National Institutes of Health (NIH)/Financial Conflict of Interest**

The regulation for NIH-funded research is formally known as the "Responsibility of Applicants for Promoting Objectivity in Research for which PHS Funding is Sought," 42 CFR 50 Subpart F.[6]

The regulation is designed to "promote objectivity in research by establishing standards that provide a reasonable expectation that the design, conduct, or reporting of research funded under the PHS [Public Health Service] grants or cooperative agreements will be free from bias by any conflicting financial interests of an Investigator…and any other person, regardless of title or position, who is responsible for the design, conduct, or reporting of research funded by PHS…"[7]

*The regulation places responsibilities upon the Institution to have in place detailed and effective conflict of interest policies, and to ensure those policies are well known and disseminated.*

The regulation at 42 CFR 50.604, named "Responsibilities of Institutions regarding Investigator financial conflicts of interest," states:

Each Institution shall:

**(a)** Maintain an up-to-date, written, enforced policy on financial conflicts of interest that complies with this subpart, and make such policy available via a publicly accessible Web site. If the Institution does not have any current presence on a publicly accessible Web site (and only in those cases), the Institution shall make its written policy available to any requestor within five business days of a request. If, however, the Institution acquires a presence on a publicly accessible Web site during the time of the PHS award, the requirement to post the information on that Web site will apply within 30 calendar days. If an Institution maintains a policy on financial conflicts of interest that includes standards that are more stringent than this subpart (e.g., that require a more extensive disclosure of financial interests), the Institution shall adhere to its policy and shall provide FCOI reports regarding identified financial conflicts of interest to the PHS Awarding Component in accordance with the Institution's own standards and within the timeframe prescribed by this subpart.

**(b)** Inform each Investigator of the Institution's policy on financial conflicts of interest, the Investigator's responsibilities regarding disclosure of significant financial interests, and of these regulations, and require each Investigator to complete training regarding the same prior to engaging in research related to any PHS-funded grant and at least every four years, and immediately when any of the following circumstances apply:

   **(1)** The Institution revises its financial conflict of interest policies or procedures in any manner that affects the requirements of Investigators;

   **(2)** An Investigator is new to an Institution; or

   **(3)** An Institution finds that an Investigator is not in compliance with the Institution's financial conflict of interest policy or management plan.

The monetary threshold at which significant financial interests require disclosure is $5000. The regulation at 42 CFR 50.603 states the following regarding "significant financial interest":

**(i)** With regard to any publicly traded entity, a *significant financial interest* exists if the value of any remuneration received from the entity in the twelve months preceding the disclosure and the value of any equity interest in the entity as of the date of disclosure, when aggregated, exceeds $5000. For purposes of this definition, remuneration includes salary and any payment for services not otherwise identified as salary (e.g., consulting fees, honoraria, paid authorship); equity interest includes any stock, stock option, or other ownership interest, as determined through reference to public prices or other reasonable measures of fair market value;

**(ii)** With regard to any non-publicly traded entity, a *significant financial interest* exists if the value of any remuneration received from the entity in the twelve months preceding the disclosure, when aggregated, exceeds $5000, or when the Investigator (or the Investigator's spouse or dependent children) holds any equity interest (e.g., stock, stock option, or other ownership interest).[8]

NIH has developed a Frequently Asked Question (FAQ) list that is extremely useful for researchers who are covered by the FCOI. The FAQ can be found here: https://grants.nih.gov/grants/policy/coi/coi_faqs.htm.

Questions regarding the applicability and/or compliance with these regulations should be directed to: FCOICompliance@mail.nih.gov.

## 2.3 CONFIDENTIALITY DISCLOSURE AGREEMENT (ALSO KNOWN AS A NON-DISCLOSURE AGREEMENT)

*Purpose of section*:

- Define a Confidentiality Disclosure Agreement (CDA)
- Introduce the Confidentiality Disclosure Agreement Template in the Appendix
- Provide tips for executing a CDA

### How the CDA/NDA works

Sponsors send a CDA/NDA to a potential Principal Investigator (PI) prior to sending to him/her a study protocol and other study documents. The purpose of the CDA/NDA is to secure the confidentiality of the Sponsor's materials and study concept. The CDA/NDA must be signed before the Sponsor will release the study documents.

### Definition

"A **Confidentiality** (Disclosure) **Agreement** (also called a Non-Disclosure **Agreement** or NDA) is a legally binding contract in which a person or business promises to treat specific information as a trade secret and promises not to disclose the secret to others without proper authorization."[9]

Please see the Confidentiality Disclosure Agreement Template in Appendix 37.

A properly written CDA/NDA will only include terms of confidentiality and will be about three (3) pages long. Longer CDAs/NDAs should be reviewed carefully.

Sometimes, terms beyond confidentiality (that belong in a research study contract) can be added into a CDA/NDA. It is prudent, therefore, to have your Legal Office or Contracts Office review the CDA/NDA and to have an Institutional officer sign it.

The signature lines in the CDA/NDA should include one for the disclosing Sponsor and one for the authorized medical institution official. The Principal Investigator's signature is optional. CDAs/NDAs with a Sponsor signature line and a PI signature line should be revised to include the Institutional Official's signature line. The reason is that a PI may sign off on a CDA/NDA and bind the medical institution to terms the institution is not willing to accept. Staff with contractual or legal expertise should be made aware that a CDA/NDA has been offered to a PI for proper due diligence and an administrative check and balance.

**Quick Turnaround**

The expectation in the clinical research industry is that the CDA/NDA will be reviewed and signed very quickly—within one business week, and typically within a few business days.

## 2.4 THE CLINICAL TRIAL CONTRACT (ALSO KNOWN AS A CLINICAL SERVICES AGREEMENT/CSA OR A CLINICAL TRIAL AGREEMENT/CTA)

*Purpose of section*:

* Provides tips for contract review and content
* Provides a Contract Contents Checklist (Checklist is provided in Appendix 4)

👍 The goal of contract language is to create a mutually beneficial document, a "win-win" agreement. Keep in mind that you could be in a professional relationship with a sponsor or funder for a long time as multiple study opportunities will arise over the years with various PIs and Departments. Therefore, you will always want a positive, respectful relationship with your Sponsors.

Your Legal Department will have a strong stance regarding the language it prefers or requires in its contracts. Therefore, only a sampling of topics is provided for consideration and guidance in your contract writing and negotiations. They include:

**1.** How a "win-win" contract can be created from a "win-lose" contract:

You will find that contracts can be written to inure to the benefit of one party only. You will want to change this. Here are two examples of the language inuring to one party only and how you can change it to inure to both:

### EXAMPLE 1

NO Termination by Sponsor: Sponsor may terminate this Agreement at any time upon giving thirty (30) days' advance written notice to Institution.

YES Termination: Sponsor or Institution may terminate this Agreement at any time upon sixty (60) days' written notice to the other, subject to the survival provisions of subsection (name the subsection, i.e., 16.2.) Principal Investigator, Sponsor, Institution, or Institution IRB may terminate the Study immediately upon written notice because of safety concerns. In the event that concerns arise regarding the safety of patients enrolled in the Study, the Institution may, in its discretion, immediately stop the enrollment of subjects into the Study, and/or follow-up visits pursuant to the Protocol, and will promptly notify the Sponsor. In such event, the parties will discuss and negotiate in good faith a mutually agreeable course of action in regard to the Study and its activities.

### EXAMPLE 2

NO Inventions: All right, title, and interest in and to all Inventions shall belong solely to the Sponsor. Hospital hereby assigns to Sponsor all of its right, title, and interest in and to such Inventions.

YES Inventions: Sponsor or Hospital, individually, shall retain title to any patent or other intellectual property rights for Inventions made solely by its employees in conducting the Study. New Inventions made jointly by the Sponsor and Hospital shall be jointly owned by the parties and each party is free to use it without restriction; provided however that neither party is required to provide an accounting to the other for revenues realized in utilizing the New Inventions. For New Inventions developed solely by the Sponsor in conducting the Study, the Sponsor shall discuss with the Hospital, consistent with the Sponsor's technology transfer policies, the terms under which Sponsor would license such New Inventions to the Hospital.

**2.** Choice of law and venue

If the Sponsor and you cannot agree on the State because your site and the Sponsor's place of business are located in different States, go silent (meaning, delete this section from the contract). You can waste A LOT of time going back and forth on this. If your Legal Office agrees, it may be better to go silent on the choice of law and venue (hoping you will never get to this point) than to lose the contract/ study.

Sample language:

> Choice of Law and Venue. This Agreement shall be interpreted, construed, and enforced in accordance with the laws of the State of _____, applied without giving effect to any conflicts of law principles. Any lawsuit that may be brought with respect to this Agreement shall be brought and tried in a court of competent jurisdiction in the State of _____.

**3.** Contract language included from guidelines set by the Association for the Accreditation of Human Research Protection Programs (AAHRPP)

If your Institution is an AAHRPP-accredited facility, you will need to include the AAHRPP language expectations into your contracts, or document how the language from the Sponsor/funder is similar and, therefore, meets the standards of AAHRP.

If your Institution wants to become AAHRPP accredited, start including their language expectations into your contracts, or document how the language from the Sponsor/funder is similar and, therefore, meets the standards of AAHRPP.

You can go to www.aahrpp.org to get information. Take a look at the "Evaluation Instrument for Accreditation" and the "AAHRPP Accreditation Procedures" found on the main web page.

Within the "Evaluation Instrument for Accreditation", Standard I-8 speaks to the content expected in a written agreement with a Sponsor. The October 3, 2016 version, currently on the AAHRPP website, manifests the following in its Table of Contents for Standard I-8 shown in Fig. 2.1.

Read each Element on the website to get the full scope.[10]

**4.** Payment for research-related injury

Element I.8.A in the AAHRPP language noted above is critically important for your medical center. Refer to your Institutional policy or Legal office first. If you need to create this language and policy, there are several possible approaches:

**(1)** The study sponsor will pay for research-related injuries.

**(2)** The medical center will provide medical care for research-related injuries and will charge the subject's insurance.

**(3)** A combination of sponsor payment and medical insurance payment

  **(a)** Spell it out.

  **1.** For example, the sponsor will pay for co-pays and deductibles only.

**(4)** A combination of insurance and free care

  **(a)** For example, the medical center will provide medical care for research-related injuries and will charge the subject's insurance, but if the medical insurer will not reimburse the medical center, the medical center will provide the services free of charge.

**(5)** The medical center will provide medical care for research-related injuries free of charge

  **(a)** The medical center may want to place a cap on this.

**FIG. 2.1**

AAHRPP Standard I-8.

---

Check with each study sponsor to learn what their policy is. The Sponsor's policy may or may not agree with your Institutional policy. If there is disagreement, it will become a matter of negotiation.

See the sample Payment for Research-Related Injury language in the Consent Form Sample in Appendix 5.

⚠ Remember: The terms stated in the contract for Research-Related Injury should match the terms stated in the consent.

🏃ICH ICH GCP has this to say about research-related injury costs:

5.8.2 The sponsor's policies and procedures should address the costs of treatment of trial subjects in the event of trial—related injuries in accordance with the applicable regulatory requirement(s).[11]

**5.** Contact information

📝 Tip: Make sure to have contact information for billing/invoicing written into the contract. This can be left out of contracts (leaving hospital invoicing personnel on a time-consuming e-mail and phone chase to find the right contact). The terms are stated, but you also need a contact to whom your invoices will be sent to request payment. Have a general billing office phone number written into the contract as well in case the billing contact named leaves the company.

**6.** Indemnification

"Indemnification" is the act of holding someone/some company harmless in the event of an infraction. Another definition is to secure (someone/some company) against legal responsibility for their actions.

*This should be in every contract.* The Sponsor should indemnify the Institution and the Principal Investigator. (Make sure the PI is indemnified. This has to be edited in at times.) The Institution and PI should indemnify the Sponsor.

Some Federal Grants will not allow indemnification. See 2 CFR 200.447 for OMB Guidance on indemnification.

ↄↄICH Here is what ICH GCP has to say about indemnification:

5.8. Compensation to Subjects and Investigators

5.8.1. If required by the applicable regulatory requirement(s), the sponsor should provide insurance or should indemnify (legal and financial coverage) the investigator/the institution against claims arising from the trial, except for claims that arise from malpractice and/or negligence.

**ICH GCP regarding contracts:**

1.17. Contract

A written, dated, and signed agreement between two or more involved parties that sets out any arrangements on delegation and distribution of tasks and obligations and, if appropriate, on financial matters. The protocol may serve as the basis of a contract.

4.5.1. The investigator/institution should conduct the trial in compliance with the protocol agreed to by the sponsor and, if required, by the regulatory authority(ies) and which was given approval/favorable opinion by the IRB/IEC. The investigator/institution and the sponsor should sign the protocol, or an alternative contract, to confirm agreement.

5.2.2. Any trial-related duty and function that is transferred to and assumed by a CRO should be specified in writing.

ICH GCP E6 R2 5.2.2 ADDENDUM

The sponsor should ensure oversight of any trial-related duties and functions carried out on its behalf, including trial-related duties and functions that are subcontracted to another party by the sponsor's contracted CRO(s).[12]

*Contract Contents Checklist*

🏢 We have provided a Contract Contents Checklist in Appendix 4. This is a tool for contract office personnel or medical center paralegals who review contracts before they go to the Legal office. The Checklist provides multiple contract terms, which can be included in a contract. The goal of the checklist is to make certain that all terms your Institution wants in a contract are written into the checklist and checked off when they are found in a contract. Where the particular term is not checked off, you will know it needs to be written into the contract being reviewed. Please note that the Checklist should be revised according to your Institution's policies.

## 2.5 CONSENT FORMS AND DOCUMENTATION

*Purpose of section*:

- Provides an explanation of why certain language is contained in the consent form
- Provides language samples for the consent form
- Provides tips from the authors' practical experience in the consenting process
- Provides a Consent Form Template in Appendix 5

What exactly is "consent?"

In the context of a clinical trial, "consent" is the voluntary permission of an individual to choose to become a participant in a clinical trial. The consent form documents the individual's voluntary permission and explains what the subject can expect to experience while in the trial. "Consenting" is a state of permission exercised throughout the trial as the subject participates "at will."

**Why is a consent form needed?**

- It documents the subject's voluntary permission;
- It provides the proper due diligence and compliance for the Institution and Sponsor;
- It informs the subject of what the study entails; and,
- It provides a written record that the subject keeps and can reference.

21 CFR 50.20 and 45 CFR 46.116:
No Investigator may involve a human being as a subject in research…unless the Investigator has obtained the legally effective informed consent of the subject or the subject's legally authorized representative.

45 CFR 46.116 (a)(1) New Common Rule
   Before involving a human subject in research covered by this policy, an investigator shall obtain the legally effective informed consent of the subject or the subject's legally authorized representative.

ᛁᏟᴵᶜᴴ Freely given informed consent should be obtained from every subject prior to clinical trial participation. ICH GCP E6 R2, 2.9

ALL consent forms must contain **full disclosure** of the "Basic elements" and may contain the "Additional elements." A best practice is to include all of the Basic elements and all of the Additional elements. It is best to have more than less where human subject protections are concerned. The FDA and HHS regulations displaying the Basic and Additional elements is provided in Table 2.1.[13]

**Table 2.1 Basic and Additional Elements of Consent**

| Consent Table |
|---|
| 45 CFR 46.116: General requirements for informed consent (and 21 CFR 50.25 a and b) |
| Basic elements |
| 1   A statement that the study involves research, an explanation of the purposes of the research and the expected duration of the subject's participation, a description of the procedures to be followed, and identification of any procedures which are experimental |
| 2   A description of any reasonably foreseeable risks or discomforts to the subject |
| 3   A description of any benefits to the subject or to others which may reasonably be expected from the research |
| 4   A disclosure of appropriate alternative procedures or courses of treatment, if any, that might be advantageous to the subject |
| 5   A statement describing the extent, if any, to which confidentiality of records identifying the subject will be maintained |

---

**Table 2.1 Basic and Additional Elements of Consent—cont'd**

**Consent Table**

6       For research involving more than minimal risk, an explanation as to whether any compensation and an explanation as to whether any medical treatments are available if injury occurs and, if so, what they consist of, or where further information may be obtained

7       An explanation of whom to contact for answers to pertinent questions about the research and research subjects' rights, and whom to contact in the event of a research-related injury to the subject; and

8       A statement that participation is voluntary, refusal to participate will involve no penalty or loss of benefits to which the subject is otherwise entitled, and, the subject may discontinue participation at any time without penalty or loss of benefits to which the subject is otherwise entitled.

Additional elements

1       A statement that the particular treatment or procedure may involve risks to the subject (or to the embryo or fetus, if the subject is or may become pregnant) which are currently unforeseeable;

2       Anticipated circumstances under which the subject's participation may be terminated by the investigator without regard to the subject's consent;

3       Any additional costs to the subject that may result from participation in the research

4       The consequences of a subject's decision to withdraw from the research and procedures for orderly termination of participation by the subject;

5       A statement that significant new findings developed during the course of the research which may relate to the subject's willingness to continue participation will be provided to the subject; and,

6       The approximate number of subjects involved in the study.

**For the New Common Rule, at 45 CFR 46.116(b), there is a 9th Basic element, which is:**
**(9) One of the following statements about any research that involves the collection of identifiable private information or identifiable biospecimens:**
**(i) A statement that identifiers might be removed from the identifiable private information or identifiable biospecimens and that, after such removal, the information or biospecimens could be used for future research studies or distributed to another investigator for future research studies without additional informed consent from the subject or the legally authorized representative, if this might be a possibility; or**
**(ii) A statement that the subject's information or biospecimens collected as part of the research, even if identifiers are removed, will not be used or distributed for future research studies.**

**For the New Common Rule, at 45 CFR 46.116(c), there are three Additional elements, which are:**
**(7) A statement that the subject's biospecimens (even if identifiers are removed) may be used for commercial profit and whether the subject will or will not share in this commercial profit;**
**(8) A statement regarding whether clinically relevant research results, including individual research results, will be disclosed to subjects, and if so, under what conditions; and**
**(9) For research involving biospecimens, whether the research will (if known) or might include whole genome sequencing (*i.e.*, sequencing of a human germline or somatic specimen with the intent to generate the genome or exome sequence of that specimen).**

---

No risk can be left out of the consent form, nor can the duration and/or significant, individual time commitments of a study visit be left out of the consent form. For example, some pharmacokinetic (PK) visits last 4–6 hours.

The focus on recruitment of a subject cannot be greater than the moral obligation to tell a potential subject the truth as to what he/she would experience in the trial.

**General Information**

**Writing at a specific grade level**

IRB As a general rule of thumb, consent forms are to be written at the 7th grade level. However, your Institution may require a different grade level. Check with your IRB.

**Following is a step-by-step breakdown of an informed consent form:**
**Investigators**
Principal Investigator, Co-Investigator, Sub-Investigators:

At the top of the form is the name of the Principal Investigator (PI) who is the managing physician of the clinical trial. The PI is responsible for the oversight and regulatory compliance of the trial and the welfare of subjects throughout the trial.

There may be a Co-Investigator (Co-I) who shares the responsibilities of the Principal Investigator or/and Sub-Investigators (Sub-I) who are under the leadership of the PI and Co-I.

An Investigator must be available 24/7 throughout the trial. The contact information must include a phone number at which the Investigator can be reached any time day or night. This is often the reason to have a Co-I or Sub-I. Another reason is if the Principal Investigator does significant traveling. Additionally, if the study is high enrolling, there will be a need for another Investigator to share in the subject evaluations.

What is the reason for the 24/7 level of contact? If an Adverse Event (AE) or Serious Adverse Event (SAE) occurs, the subject must be able to reach an Investigator who can determine whether the AE/SAE is expected or unexpected and whether it is urgently actionable or not.

Having the Investigator contact information on the first page is a best practice. In the event of an emergency or subject concern, the subject has the contact information readily available without having to search through the pages of the consent when under duress to find the Investigator's phone number.

**Research coordinator or other study team members**
Because study team members may turnover, you do not want their name on the consent form so that you do not have to revise the consent each time there is turnover (thus necessitating additional IRB reviews).

**Study title**
Following is the study title along with its short title.

**Site address**
Then, name and address of the facility

**Sponsor name**
Followed by the sponsor's name and address.

In this Internet-savvy era, the subject and family will likely go online to locate and assess the sponsor.

**Initial question**
There is no regulation limiting an individual from enrolling in more than one clinical trial concurrently. However, in drug and device trials, co-enrollment can confound results, because it will not be known to which study a side effect is attributed. Additionally, there can be drug interactions that could pose a safety risk to a subject. If one study is observational and another interventional, your Institution may approve this. You must know your IRB's policy regarding co-enrollment. If your Institution does not allow co-enrollment, it is best to have a statement confirming this at the beginning of the consent form process, below the contact information, with wording such as "I am not currently enrolled in any other research study" followed by an initial line to the right of it. (There have been some instances in which an RC goes through the consenting process only to learn at the conclusion that an individual is already in a trial.) It is important to address this up front in order to save everyone's time. Potential subjects often do not know they cannot be in more than one trial at a

time per your IRB policy or as a matter of safety determined by the PI, so you must guide the conversation.

### Footer—Subject initials

👍 Having the subject initial the bottom of each page of the consent form is a suggestion. From experience, it is helpful to document that the subject has read and approved each page of the consent form. If there is a subject injury or misunderstanding as the trial moves along, this holds up very well in court and helps the subject be purposeful in their reading.

### Footer—Consent version number and date

It is important that the PI and his/her team are diligent about keeping a close eye on "versioning" of the consent form. What does this mean? There may well be changes—major or minor—to the protocol as the study progresses, necessitating protocol amendments. Some amendments will alter the consent form, such as the addition or deletion of a test, or a change in the risks. Ensure that when you revise the consent form, you update the date on the consent form and write the next version number on the consent form. Creating a bottom-of-the-page footer for versioning is a best practice.

👍 Make sure you are always working with the current version of the consent form. Monitors from the Sponsor or CRO will watch this closely. Make sure you remove, then shred old versions, and change them out with the newest version from the places where you keep consent forms to be ready to speak with prospective subjects, such as at the Emergency Room, Operating Suite or Cath Lab.

### Footer—IRB Stamp of Approval and valid dates

Another best practice is to have the IRB's stamp of approval in the footer along with the date of IRB approval and the date of expiration.

Note: If a subject signs an old version (invalid) consent form, the study team will have to re-consent the subject with the new consent form. Try to avoid this situation; it damages the study team's credibility in the subject's eyes and may require an extra visit, which subjects will not be happy about.

### Opportunity to ask questions

Write in the consent that it is important that the subject or subject representative reads the consent form and asks questions. This represents a lack of coercion and an interest in the subject's welfare.

For example, here is a helpful statement to use: "It is important that you read this consent form carefully before deciding whether or not to take part in the study. If you do not understand anything on this form, please ask one of the investigators or the study coordinator to explain it to you."

### Voluntary nature

Basic element #8 must be written in your consent form. Sample language is, "Taking part in this study is entirely voluntary. If you choose not to take part, your choice will not affect the quality of your medical care and will involve no penalty or loss of benefits to which you are otherwise entitled."

### Subject must pass screening

The subject needs to know that they have to pass a screening after signing the consent in order to go forward in the study and that they may be disqualified. (Conducting a thorough medical chart review as a part of your "activities preparatory to research" will help you to screen candidates who meet the exclusion and inclusion criteria to avoid disqualification, but there is a chance that their health on the day you screen has changed.) Sample language is, "In order to take part in the study, you will have to meet certain conditions. If you sign this consent form, but do not meet the conditions, a Study Coordinator will let you know." For example, the subject may have high blood pressure, which would disqualify the subject from a study when "high blood pressure" is found in the exclusion criteria.

**Introduction**

You must explain why the subject is being chosen for this study. Here's an example: "You have acute coronary syndrome and this study is examining how an experimental drug [name of IND] will treat this condition."

**Purpose of the study**

Refer to your protocol to write the purpose(s).

**Number of participants**

This section helps the subject feel comfortable about joining the study. They will learn here that they are not alone, that there are other people in the study with the same affliction that are undergoing the same procedures and investigational testing at your site and in other centers.

**Duration and number of visits**

Another part of the consent is to state:

- how long subjects will be in the study (total time)
- how many visits will be required
- the amount of time per visit
  - o Make sure to be up front about long PK visits. Some may last 6 hours, for example.

Providing this information up front is extremely helpful in minimizing subject withdrawals from the study, helping compliance, and setting expectations. The subject needs to determine whether he or she can commit to the time requirements of the study.

It is helpful for the subject's consideration and your enrollment, to break down how many visits will occur within a time period. For example, a subject will hear from you that the study lasts two (2) years, for example, but there are only six visits in that timeframe. A 2-year commitment sounds a lot larger than 6 visits.

**Procedures**

⚠ **TIP**: Next to each procedure on the form, it is useful to have a parenthetic "standard of care" or " research." From the subject's point of view, this will help recruitment because the subject understands that the experimental portion is small in relation to the routine or standard of care to be provided. This is also a useful tool for the Institution's billing department and assists the research coordinator in filling out billing forms/entering billing information into a CTMS or other electronic solution to distinguish between what the sponsor pays vis-a-vis what the insurance pays for qualifying clinical trials. This is also a critical compliance aid to avoid double billing.

*TIP*: When you are mentioning samples, state the amount. For example, when talking about blood draws, say how much, e.g. three teaspoons, rather than leaving it open as to how much in order to alleviate the subject's fears (which may be unspoken).

**Randomization tip**

When Randomization is a part of the study design, the subject will need to know what randomization means. Explain it in terms that are familiar, such as "the flipping of a coin." Here is useful language for your consent form:

"Randomization means that you are put into a group by chance. It is like flipping a coin. Neither you nor the investigator will choose what group you are in. There will be an active study medication group and a placebo group. You will have an equal chance of being placed into either group. Please note that because a placebo is inactive, it will have no effect on your condition. If you are assigned to either group—active or placebo—your condition might not improve or may become worse."

Please note, every study is different. If you have a subject that has to take a certain medication to remain stable in his condition, the experimental agent will be taken in addition to that medication. When applicable, it is important to write this into the consent form.

*TIP*: Medical personnel are accustomed to the procedures they perform and terms they use. They may not think twice about defining procedures or terms to subjects. You will need to be aware of this and define any medical jargon.

An example: Don't state that you are giving them a physical exam. You want to state that you are taking their blood pressure, heart rate, temperature, and weight. Subjects are always worried about shots and needle pricks, so be aware that this fear may be unspoken. Make this a talking point when you are discussing the informed consent form. If there are no shots or needle sticks in a visit, let the potential subject know. State up front there will be no gynecological exams for women. All of this alleviates subjects' (often unspoken) fears and helps recruitment.

Ask questions of the subject. Elicit conversation and provide an opportunity for open discussion with the subject.

*TIP*: On the summary at the end of the consent form, outline a list of the procedures that are Standard of Care (SOC) and a list of the research procedures and the experimental procedures so that the subject has a quick glance at all the procedures.

See the Consent Form Template, pp. 2 and 4, in Appendix 5.

Definition for **standard of care:** In legal terms, the level at which the average, prudent provider in a given community would practice. It is how similarly qualified practitioners would have managed the patient's *care* under the same or similar circumstances.[14]

**Risks and discomforts**

TIP: Required: A list of the risks and discomforts of the study. This is a description of reasonably foreseeable risks or discomforts to the subject. Risks can be found in the protocol, and if an IND or IDE study, in the Investigator's Brochure or Instructions For Use.

*TIP*: A statement placed in the consent form about unknown risks or side effects is smart:

👍 "As with any experimental procedure, there may be risks or side effects that are currently unknown."

*TIP*: For the "additional element" of significant new findings, here is sample language: "If we learn of any risks or findings that might affect your willingness to be in the study, we will discuss these with you. You will be promptly told if during the study any new information develops which may cause you to change your mind about continuing in the study."

👍 **TIP:** Break down the risks from the Investigators' Brochure or Instructions for Use as to which risks and side effects:

1. May occur
2. Are less likely to occur
3. Rarely occur

This provides greater clarity for the subject and aids your recruitment by providing probabilities for the discerning potential subject.

See the Consent Sample for language ideas in the following sections:

**Avoidance of pregnancy**

**Benefits**

**Alternatives**
**Payment**
**Subject Payment for participation**

*TIP*: Will your potential study population have trouble with transportation to your site? Will bus fare, or gas money, help them make it to appointments? If so, let your sponsor/funder know and ask to have a payment for your subjects added to your budget and consent form. If visits are particularly long, request a lunch payment as well.

When adding language into the consent form for a payment, write that it will be given AFTER visit completion. (There have been subjects who have taken the payment and left the study visit early, creating an incomplete visit.)

**Charging**

Tip: Be very cautious about statements offering "free" care. Make it clear that the charges sent to the subject's medical insurance still require a co-pay, co-insurance, and deductible from the patient.

Additionally, when you wish to express that care is "free" to the subject because the Sponsor is paying for it, more prudent language is the following: "The study sponsor, (name the sponsor), is paying for the 'research' and 'experimental' procedures performed in this study. These costs will not be billed to your insurance company or you."

**Think in terms of a court case and whether your language in this section could withstand legal scrutiny.**

**Subject injury**

Your medical center should have its own language for this section. Check with your Legal Department or IRB.

See the sample subject injury language in the Consent Form Template in Appendix 5 and in the Contract language section in Section 2.4 of this chapter.

**Are researchers being paid?** See Consent Form Template in Appendix 5.

**Privacy and Confidentiality (HIPAA)**

Your Medical Center should have its own HIPAA statement. It can be included in the consent form or provided as a separate document. Refer to your IRB for their preference.

There is a HIPAA Statement sample within the Consent Form Template in Appendix 5.

See the Consent Form Template for **Withdrawal** language.

**Contact information**

Fill in the Investigator's 24/7 contact information.

**ClinicalTrials.gov**

The following, exact statement must be included in the informed consent documents of "applicable clinical trials" as stated in 21 CFR 50.25 (c):

"A description of this clinical trial will be available on http://www.ClinicalTrials.gov, as required by U.S. Law. This Web site will not include information that can identify you. At most, the Web site will include a summary of the results. You can search this Web site at any time."[15]

**Placing the Schedule of Events in the Consent Form**

This is a preference of a site and Sponsor. Some like it in the consent form, some do not. Check with your Sponsor and IRB.

### Research Subject's Bill of Rights

IRB Your Medical Center should have its own Research Subject's Bill of Rights. It can be included in the consent form or provided as a separate document. Refer to your IRB for their preference. Note that in the Consent Form Template in Appendix 5, the subject signature language states that the subject has received the "Research Subject's Bill of Rights."

### Consent Extras

Your study may utilize a Certificate of Confidentiality, or offer the archiving of tissue in a biorepository, or you may be capturing genetic information, or you may want to store PHI in a database, or you may want to emphasize or clarify a section in the consent. Here is information and sample language for these scenarios:

### Certificate of Confidentiality (CoC)

CoCs allow researchers to refuse to disclose names or other identifying characteristics of research subjects in response to legal demands. Certificates are issued by NIH to researchers to help protect the privacy of human subjects enrolled in <u>sensitive</u>, health-related research. NIH defines a CoC this way:

Certificates of Confidentiality are issued by the National Institutes of Health (NIH) to protect identifiable research information from forced disclosure. They allow the investigator and others who have access to research records to refuse to disclose identifying information on research participants in any civil, criminal, administrative, legislative, or other proceeding, whether at the federal, state, or local level. Certificates may be granted for studies collecting information that if disclosed could have adverse consequences for subjects or damage their financial standing, employability, insurability, or reputation.[16]

The following link below is to NIH's Certificate of Confidentiality (CoC) kiosk webpage. Click here for more information or to apply for a CoC for your study: https://humansubjects.nih.gov/coc/index. Also, see Chapter 8, Section 5 for the new changes to Certificates of Confidentiality.

**Here is sample consent language if you are using a Certificate of Confidentiality in your study:**

Because of the sensitive nature of this study, the study team has received a "Certificate of Confidentiality" (CoC) from the National Institutes of Health (NIH) to protect your privacy and personal information.

CoCs allow researchers to refuse to disclose names or other identifying characteristics of research subjects in response to legal demands.

This means that the study team cannot be forced by legal action, such as a court order or subpoena, to turn over your personal, identifying information from this study.

It does not prevent the U.S. Department of Health and Human Services (DHHS) from auditing this study, if they choose to, which means that your personal, identifying information will be seen by the DHHS in such an audit. DHHS keeps the results of such audits within the DHHS. No personal, identifying information about you would be released in a report of audit findings.

You must actively protect your own privacy as well by not allowing permission to employers or your health insurance to receive information from this study about you. Read the general medical center consent to procedures or/and billing consent carefully regarding this disclosure and only sign what you agree to.

Please know that the study team is not prevented from responding to and reporting concerns of serious harm to you or others when a CoC is received for a study. For example, if you or anyone you know may be in danger, the study team is required to report this to the authorities and to get emergency help if needed.

### Genetic Information Non-Discrimination Act (GINA)

The **Genetic Information Non-Discrimination Act** of 2008 (Pub.L. 110–233, 122 Stat. 881, enacted May 21, 2008, GINA, pronounced Gee-na) is an Act of the U.S. Congress designed to prohibit the use of genetic information in health insurance and employment. Title II of GINA, which prohibits genetic information discrimination in employment, took effect on November 21, 2009.[17]

GINA defines *genetic information* as information about:

- An individual's genetic tests (including genetic tests done as part of a research study);
- Genetic tests of an individual's family members (defined as dependents and up to and including 4th-degree relatives);
- Genetic tests of any fetus of an individual or family member who is a pregnant woman, and genetic tests of any embryo legally held by an individual or family member utilizing assisted reproductive technology;
- The manifestation of a disease or disorder in an individual's family members (family history); or,
- Any request for, or receipt of, genetic services or participation in clinical research that includes genetic services (genetic testing, counseling, or education) by an individual or an individual's family members.

Genetic information does not include information about the sex or age of any individual.

The Office of Human Research Protections (OHRP, U.S. Department of Health and Human Services) recommends that for genetic research undergoing initial or continuing review, investigators and IRBs consider whether consent processes and documents should include language regarding the protections provided by GINA, and if so, ensure that such language accurately describes the impact of GINA on the risks and confidentiality protections for such research.

The following is one example of sample language regarding the protections provided under GINA that investigators and IRBs may consider including in informed consent documents for such research, if it is determined that including such language is appropriate:

*A new Federal law, called the Genetic Information Non-Discrimination Act (GINA), generally makes it illegal for health insurance companies, group health plans, and most employers to discriminate against you based on your genetic information. This law generally will protect you in the following ways:*

- *Health insurance companies and group health plans may not request your genetic information that we get from this research.*
- *Health insurance companies and group health plans may not use your genetic information when making decisions regarding your eligibility or premiums.*
- *Employers with 15 or more employees may not use your genetic information that we get from this research when making a decision to hire, promote, or fire you or when setting the terms of your employment.*

*Be aware that this new Federal law does not protect you against genetic discrimination by companies that sell life insurance, disability insurance, or long-term care insurance.*

IRBs should feel free to revise the sample language above as appropriate based on the nature of the research and the types of human subjects involved.

If you have specific questions about how to apply this guidance, please contact OHRP by phone at (866) 447-4777 (toll-free within the U.S.) or (240) 453-6900, or by e-mail at ohrp@hhs.gov.[18]

**FYI**

- Health Insurance—Insurers may not discriminate against individuals based on family medical history or individuals' and family members' genetic tests and services.
  - Health insurers may not use genetic information to make eligibility, coverage, underwriting, or premium-setting decisions.
  - Health insurers may not request or require individuals or their family members to undergo genetic testing or to provide genetic information.
  - Insurers cannot use genetic information obtained intentionally or unintentionally in decisions about enrollment or coverage.
  - The use of genetic information as a pre-existing condition is prohibited in both the Medicare supplemental policy and individual health insurance markets.
  - Narrow exceptions to the rules for health insurers are summarized online[19]
- Employment—GINA makes it illegal to discriminate against employees or applicants because of genetic information.
  - Employers may not discriminate on the basis of genetic information when it comes to any aspect of employment.
  - Whether by a supervisor, co-worker, client, or customer, harassment because of someone's genetic information is illegal.
  - It is illegal for an employer to fire, demote, harass, or otherwise "retaliate" against an applicant or employee who has filed a charge of discrimination, participates in a discrimination proceeding, or opposes genetic discrimination.
  - GINA makes it illegal for an employer to obtain genetic information, including family medical history, except under certain exceptions. Employers are forbidden from disclosing genetic information about applicants or employees.[20]
- GINA sets a minimum standard of protection that must be met across the country. It does not weaken the protections provided by any state law.
- The law does not cover life insurance, disability insurance, or long-term care insurance.[21]

### Genetic Studies

For sample consent language regarding the permission to perform genetic studies, state whether the subject will be identified or whether the samples will be de-identified—in 7th-grade language, or in the grade level approved by your IRB.

**Sample consent language for permission:**

**Biological sample genetic studies**: DNA, RNA, proteins, and other materials may be separated from your tissue samples and used for genetic studies.

Yes No _____ initials. Have the research subject circle either "Yes" or "No".

If you are offering test result information (from identifiable tissue samples), your consent language can continue to read:

You or your physician may contact the study doctor to request available genetic study results. If the information may be helpful for decisions regarding your health care, the genetic study results may be released to your treating physician. Your treating physician will speak with you about the suggested use of the information for your medical care.

### Banking of Tissue Specimens

Sample consent language:

We would like to store tissue specimens collected from you in this study in a tissue bank for future research as noted below. The tissue specimens consist of [specify, e.g., tissue, blood, and other body fluids, as well as DNA and RNA from these biological specimens]. The tissue bank is housed by [insert name of Institution. If tissue bank is maintained at your Medical Center, specify the responsible Department].

**Please indicate your approval of each of the following by initialing on the lines below:**

My tissue may be stored in the above-named tissue bank for future analysis related to [insert name of specific study]. Yes No _____ initials

My tissue may be stored in the above-named tissue bank. Researchers may contact me to request my authorization for future studies that are not related to this study or the disease named above. Yes No _____ initials

My tissue may be stored without any of my identifying information for use in other studies of other diseases. Yes No _____ initials

I may change my mind at a later time and request that my tissue specimen be destroyed. If I change my mind and want to request that my tissue be destroyed, I must do so in writing to [Insert name and contact information of PI].

**For tissue extraction and storage, consent language may read as follows:**

**Storage and use of leftover tissue removed at the time of a surgical procedure:** If you have surgery to remove tissue as a part of your routine medical care, there can be a small amount of tissue leftover. This leftover tissue is not needed for your clinical care and may be thrown away. We would like permission to store it for research instead. Your routine medical surgery will not change if you agree to take part in this repository.

Yes No _____ initials

**Storage of PHI in a Database:**

We would like to store personal health information collected from you in this study in a database for future research. The database is housed by [Insert name of Institution. If database is maintained at your Medical Center, specify the responsible Department].

**Please indicate your approval of each of the following by initialing on the lines below**:

My personal health information may be stored in the above-named database for future analysis related to [Insert name of specific study]. Yes No _____ initials

My personal health information may be stored in the above-named database. Researchers may contact me to request my authorization for future studies that are not related to this study or the disease named above. Yes No _____ initials

My personal health information may be stored without any of my identifying information for use in other studies. Yes No _____ initials

**Notice of Privacy Practices and Privacy Officer Contact**

If you DO NOT include the HIPAA statement <u>IN</u> your consent form, you must find out if your potential research subjects have obtained the HIPAA information from your medical center at a previous clinical visit, or you must give it to them as a separate document.

**Sample consent language:**

If you have not already received a Notice of Privacy Practices from (Name of your Medical Center), you may request a copy from a study team member and will be given one. If you have any questions or concerns about your privacy rights, you may contact the (Name of your Medical Center) Privacy Officer at phone number xxx-xxx-xxxx.

**Dietary supplements**

**Sample consent language:**

At the study screening, you will need to tell a study team member about all of the prescription and over-the-counter drugs, vitamins, herbs, supplements, and alternative medicines you are taking. Any of these can interact with the study agent, so it is important you tell us about them.

A study team member will review all of these with you and will let you know if you can take part in the study.

During the course of the study, if you want to add a new over-the-counter drug, a vitamin, or other supplement to your diet, you agree to talk about this with your study doctor before taking it.

**If media such as video or audio tapes/DVDs/digital recordings, or photographs are being used for the research study:**

**Write in your consent form:**

- Whether the subjects will be identifiable (voice recognition, facial images, etc.)
- Whether transcripts of the video or audio recordings will be made and the tapes destroyed, thus de-identifying the subjects
  - What will happen to the media at the end of the study?
- Will the recordings be stored as is? If so, consent for PHI use will be needed.
- How long will the recordings or photos be stored and where?
- If the media will be displayed in a public setting such as at conferences or for teaching, or for advertisement, or publication, you will need to prepare an additional Media Consent Form.

A modification to the National Center for Research Resources (NCRR) **RFA-RM-10-001 released on March 16, 2010 states:**

*Regulatory support should include research subject advocacy functions through a designated department or office independent of the IRB function, to serve as an advocate for research participants, and work with investigators, trainees, and research teams to ensure that research involving human subjects accords the highest priority to human subject protections.*[22]

Reference your Medical Center's policy on Research Subject Advocates (RSAs) to learn the duties assigned to this position. For example, RSAs can serve as an impartial witness during consenting, or/and RSAs can meet with research subjects individually to address their concerns, or/and RSAs can review protocols and amendments for human subjects protections, and other duties.

Should you offer a Research Subject Advocate for your study, here is sample consent language:

**Research Subject Advocate:**

The National Institutes of Health supports a Research Subject Advocate or RSA for the research study that you are being asked to join. The RSA for (name your Medical Center) is (Title and name of person or Department). He/She/The Department can be called to answer your questions or concerns about taking part in this research study. He/She/The Department does not work for the Investigator(s) who are doing this research and he/she/they do(es) not pay him/her/the Department. He/She/The Department will help to protect your research subject rights during this research study if you would like to ask for the Department's support.

You can call (Title and name of person or Department) at XXX-XXX-XXXX or reach the Department/Office by e-mail at (e-mail address).

For studies involving interviews, questionnaires, surveys, or other procedures revealing sensitive information, include in your consent language: Under (Name your State) Law, suspected child or elder abuse must be reported to the appropriate authorities. (Know your State law before including this statement in a consent form.)

**Signature of language interpreter (if applicable)**
Printed Name of Interpreter:

Interpreter's Signature:
Language: ___
Date and Time: a.m./p.m. (circle one)
**WITNESS**
See the "Witness" section of the book.

If the subject cannot read or speak or write, the signature of an impartial witness is required:

The witness signature line should be the last signature line on the consent form.
Include:
The method used for communicating with the subject was:

The specific means by which the prospective subject communicated agreement to participate in the study was:

Printed Name of Witness          Date
Signature of Witness               Time AM/PM (circle one)

**If you will need to consent over the phone or via video conferencing, here are the steps:**

1. Place in a large envelope in the mail or via courier:
   **a.** Two copies of the informed consent form with a self-addressed stamped envelope (SASE).
   **b.** Instructions for calling the PI or Research Nurse or Study Coordinator (your choice) when the consent forms are received
2. The PI or Research Nurse or Study Coordinator will read through and explain the consent and study over the phone or video conference.
3. The potential subject will be given the opportunity to ask any and all questions they would like.
4. The potential subject can be given time to discuss the study with their family or their primary care physician or they may tell you their decision during the phone call. It is up to the potential subject.
5. If the potential subject decides to consent, have him/her sign one consent form and send it back in the SASE. Have him/her keep the second consent form for his/her own records.
6. The study team will receive the signed consent form in the mail or via courier and will have it signed by the PI.

**Research Subject Card**
The study team will need to create a Research Subject Card if they want to use cards in a study. The card is created for the purpose of notifying anyone to whom the card is presented (such as a physician or emergency room doctor or dentist) that the patient is in a medical research study. It should contain

the contact information of the Principal Investigator in case of an emergency, and whether an IND or IDE or other intervention is being used. If the trial is a qualifying clinical trial, write the NCT number from www.clinicaltrials.gov on the card so that the exact study information may be referenced.

ICH **ICH GCP states the following regarding informed consent:**

**4.6. Informed Consent of Trial Subjects**

4.8.1. In obtaining and documenting informed consent, the investigator should comply with the applicable regulatory requirement(s), and should adhere to GCP and to the ethical principles that have their origin in the Declaration of Helsinki. Prior to the beginning of the trial, the investigator should have the IRB/IEC's written approval/favorable opinion of the written informed consent form and any other written information to be provided to subjects.

4.8.2. The written informed consent form and any other written information to be provided to subjects should be revised whenever important new information becomes available that may be relevant to the subject's consent. Any revised written informed consent form, and written information should receive the IRB/IEC's approval/favorable opinion in advance of use. The subject or the subject's legally acceptable representative should be informed in a timely manner if new information becomes available that may be relevant to the subject's willingness to continue participation in the trial. The communication of this information should be documented.

4.8.3. Neither the investigator, nor the trial staff, should coerce or unduly influence a subject to participate or to continue to participate in a trial.

4.8.4. None of the oral and written information concerning the trial, including the written informed consent form, should contain any language that causes the subject or the subject's legally acceptable representative to waive or to appear to waive any legal rights, or that releases or appears to release the investigator, the institution, the sponsor, or their agents from liability for negligence.

4.8.5. The investigator, or a person designated by the investigator, should fully inform the subject or, if the subject is unable to provide informed consent, the subject's legally acceptable representative, of all pertinent aspects of the trial including the written information and the approval/ favorable opinion by the IRB/IEC.

4.8.6. The language used in the oral and written information about the trial, including the written informed consent form, should be as non-technical as practical and should be understandable to the subject or the subject's legally acceptable representative and the impartial witness, where applicable.

4.8.7. Before informed consent may be obtained, the investigator, or a person designated by the investigator, should provide the subject or the subject's legally acceptable representative ample time and opportunity to inquire about details of the trial and to decide whether or not to participate in the trial. All questions about the trial should be answered to the satisfaction of the subject or the subject's legally acceptable representative.

4.8.8. Prior to a subject's participation in the trial, the written informed consent form should be signed and personally dated by the subject or by the subject's legally acceptable representative, and by the person who conducted the informed consent discussion.

4.8.9. If a subject is unable to read or if a legally acceptable representative is unable to read, an impartial witness should be present during the entire informed consent discussion. After the written informed consent form and any other written information to be provided to subjects, is read and explained to the subject or the subject's legally acceptable representative, and after the subject or the subject's legally acceptable representative has orally consented to the subject's participation in the trial and, if capable of doing so, has signed and personally dated the informed consent form, the witness should sign and personally date the consent form. By signing the consent form, the witness attests that the information in the consent form and any other written information was accurately explained to, and apparently understood by, the subject or the subject's legally acceptable representative, and that informed consent was freely given by the subject or the subject's legally acceptable representative.

4.8.10. Both the informed consent discussion and the written informed consent form and any other written information to be provided to subjects should include explanations of the following:

**(a)** That the trial involves research.
**(b)** The purpose of the trial.
**(c)** The trial treatment(s) and the probability for random assignment to each treatment.
**(d)** The trial procedures to be followed, including all invasive procedures.
**(e)** The subject's responsibilities.
**(f)** Those aspects of the trial that are experimental.
**(g)** The reasonably foreseeable risks or inconveniences to the subject and, when applicable, to an embryo, fetus, or nursing infant.
**(h)** The reasonably expected benefits. When there is no intended clinical benefit to the subject, the subject should be made aware of this.
**(i)** The alternative procedure(s) or course(s) of treatment that may be available to the subject, and their important potential benefits and risks.
**(j)** The compensation and/or treatment available to the subject in the event of trial-related injury.
**(k)** The anticipated prorated payment, if any, to the subject for participating in the trial.
**(l)** The anticipated expenses, if any, to the subject for participating in the trial.
**(m)** That the subject's participation in the trial is voluntary and that the subject may refuse to participate or withdraw from the trial, at any time, without penalty or loss of benefits to which the subject is otherwise entitled.
**(n)** That the monitor(s), the auditor(s), the IRB/IEC, and the regulatory authority(ies) will be granted direct access to the subject's original medical records for verification of clinical trial procedures and/or data, without violating the confidentiality of the subject, to the extent permitted by the applicable laws and regulations and that, by signing a written informed consent form, the subject or the subject's legally acceptable representative is authorizing such access.
**(o)** That records identifying the subject will be kept confidential and, to the extent permitted by the applicable laws and/or regulations, will not be made publicly available. If the results of the trial are published, the subject's identity will remain confidential.
**(p)** That the subject or the subject's legally acceptable representative will be informed in a timely manner if information becomes available that may be relevant to the subject's willingness to continue participation in the trial.
**(q)** The person(s) to contact for further information regarding the trial and the rights of trial subjects, and whom to contact in the event of trial-related injury.
**(r)** The foreseeable circumstances and/or reasons under which the subject's participation in the trial may be terminated.
**(s)** The expected duration of the subject's participation in the trial.
**(t)** The approximate number of subjects involved in the trial.

4.8.11. Prior to participation in the trial, the subject or the subject's legally acceptable representative should receive a copy of the signed and dated written informed consent form and any other written information provided to the subjects. During a subject's participation in the trial, the subject or the subject's legally acceptable representative should receive a copy of the signed and dated consent form updates and a copy of any amendments to the written information provided to subjects.

4.8.12. When a clinical trial (therapeutic or non-therapeutic) includes subjects who can only be enrolled in the trial with the consent of the subject's legally acceptable representative (e.g., minors, or patients with severe dementia), the subject should be informed about the trial to the extent compatible with the subject's understanding and, if capable, the subject should sign and personally date the written informed consent.

4.8.13. Except as described in 4.8.14, a non-therapeutic trial (i.e., a trial in which there is no anticipated direct clinical benefit to the subject) should be conducted in subjects who personally give consent and who sign and date the written informed consent form.

4.8.14. Non-therapeutic trials may be conducted in subjects with consent of a legally acceptable representative provided the following conditions are fulfilled:

**(a)** The objectives of the trial cannot be met by means of a trial in subjects who can give informed consent personally.
**(b)** The foreseeable risks to the subjects are low.
**(c)** The negative impact on the subject's well-being is minimized and low.
**(d)** The trial is not prohibited by law.
**(e)** The approval/favorable opinion of the IRB/IEC is expressly sought on the inclusion of such subjects, and the written approval/ favorable opinion covers this aspect. Such trials, unless an exception is justified, should be conducted in patients having a disease or condition for which the investigational product is intended. Subjects in these trials should be particularly closely monitored and should be withdrawn if they appear to be unduly distressed.

4.8.15. In emergency situations, when prior consent of the subject is not possible, the consent of the subject's legally acceptable representative, if present, should be requested. When prior consent of the subject is not possible, and the subject's legally acceptable representative is not available, enrollment of the subject should require measures described in the protocol and/or elsewhere, with documented approval/favorable opinion by the IRB/IEC, to protect the rights, safety and well-being of the subject and to ensure compliance with applicable regulatory requirements. The subject or the subject's legally acceptable representative should be informed about the trial as soon as possible and consent to continue and other consent as appropriate (see 4.8.10) should be requested.

## 2.5.1 WAIVER OR ALTERATION OF CONSENT

*Purpose of section*:

• Explains when a waiver or alteration of consent applies
• Explains what the short form consent is and when it applies
• Explains a waiver of documentation of consent
• Provides a short form consent sample

### Waiver or alteration of consent—Common rule
The Code of Federal Regulations that permit informed consent to be waived are found here: 45 CFR 46.116 (c) and (d)

(c) An IRB may approve a consent procedure which does not include, or which alters, some or all of the elements of informed consent set forth above, or waive the requirement to obtain informed consent provided the IRB finds and documents that:

**(1)** The research or demonstration project is to be conducted by or subject to the approval of state or local government officials and is designed to study, evaluate, or otherwise examine: (i) Public benefit of service programs; (ii) procedures for obtaining benefits or services under those programs; (iii) possible changes in or alternatives to those programs or procedures; or (iv) possible changes in methods or levels of payment for benefits or services under those programs.
**(2)** The research could not practicably be carried out without the waiver or alteration.

(d) An IRB may approve a consent procedure which does not include, or which alters, some or all of the elements of informed consent set forth in this section, or waive the requirements to obtain informed consent provided the IRB finds and documents that:

**(1)** The research involves no more than minimal risk to the subjects;
**(2)** The waiver or alteration will not adversely affect the rights and welfare of the subjects;
**(3)** The research could not practicably be carried out without the waiver or alteration; and
**(4)** Whenever appropriate, the subjects will be provided with additional pertinent information after participation.[23]

An example of C is your State's Food Stamp program. If a study is conducted to determine the number of families in the State needing food stamps, what their median household income is, and how people access the program, informed consent could be waived to access this family information before it is de-identified and aggregated for evaluation.

An example of D is retrospective chart reviews to gather information when studying the natural history of a disease. Trying to find the current contact information for hundreds of patients and requesting the use of their medical chart information could render the study inoperable.

A waiver of HIPAA authorization will also be required for studies accessing or using PHI.

For other situations in which informed consent can be waived or altered, also see "Emergency Use of a Test Article" in Chapter 6, Section 6.3, which falls under the FDA regulations found in 21 CFR 50. Also, see a Short form consent sample in Appendix 5. See your IRB for their process.

---

Waiver or Alteration of Consent—New Common Rule
45 CFR 46.116 (f) (1), (2), and (3)
(f) *General waiver or alteration of consent*:
(1) *Waiver.* An IRB may waive the requirement to obtain informed consent for research under paragraphs (a) through (c) of this section, provided the IRB satisfies the requirements of paragraph (f)(3) of this section. If an individual was asked to provide broad consent for the storage, maintenance, and secondary research use of identifiable private information or identifiable biospecimens in accordance with the requirements at paragraph (d) of this section, and refused to consent, an IRB cannot waive consent for the storage, maintenance, or secondary research use of the identifiable private information or identifiable biospecimens.
(2) *Alteration.* An IRB may approve a consent procedure that omits some, or alters some or all, of the elements of informed consent set forth in paragraphs (b) and (c) of this section provided the IRB satisfies the requirements of paragraph (f)(3) of this section. An IRB may not omit or alter any of the requirements described in paragraph (a) of this section. If a broad consent procedure is used, an IRB may not omit or alter any of the elements required under paragraph (d) of this section.
(3) *Requirements for waiver and alteration.* In order for an IRB to waive or alter consent as described in this subsection, the IRB must find and document that:

(i) The research involves no more than minimal risk to the subjects;
(ii) The research could not practicably be carried out without the requested waiver or alteration;
(iii) If the research involves using identifiable private information or identifiable biospecimens, the research could not practicably be carried out without using such information or biospecimens in an identifiable format;
(iv) The waiver or alteration will not adversely affect the rights and welfare of the subjects; and
(v) Whenever appropriate, the subjects or legally authorized representatives will be provided with additional pertinent information after participation.

## 2.5.2 WAIVER OF DOCUMENTATION OF CONSENT

*Purpose of section*:

- Explains why and when a Waiver of Documentation of Consent is used
- Provides an overview of Regulations concerning a Waiver of Documentation of Consent

Waiver of the documentation of consent occurs when potential research subjects read through and consider the written consent form, but the consent form is not signed because the IRB has allowed for consent without the subject's signature.

The regulation:

45 CFR 46.117 (c) (This is the U.S. Health and Human Services regulation.)

"An IRB may waive the requirement for the investigator to obtain a signed consent form for some or all subjects if it finds either:

**(1)** That the only record linking the subject and the research would be the consent document and the principal risk would be potential harm resulting from a breach of confidentiality. Each subject will be asked whether the subject wants documentation linking the subject with the research, and the subject's wishes will govern; or

**(2)** That the research presents no more than minimal risk of harm to subjects and involves no procedures for which written consent is normally required outside of the research context.

In cases in which the documentation requirement is waived, the IRB may require the investigator to provide subjects with a written statement regarding the research."[24]

---

45 CFR 46.117 (c) New Common Rule

(c)(1) An IRB may waive the requirement for the investigator to obtain a signed informed consent form for some or all subjects if it finds any of the following:

(i) That the only record linking the subject and the research would be the informed consent form and the principal risk would be potential harm resulting from a breach of confidentiality. Each subject (or legally authorized representative) will be asked whether the subject wants documentation linking the subject with the research, and the subject's wishes will govern;

(ii) That the research presents no more than minimal risk of harm to subjects and involves no procedures for which written consent is normally required outside of the research context; or

(iii) If the subjects or legally authorized representatives are members of a distinct cultural group or community in which signing forms is not the norm, that the research presents no more than minimal risk of harm to subjects and provided there is an appropriate alternative mechanism for documenting that informed consent was obtained.

(2) In cases in which the documentation requirement is waived, the IRB may require the investigator to provide subjects or legally authorized representatives with a written statement regarding the research.

Examples of number (1) above (for both the Common Rule and New Common Rule) is HIV research, or research that enrolls homosexual persons who have not gone public with their sexual orientation, or any study that collects information considered sensitive. For example, a study subject may have concerns that his/her HIV diagnosis could become known if a "breach" or mistake is made in holding their information confidential.

An example of number (2) above (for both the Common Rule and New Common Rule) is a study that interviews research subjects either in person or via phone, or a study that administers mailed or online surveys. (There are no invasive procedures, for example, and the greatest risk is the risk of a breach in confidentiality.)

⚠ Please note, the FDA regulations at 21 CFR 50 do not allow for a waiver of the documentation of consent. The FDA regulations expect a signature on a consent form or the use of the short form and summary. What does this mean? Here are two examples: If you are conducting research under the FDA regulations, such as an IND or IDE clinical trial, you cannot waive the documentation of consent. If you are conducting Investigator Initiated research under the HHS regulations, you can.

**When utilizing the waiver of documentation of consent, HIPAA requirements have to be taken into account. This means that a waiver or alteration of HIPAA authorization HAS TO accompany a waiver of documentation of consent WHEN protected health information (PHI) will be used or shared in your research study.**

IRB **Your IRB will have a process for this review and authorization.**

## 2.5.3 SHORT FORM CONSENT

*Purpose of section*:

- Explains the short form consent document

The relevant regulations for short form consent are: 21 CFR 50.27(b) (2) and 45 CFR 46.117 (b) (2) [These two regulations have the exact same wording except for the CFR reference. The 21 CFR 50 regulation is the FDA regulation. The 45 CFR 46 regulation is the HHS Common Rule regulation.

What these regulations say:

A *short form* written consent document stating that the elements of informed consent required by 50.25 (46.116) have been presented orally to the subject or the subject's legally authorized representative. When this method is used, there shall be a witness to the oral presentation. Also, the IRB shall approve a written summary of what is to be said to the subject or the representative. Only the short form itself is to be signed by the subject or the representative. However, the witness shall sign both the short form and a copy of the summary, and the person actually obtaining the consent shall sign a copy of the summary. A copy of the summary shall be given to the subject or the representative in addition to a copy of the short form.[25]

---

45 CFR 46.117 (b) (2) New Common Rule

(2) A short form written informed consent form stating that the elements of informed consent required by §ll.116 have been presented orally to the subject or the subject's legally authorized representative, and that the key information required by §ll.116(a)(5)(i) was presented first to the subject, before other information, if any, was provided. The IRB shall approve a written summary of what is to be said to the subject or the legally authorized representative. When this method is used, there shall be a witness to the oral presentation. Only the short form itself is to be signed by the subject or the subject's

legally authorized representative. However, the witness shall sign both the short form and a copy of the summary, and the person actually obtaining consent shall sign a copy of the summary. A copy of the summary shall be given to the subject or the subject's legally authorized representative, in addition to a copy of the short form.

In support of this regulation, here is 45 CFR 46.116 (a)(5)(i) in the New Common Rule:

Informed consent must begin with a concise and focused presentation of the key information that is most likely to assist a prospective subject or legally authorized representative in understanding the reasons why one might or might not want to participate in the research. This part of the informed consent must be organized and presented in a way that facilitates comprehension.

| Table 2.2 Short Form Consenting Signatures Table | | | |
|---|---|---|---|
| | **Subject/LAR** | **Witness** | **Person obtaining consent** |
| Short form | X | X | |
| Summary | | X | X |

Required Signatures for Short Form consenting (according to the Common Rule and New Common Rule) is shown in Table 2.2.

Presenting a consent orally to a subject or LAR may be necessary because a subject may be illiterate. If the potential subject cannot read or write, but understands spoken English, he or she may sign the short form with an "X" or other mark unique to him or her (something of their own design) in the presence of a witness.

Another example is a potential subject who does not speak English. The short form must be translated into the language of the potential subject. If you have a study into which you will be recruiting English-speaking persons, but you may get a few who do not speak English, the short form consent and summary translated into the relevant language(s) can be used. If you will potentially be able to recruit a number of persons who speak another language, it is best to translate a full consent form and to go through the regular consenting process.

IRB Refer to your IRB's policy on subjects who speak languages other than English if they have one. (Otherwise, use this Section to help guide you.) When the short form is translated, you will also need an interpreter to answer questions and ascertain the potential subject's understanding of the research study.

A sample short form consent by the Office for Human Research Protections within the U.S. Health and Human Services (HHS) found at: https://www.hhs.gov/ohrp/regulations-and-policy/guidance/obtaining-and-documenting-infomed-consent-non-english-speakers/index.html

**SAMPLE SHORT FORM WRITTEN CONSENT DOCUMENT FOR SUBJECTS WHO DO NOT SPEAK ENGLISH**

***THIS DOCUMENT MUST BE WRITTEN IN A LANGUAGE UNDERSTANDABLE TO THE SUBJECT***

Consent to Participate in Research

You are being asked to participate in a research study.

Before you agree, the investigator must tell you about (i) the purposes, procedures, and duration of the research; (ii) any procedures, which are experimental; (iii) any reasonably foreseeable risks, discomforts, and benefits of the research; (iv) any potentially beneficial alternative procedures or treatments; and (v) how confidentiality will be maintained.

Where applicable, the investigator must also tell you about (i) any available compensation or medical treatment if injury occurs; (ii) the possibility of unforeseeable risks; (iii) circumstances when the investigator may halt your participation; (iv) any added costs to you; (v) what happens if you decide to stop participating; (vi) when you will be told about new findings which may affect your willingness to participate; and (vii) how many people will be in the study.

If you agree to participate, you must be given a signed copy of this document and a written summary of the research.

You may contact (**name**) at (**phone number**) any time you have questions about the research.

You may contact (**name**) at (**phone number**) if you have questions about your rights as a research subject or what to do if you are injured.

Your participation in this research is voluntary, and you will not be penalized or lose benefits if you refuse to participate or decide to stop.

Signing this document means that the research study, including the above information, has been described to you out loud, and that you voluntarily agree to participate.

Signature of participant _____

date_____

Signature of witness _____

date_____

The summary is to be read out loud to the potential subject and will include the specifics of your study that match what is mentioned in the short form (which all match the basic and additional elements of informed consent from the CFR, provided in the table earlier in the chapter). For example, taking "i" from the short form above:

Before you agree, the investigator must tell you about (i) the purposes, procedures, and duration of the research.

The purpose of this research is to determine whether an investigational drug, named AHQ123, will reduce blood sugar levels in diabetics. The procedures are:

Name ALL of the procedures that are to occur at each visit. For example, a physical exam, which will entail a medical history, height, weight, vital signs, and a review of any medications you are taking. A blood sample will be taken to measure… (and continue this way).

If you agree to participate, you will be in the study for 2 years. There will be 8 visits total within the 2 years.

## 2.5.4 ASSENT

*Purpose of section*:

- Defines Assent
- The IRB determination of whether assent is required
- Clarifies parental permission and child assent and which takes precedence

To begin, here are some useful definitions:

*Assent* means a child's affirmative agreement to participate in research. Mere failure to object should not, absent affirmative agreement, be construed as assent (45 CFR 46.402 (b)).[26]

*Children* are persons who have not attained the legal age for consent to treatments or procedures involved in the research, under the applicable law of the jurisdiction in which the research will be conducted (45 CFR 46.402 (a)).[27]

*Permission* means the agreement of parent(s) or guardian to the participation of their child or ward in research. (45 CFR 46.402 (c)).[28]

The IRB of record will determine whether children need to be assented or not:

"…In determining whether children are capable of assenting, **the IRB shall take into account the ages, maturity, and psychological state of the children involved. This judgment may be made for all children to be involved in research under a particular protocol, or for each child, as the IRB deems appropriate**. If the IRB determines that the capability of some or all of the children is so limited that they cannot reasonably be consulted or that the intervention or procedure involved in the research holds out a prospect of direct benefit that is important to the health or well-being of the children and is available only in the context of the research, the assent of the children is not a necessary condition for proceeding with the research. Even where the IRB determines that the subjects are capable of assenting, the IRB may still waive the assent requirement under circumstances in which consent may be waived in accord with §46.116 of Subpart A" (45 CFR 46.408 (a)).[29]

**The Assent Form method of providing Assent:**

When the IRB determines that assent is required, it shall also determine whether and how assent must be documented (45 CFR 46.408 (e)).[30]

Assent Forms are typically used to acquire the assent of children. There are two Template Assent Forms in Appendix 27 for your use. One form is for children from 12-17 years of age. The other is for children from 7 to 11 years of age.

When a child reaches the age of adulthood as defined by your State (which is 18 years of age in most States) consenting with an adult consent form or other means of consenting as required by your IRB must take place.

**Regulatory Requirements for Parent/Guardian Permission**

Permission from parent(s) or guardian(s) must be obtained prior to enrolling a child in research. This permission must meet the requirements for informed consent found in 45 CFR 46.116. (This same regulation reference applies to both the Common Rule and the New Common Rule.) The parent permission form is an adult consent form. See "Consent Forms and Documentation" in Section 2.5.

- The permission of one parent may be sufficient for research to be conducted under 45 CFR 46.404 or 46.405.
- Where research is covered by 45 CFR 46.406 and 46.407 and permission is to be obtained by parents, both parents must give their permission unless:
  - One parent is deceased, unknown, incompetent, or not reasonably available; or
  - Only one parent has legal responsibility for the care and custody of the child. 45 CFR 46.408(b).[31]

**The following two Questions and Answers are very helpful points from HHS.gov *Research with Children FAQs:***

Do parental permission and child assent for research involving children have to occur at the same time or in any particular order?

The HHS regulations do not specify the order in which parental or guardian permission and child assent should be sought. Therefore, Institutional Review Boards (IRB) have the discretion to determine the appropriate order given the research and the context in which it will be conducted.

In general, parental or guardian permission should be sought before seeking the assent of a child, particularly in more than minimal risk research, unless the requirement for obtaining parental or guardian permission can be waived. There might be some cases, however, involving minimal risk research, where it would be reasonable to seek child assent prior to seeking parental permission.

For example, a school-based study of minimal risk (e.g., investigating children's responses to music), could be posed to children in the school setting. Children could be asked if they wanted to participate and, if so, sent home with a request for parental or guardian permission. In all cases, except when the requirement for obtaining parental or guardian permission can be waived, parental or guardian permission, even if sought after child assent is provided, is required before the child can be enrolled in the study.

<u>What happens when there is disagreement between a child and his/her parents about research participation?</u>

If a child is capable of assent and the Institutional Review Board (IRB) requires that assent be sought, it must be obtained before the child can participate in the research activity. Thus, if the child dissents from participating in research, even if his or her parents or guardian have granted permission, the child's decision prevails.

However, the regulations state at <u>45 CFR 46.408(a)</u> that the IRB may waive the assent requirements if the intervention or procedure involved in the research holds out the prospect of direct benefit that is important to the health or well-being of the children and is available only in the context of research. Conversely, if a child assents to participate in research, and parental permission has not been waived by the IRB, the permission of the parents or guardian is also required before the child can be enrolled in the research.[32]

## 2.6 THE CLINICAL TRIAL BUDGET

*Purpose of section*:

- Explains how to create a clinical trial per patient budget
- Explains invoiceable fees and their budgeting
- Explains non-procedures and their budgeting
- Describes the Cost Reimbursable Budget

### The Clinical Trial Per Patient Budget

Following are the step-by-step instructions for creating a Per-Patient Budget:

**(1)** Start with the Schedule of Events in the protocol. (Of note, every Industry Sponsor will have its own name for this table. It can be called the Schedule of Assessments or the Visit Table, etc. It is the grid manifesting the procedures to be performed in the study and the visits at which they will occur.)

**(i)** Example:

This "schedule" continues through the length of the study for every visit. (See Table 2.3.)

If you are not conducting an Industry-sponsored study, and the funder is not providing a Schedule of Events, create one yourself! This one was created in Microsoft Excel. The "x" indicates that the procedure or activity is to occur at the visit in which the "x" is found. This table will keep you organized and will make sure you are providing the same tests/procedures/activities for every research subject.

**(ii)** 👍 Read through the procedure section in the protocol to make sure the Schedule of Events has captured all procedures and activities for a trial. There can be different teams within a Sponsor's company that work on the written and financial parts of a study. The documents do not always agree, because the teams do not always coordinate. Therefore, do a "congruency review" to make sure the protocol's written procedure section, the budget template, and the Schedule of Events match. If not, call the Sponsor and talk it through. Sometimes, an amendment is required to fix what has been missed or is not in a budget template or protocol.

**Table 2.3  Per Patient Budget Sample 1**

| Procedures/Activities | Screening | Visit 1 | Visit 2 | Visit 3 |
|---|---|---|---|---|
| Consent | X | | | |
| Inclusion/exclusion criteria | X | | | |
| Concomitant medications | X | X | X | X |
| Vital signs | X | X | X | X |
| Physical exam | X | | | |
| Lab tests: AST, ALT, Bilirubin, CBC | X | | X | |
| 12 Lead EKG | | X | | X |
| AE/SAE assessment | | | X | X |
| IND dispensing | | X | | |
| PK | | | X | |
| Quality-of-life survey | | | | X |

    **(iii)** 👍 If you are writing the protocol, budget, and Schedule of Events, make sure they match. Do your own congruency review.

**(2)** Identify the CPT codes for each procedure. CPT coders work in the Hospital Billing Department. You may need to work in collaboration with a designated clinical research coder in Hospital Billing, if your Institution has one, or with a general coder in Hospital Billing.

    **(a)** Most Finance Department employees who perform budgeting do not have a CPT coding certificate or CPT coding expertise. And most CPT coders do not have budgeting experience or expertise, so collaboration is essential.

    **(b)** You may find an individual who has both a CPT coding certification and budgeting experience who can create your clinical research budgets, but this is extremely rare, so plan on collaborating or training to get the required skill sets needed.

**(3)** Everywhere there is an "x," replace it with a dollar value for the charge of the procedure at your medical center.

    **(a)** Every hospital has a "ChargeMaster," which is a list of every procedure, and its CPT code, and every supply offered at the hospital and what the hospital charges for it. Use the Chargemaster to plug in the charges for the procedures/activities.

        **(i)** Be aware that there are technical fees and professional fees. Your Institution may bundle them together or separate them. If they are separated, you will need to add the technical fee and the professional fee together for each procedure to arrive at your final dollar value.

        **(ii)** Non-procedural activities will have professional fees only, such as consenting, and analyzing inclusion/exclusion criteria, and performing AE/SAE assessments.

    **(b)** 🏥 Your medical center may have a reduced rate or discount for research procedures/activities. Find out if they do and apply this rate if it pertains.

        **(i)** Now your table will look like this: (Each value for a procedure is your technical and professional fee added together minus the research discount. Each non-procedural activity is the professional fee only minus the research discount.) (See Table 2.4.)

    (Of note, Industry sponsors typically pay for all trial procedures and activities indicated in the protocol's Schedule of Events.)

**Table 2.4  Per Patient Budget Sample 2**

| Procedures/Activities | Screening | Visit 1 | Visit 2 | Visit 3 |
|---|---|---|---|---|
| Consent | 100 | | | |
| Inclusion/exclusion criteria | 50 | | | |
| Concomitant medications | 25 | 25 | 25 | 25 |
| Vital signs | 55 | 55 | 55 | 55 |
| Physical exam | 245 | | | |
| Lab tests: AST, ALT, Bilirubin, CBC | 315 | | 315 | |
| 12 Lead EKG | | 403 | | 403 |
| AE/SAE assessment | | | 40 | 40 |
| IND dispensing | | 33 | | |
| PK | | | 500 | |
| Quality-of-life survey | | | | 35 |

**(ii)** If some of the procedures will be paid by the subject's medical insurance from a Coverage Analysis, which determined that the Clinical Trial qualified for medical insurance coverage for routine costs (See Medicare Coverage Analysis in Section 2.8 of this chapter), your budget will need to be broken down into what is Standard of Care that will be paid by insurance, and what is considered "research" that will be paid by the sponsor/funding source. For qualifying trials, you will want to do this step before filling in values. The budget will then look something like this (Table 2.5). If the person/Department that is performing the Coverage Analysis is separate from the person/Department writing the budget, you can write "RES" for Research instead of putting a dollar value directly in a cell. "RES" will convey that a dollar amount needs to be written in the cell because the Sponsor or funder will be paying.

**Table 2.5  Per Patient Budget Sample 3**

| Procedures/Activities | Screening | Visit 1 | Visit 2 | Visit 3 |
|---|---|---|---|---|
| Consent | 100 | | | |
| Inclusion/exclusion criteria | 50 | | | |
| Concomitant medications | SOC | SOC | SOC | SOC |
| Vital signs | SOC | SOC | SOC | SOC |
| Physical exam | SOC | | | |
| Lab tests: AST, ALT, Bilirubin, CBC | 315 | | SOC | |
| 12 Lead EKG | | SOC | | SOC |
| AE/SAE assessment | | | 40 | 40 |
| IND dispensing | | 33 | | |
| PK | | | 500 | |
| Quality-of-life survey | | | | 35 |

**(4)** Add fees to the budget that are not present through the Schedule of Events. These include:
- **(a)** Overhead
  - **(i)** This will typically be a row near the bottom of your budget with a formula to add overhead to every visit column subtotal.
    - **(1)** For example: (In this example, the Sponsor is paying for all procedures.) (See Table 2.6.)
- **(b)** PI Fee
- **(c)** RC Fee
- **(d)** Data Analyst Fee (if you have a Data Analyst)
- **(e)** Charges for any Ancillary Departments that will be providing services for your trial, such as: (Project Management is required to coordinate with the Ancillary Departments to obtain their budgets and then add them to the overall study budget.)
  - **(i)** Anesthesia and Recovery Room
  - **(ii)** Research Pharmacy/Investigational Drug Services (IDS)
  - **(iii)** Staff from other Departments who are providing patient services, such as Research Nurses performing PKs with multiple sticks over several hours.
  - **(iv)** Physical Therapy or Occupational Therapy
  - **(v)** Psychiatry
  - **(vi)** Ophthalmology
  - **(vii)** Pulmonary Department
  - **(viii)** Any others that pertain to your study procedures
- **(f)** Create a "Conditional Procedures" or "Invoiceables" table for procedures that:
  - **(i)** May occur/ that do not occur with every subject. For example:
    - **(2)** Urine Pregnancy Test
      - **(a)** This test will only apply to females after a certain age. For any males in your study, this test will not be run. Therefore, it goes on the Conditional Procedures/ Invoiceables table.

**Table 2.6 Per Patient Budget Sample 4**

| Procedures/Activities | Screening | Visit 1 | Visit 2 | Visit 3 |
|---|---|---|---|---|
| Consent | 100 | | | |
| Inclusion/exclusion criteria | 50 | | | |
| Concomitant medications | 25 | 25 | 25 | 25 |
| Vital signs | 55 | 55 | 55 | 55 |
| Physical exam | 245 | | | |
| Lab tests | 315 | | 315 | |
| 12 Lead EKG | | 403 | | 403 |
| AE/SAE assessment | | | 40 | 40 |
| IND dispensing | | 33 | | |
| PK | | | 500 | |
| Quality-of-life survey | | | | 35 |
| PI Fee | 250 | 200 | 200 | 200 |
| RC Fee | 200 | 150 | 150 | 150 |
| Subtotal | 1240 | 866 | 1285 | 908 |
| Overhead—25% | 310 | 216.50 | 321.25 | 227 |
| Total | 1550 | 1082.50 | 1606.25 | 1135 |

**Table 2.7  Invoiceables Table**

| Invoiceables | Charge | 25% Overhead | Total |
|---|---|---|---|
| Urine pregnancy test | 73.00 | 18.25 | 91.25 |
| Screen failures | 2351.00 | 587.75 | 2938.75 |
| Unscheduled visits | 356.00 | 89.00 | 445.00 |

      **(3)** Screen Failures
      **(4)** Unscheduled Visits
   **(ii)** For example, see Table 2.7.

**(g)** Create a non-procedures table. This may include charges for:
   **(1)** Local or Central IRB initial review
   **(2)** Local or Central IRB continuing review
   **(3)** Local or Central IRB amendments
   **(4)** Off-site Document Storage
   **(5)** PI travel for meetings or conferences required for the protocol
   **(6)** Monitoring Visit (for the time and effort of the Coordinator to be available while the Monitor is visiting and requesting information)
   **(7)** Site Initiation Visit—for the time of all study team members that will be present
   **(8)** Administrative Start-up Fee
      **(a)** This includes the Legal review of the contract, the study team's regulatory and administrative work to begin the trial and prepare documents for the IRB, any administrative office that manages Industry contracts and grant awards and budgets, and any other service or Department responsible for tasks when starting a study.
      **(b)** 🏛 Fees can range from $4000 to $30,000. Consult your medical center's policy.
   **(9)** SAE reporting
      **(a)** ✏ Create this as a "per-occurrence" fee. You never know how many SAEs a trial may have. We had one study that filled 4 binders due to suicidal ideation the subjects were experiencing. Other trials may have a few SAEs only. Allow for this unforeseen variability by not accepting a cap for SAE reporting.
   **(10)** IDS/research pharmacy start-up, drug maintenance/inventory control and close-out fees
   **(11)** Coverage Analysis
   **(12)** Advertising (Make sure you do your homework prior to budgeting to know what kind of media you want to advertise through and what the costs of vendors are.)
   **(13)** Study closure
   **(14)** For example:

| Non-Procedures | Charge | 25% Overhead | Total | Frequency |
|---|---|---|---|---|
| Administrative start-up fee | 10,000 | 2500 | 12,500 | One time |
| Off-site document storage | 75 | 18.75 | 93.75 | Per year |
| SAE reporting | 100 | 25 | 125 | Per occurrence |

**(5)** Depending upon the size of the medical center, the PI or/and RC will create the budget or there will be a Department dedicated to finance and budgeting that will prepare and negotiate the budget for the study team.

  **(a)** If your situation is the latter, the Finance Department should send the draft budget to the PI and RC before it is finally approved with the funder.

    **(i)** This will allow the study team the opportunity to revise anything on the budget. For example, they may know that anesthesia is required for a procedure that is not stated in the protocol.

Budget Discussion

You must have the protocol or a document that outlines the procedures for the trial in order to budget. DO NOT attempt to budget until you have this. A lot of lost time and misunderstandings about what a PI wants to do in a study can ensue without a procedural document.

For Industry studies, the Sponsor will send a template budget that the medical center can review and revise. Negotiations are expected until a final budget is approved. One budget is created for Industry studies that last until the trial is over.

For grants, the study team or the medical center grants department will typically need to create a draft budget for the study. For grants, there is usually a set dollar amount awarded that the medical center needs to fit their charges into. Negotiation is not expected for a grant award; you accept the amount awarded. Grant budgets are typically created in one year increments and the budget numbers may change from year-to-year.

When you receive an Industry budget template, note that there are little footnotes at the bottom of the Schedule of Events. These will provide helpful information, such as how many times blood must be drawn for PK analysis, or whether a central lab or local lab will analyze the results. Each note could affect your budget amounts, so be sure to read them.

Of note, the Schedule of Events and main budget should have an Early Withdrawal visit in it to capture the procedures and return of an investigational drug or device, if applicable, and the charges for the visit.

In the contract for the trial, make certain there is language indicating whether the sponsor will pay automatically from eCRFs being completed with all queries resolved, or whether the medical center will need to invoice the sponsor for payment. There may also be a Data Center that reviews a database and releases approval for a medical center to invoice for subject visits, for which the data were found to be clean and complete.

If you know the CPT codes for the procedures in your budget, write them on your budget for clarity. This will help your medical center's billing office as well as the study team and medical center finance and contract departments.

The expenses that do not have a CPT code in the American Medical Association CPT manual are considered activities. An example is consenting. To figure out what to charge, find out the salary of the person who will be consenting research subjects. Decide how much time consenting will take, e.g., 2 h. Divide the yearly salary by 2080 to get the hourly rate. Use that figure in your budget.

For example, if a Research Coordinator (RC) will be consenting research subjects: The RC makes $55,000/year. The hourly rate is (55,000/2080 = 26.44). For 2 hours, the rates is 26.44 x 2 = 52.88. Therefore, you can write $52.88 in your budget (and apply your research discount if applicable).

When figuring out what to charge for a PI who performs activities, but the PI does not want to divulge his/her salary, use the NIH Cap. You can find the NIH Cap here: https://grants.nih.gov/grants/policy/salcap_summary.htm.

For studies with multiple arms, set up an Excel budget for each arm as the procedures can differ; use a new tab at the bottom of the spreadsheet for each additional arm. Copy and paste your main budget to a new tab to save time. Then revise it according to the specifications of the arm.

Write the "Total Cost Per Subject" in a cell to get your total amount for the charges requested for the study for each research subject. Create a sum formula. See the budget template.

To know whether your budget will provide a profit, a loss, or will break even, it is advisable to write the sponsor payments in a row and the variance from your medical center's total in another row. See the budget template. Adjust your budget negotiations accordingly so that you do not operate at a loss.

A Notes section is helpful for any particular comments you wish to make regarding the budget. See the Per-Patient Budget Template in Appendix 6. Use it to create your own budgets.

Of note, there are other kinds of budgets. Again, the section above outlines the itemized per patient budget.

The next most common type of budget is a cost-reimbursable budget for a grant. Grants follow 2 CFR 200. It is lengthy and detailed. Contact your Grant Administrator at your Institution to create your cost-reimbursable budget and to manage your grant award. To help your Grant Administrator, the next section has been developed:

*Cost-Reimbursable Budgets for Grants*

Many details are needed in order to create a realistic cost-reimbursable (salary support and expense) budget. You can significantly help and partner with your Grant Administrator by having the following details available as listed below. This list will not be all inclusive dependent upon the type of research you are doing. Add or revise it as needed per your protocol. (Of note, the study protocol should include the majority of the information below when it is written to the detail necessary, not including costs or salaries, but inclusive of the level of staff, logistics, procedures and locations inherent in this information.)

1. How much time will every procedure take at every visit that is conducted by the study team? (This will not be in a protocol. You will need to contact the study team for time allocations.)
2. Who will be performing the procedure?
   a. PI
   b. Co-I
   c. RC
   d. Data Entry Specialist
   e. Research Nurse
      i. Each person has a different salary, so their salary will be broken down into the number of hours they will be working on the study.
3. Plan for the number of years of the study, whether it is 4 years or 15 years. Each year has to be budgeted out in all detail.
4. Add 3% Cost of Living (COL) increase for each year beginning at Year 1 (or 12 months into the study).
   a. For example, if visit 3 is at 12 months, add 3% to all of your procedural costs in the budget. At year 5, you will be at a 15% COL increase.
5. Figure out the number of anticipated subjects per year (for each arm or sub-study if applicable).
6. Expenses will need to be tallied according to the number of patients anticipated each year.
7. At what time point or range does each visit fall? For example, visit 1 is at week 1, whereas Visit 12 is at 14 months. Visit 13 is at 17–19 months.
   a. Know these time points or ranges so that you can properly fit them into each year for which you are budgeting.

8. How many records will you prescreen?
   a. Determine the amount of time you anticipate spending to review each chart times the number of charts.
9. How many patients do you anticipate trying to recruit?
   a. Quantify this by the amount of time it will take and which study team members will be recruiting.
10. What do you realistically think your enrollment will be?
11. How long will your study last?
12. How long is your accrual period?
13. Will any visits occur in locations outside of your institution?
14. Will lab analysis occur locally or centrally?
15. What courier service will you use and what are the anticipated costs of shipping?
    a. Include dry ice, cooler, or other container, etc.
16. Will other Departments at your hospital be assisting you with procedures? If so, what are their technical and professional fees per procedure?
17. What are the salaries of each study team member? (This will be needed to calculate their remuneration for their % of effort.)
    a. If a study team member makes $80,000 and 5% of their time will be spent on the study per year, that is a $4000 per year salary allocation.
18. What costs will you incur? (Get as specific pricing as you can.)
    a. Purchase or licensing for survey instruments/Behavioral tests
    b. Research subject payments: travel, food, gas, gift cards, etc.
    c. Recruitment/Advertising materials and media
    d. Biobanking services if applicable
    e. Assays—per each
    f. Supplies
       i. Phlebotomy—needles, tubes, alcohol swabs
       ii. Other procedural supplies
    g. New/used computer or laptop or iPad
19. Data entry fees
20. Biostatistician fees
21. IRB or Central IRB review costs
22. Archiving fee per year
23. Include in your time and effort calculation, the time for:
    a. Monitoring visits
    b. Audits
    c. Regulatory paperwork preparation
    d. SAE reporting
24. Equipment cost or rental
25. Pharmacy fees
26. Yearly conference costs
27. F&A (overhead) percentage to apply
    *See Appendix 7 for a Cost-Reimbursable Budget Template.*
    ꝕ<sup>ICH</sup> **ICH GCP has the following to say about financing:**

5.9. Financing

The financial aspects of the trial should be documented in an agreement between the sponsor and the investigator/institution.

The clinical trial protocol should include:

6.14. Financing and Insurance

Financing and insurance if not addressed in a separate agreement.[33]

## 2.7 STUDY START-UP AND SPONSOR DOCUMENTATION REQUIREMENTS

*Purpose of this section*:

- Provides tips on study start up
- Introduces tools in the Appendix that will aid study start-up efforts
- Provides advice on Form FDA 1572, Statement of Investigator

There are several useful tools to assist you in the administrative tasks required to commence a research study. It is important to be organized.

First, if you are conducting a study with an Industry Sponsor, the Sponsor will provide documents that will guide you through the study start-up process. The **Regulatory Binder Checklist** from NIH in Appendix 14 and the Essential Documents for the Conduct of a Clinical Trial, Section 8 in ICH GCP E6 R2, specifically Section 8.2 for the Essential Documents required for Good Clinical Practice "Before the Clinical Phase of the Trial Commences" will provide the information for what documentation you will need.[34]

Note: The Regulatory Binder Checklist will have study start-up documents and documents used beyond startup.

Regardless of the type of Sponsor (federal, non-profit, Industry, internal, philanthropic), the Research Coordinator will benefit from using the **Study Start-up Checklist** in Appendix 26 to identify all study start-up tasks and documents and to track their completion.

Additionally, the Research Coordinator will find the **Research Coordinator Work Queue** in Appendix 24 very helpful, if not necessary, to keep track of ALL the studies for which the Coordinator is responsible. The Queue includes Sponsor and CRO contact information, deadline dates, number of enrollments, and more. The goal is to always keep this Queue updated with current statuses.

If your Institution has a Clinical Trials Management System (CTMS), much of the tracking needed will be available through this system. Even with a CTMS, you may still benefit from the Study Start-up Checklist .The fields in the Research Coordinator Work Queue should all be available in your CTMS.

**Investigational New Drug studies and FDA Form 1572**

For IND studies, you will need to fill out FDA Form 1572 and provide it to your Sponsor or CRO (Please see Chapter 4, Section 4.5 regarding Forms). The current version of FDA Form 1572 is here: https://www.fda.gov/downloads/AboutFDA/ReportsManualsForms/Forms/UCM074728.pdf.

## AUTHOR'S CORNER

From experience, we can tell you that the names of the Principal Investigator and any Co-Investigators or/and Sub-Investigators MUST be written on Form FDA 1572 EXACTLY as their names appear on their medical licenses. If the names do not match, the 1572 will be returned to you for correction.

In addition, the expiration date of FDA Form 1572 is written in the top, right corner of the Form. Make sure you are using the current version. If you complete an outdated form, it will be returned to you and you will have to fill it out again on the current form. (Always go online to get the Form. Relying on a saved form in your electronic files will become outdated.)

The more organized you are, and the better you keep track of every document needed, its status, and have records of what you have sent to the Sponsor, the more efficient your operation will be, and the more valuable you will be to a Sponsor. The Sponsor has deadlines for study startup, which typically are pressing. The faster your study team navigates through study startup with all tasks completed, along with ethical, compliant, and efficient study conduct during the research, the greater the chance the Sponsor or funder will ask your study team to be a site for future studies.

Moreover, it is to your advantage to stay on top of other Departments that are reviewing study documents in order to keep the paperwork moving; for example, the Legal Department reviewing your contract and the Finance or Clinical Trials/Clinical Research Department reviewing your budget. The Research Coordinator should always know who (and what department) has which document at any given time. (You do not want two different departments to each think the other is reviewing a document, losing time as a result.) This is one example of how a CTMS or the Study Start-up Checklist in Appendix 26 will be useful.

## 2.8 THE MEDICARE COVERAGE ANALYSIS

*Purpose of section*:

- Defines Medicare Coverage Analysis (MCA) for drug trials
- Introduces the National Coverage Determination (NCD) 310.1
- Explains a Qualifying trial vis-à-vis a Non-Qualifying trial under MCA
- Explains "Routine" and "Research only" costs
- Explains Medicare Coverage Analysis for Investigational Device Exemptions (IDEs)

### What is the Medicare Coverage Analysis?

Medicare Coverage Analysis (MCA) is the process used to determine whether a trial qualifies for routine costs within a clinical trial to be paid by Medicare. Because Medicare sets the standard for medical reimbursements, health insurance companies typically follow the actions of Medicare. Thus, the MCA can also be used to determine whether routine costs within a clinical trial may be paid by a subject's medical insurance (rather than the sponsor/funder).

Medicare Coverage Analysis can be found through the National Coverage Determination (NCD) for Routine Costs in Clinical Trials 310.1 (or NCD 310.1). The url is: https://www.cms.gov/medicare-coverage-database/details/ncd-details.aspx?NCAId=248&NcaName=Intensive+Behavioral+Therapy+for+Cardiovascular+Disease&ExpandComments=y&ver=2&NCDId=1&ncdver=2&bc=BEAAAAA AEEAAAA%3D%3D&[35]

As you will see in the NCD 310.1, a "qualifying trial" is one in which the MCA has been performed and the analysis has determined that routine costs <u>can</u> be paid by the research subject's medical insurance or by the research subject's Medicare plan.

### AUTHORS CORNER

Of note, while one of the authors was performing Medicare Coverage Analysis, many study teams did not understand that once a trial qualifies, the budget has to be broken down into 1. What the routine costs are and 2. What the research costs are. The study teams thought that all charges could be paid by medical insurance for the trials that qualified. It is important to be aware of this misconception and to be able to explain how coverage analysis works.

Financial/Operational hospital staff will need the PI of the trial to identify what the standard of care procedures are for the particular diagnosis in the study. From this knowledge base along with consent form language (speaking to what the "research" charges are), you can divide the routine costs from the research costs.

Additionally, the reasonable and necessary items and services used to diagnose and treat complications arising from participation in all clinical trials are covered by Medicare (and may be covered by medical insurance) under the NCD (National Coverage Determination) 310.1.

**Routine Costs**

The routine costs of a clinical trial include all items and services that are otherwise generally available to Medicare beneficiaries.

Routine costs in clinical trials include:

- Items or services that are typically provided absent a clinical trial (e.g., conventional care);
- Items or services required solely for the provision of the investigational item or service (e.g., administration of a non-covered chemotherapeutic agent), the clinically appropriate monitoring of the effects of the item or service, or the prevention of complications; and
- Items or services needed for reasonable and necessary care arising from the provision of an investigational item or service--in particular, for the diagnosis or treatment of complications.

Routine Costs Do Not Include:

- The investigational item or service, itself unless otherwise covered outside of the clinical trial;
- Items and services provided solely to satisfy data collection and analysis needs and that are not used in the direct clinical management of the patient (e.g., monthly CT scans for a condition usually requiring only a single scan); and
- Items and services customarily provided by the research sponsors free of charge for any enrollee in the trial.

If a clinical trial does NOT qualify, all charges must be paid by a sponsor/funder. Charges are not allowed to be paid by Medicare or a research subject's medical insurance when the clinical trial does not qualify.[36]

*How to conduct a Medicare Coverage Analysis:*

First, recognize this is the National Coverage Determination for Routine Costs in <u>Clinical Trials</u>. Note, the title is not "Clinical Research." This means, and has been confirmed by Centers for Medicare and Medicaid Services (CMS)' refusal to revise the policy for clinical research, that the policy pertains to clinical trials only. (See the definition for a clinical trial in the Glossary.)

There are three (3) levels of analysis that must be conducted.

*The First Level*

Referring to the study protocol or Statement of Work (SOW), budget, contract or award, and the consent form, ask the following questions using these documents to determine whether the clinical trial meets the following three requirements in the first level of the analysis. All three must be met:

**(1)** The subject or purpose of the trial must be the evaluation of an item or service that falls within a Medicare benefit category (e.g., physicians' service, durable medical equipment, diagnostic test) and is not statutorily excluded from coverage (e.g., cosmetic surgery, hearing aids).

**(2)** The trial must not be designed exclusively to test toxicity or disease pathophysiology. It must have therapeutic intent.

**(a)** Therapeutic intent must be a primary objective.

  **(i)** Of note, this has been controversial. However, CMS has stated that therapeutic intent must be a primary objective, while CMS has decided not to change the wording (for further clarification) in the written policy.

  **(ii)** There is supporting verbiage for the primary objective/principal purpose in the first characteristic within the 3$^{rd}$ level of the analysis.

**(3)** Trials of therapeutic interventions must enroll patients with diagnosed disease rather than healthy volunteers. Trials of diagnostic interventions may enroll healthy patients in order to have a proper control group.

*The Second Level*

The second level of the Medicare Coverage Analysis automatically qualifies a clinical trial if any ONE of these characteristics apply (in addition to all three requirements in the first level of the analysis):

**1.** Trials funded by the following government organizations: National Institutes of Health (NIH); Centers for Disease Control (CDC); Agency for Healthcare Research and Quality (AHRQ); Centers for Medicare and Medicaid Services (CMS); U.S. Department of Defense (DOD); and U.S. Department of Veterans Affairs (VA);

**2.** Trials supported by centers or cooperative groups that are funded by the NIH, CDC, AHRQ, CMS, DOD, and VA;

**3.** Trials conducted under an investigational new drug application (IND) reviewed by the FDA; and

**4.** Drug trials that are exempt from having an IND under 21 CFR 312.2(b)(1). (See below.)

If ONE of these applies, there is no need to go to the 3rd level of analysis. AHRQ and the multi-agency panel that created the National Coverage Determination (NCD) 310.1 presume the trial meets the seven characteristics below when one of these applies. The clinical trial becomes automatically qualified to receive Medicare coverage.

In order to understand characteristic 4 regarding IND exemption, you will need to reference The Investigational New Drug (IND) Exemption regulation at 21 CFR 312.2(b)(1), which is:

(b) *Exemptions.* (1) The clinical investigation of a drug product that is lawfully marketed in the United States is exempt from the requirements of this part if all the following apply:

 **(i)** The investigation is not intended to be reported to FDA as a well-controlled study in support of a new indication (a health problem or disease for which the drug has not been FDA approved) for use nor intended to be used to support any other significant change in the labeling for the drug;

 **(ii)** If the drug that is undergoing investigation is lawfully marketed as a prescription drug product, the investigation is not intended to support a significant change in the advertising for the product;

 **(iii)** The investigation does not involve a route of administration or dosage level or use in a patient population or other factor that significantly increases the risks (or decreases the acceptability of the risks) associated with the use of the drug product;

 **(iv)** The investigation is conducted in compliance with the requirements for institutional review set forth in 21 CFR 56 and with the requirements for informed consent set forth in 21 CFR 50; (See the regulations list in the first chapter.) and

 **(v)** The investigation is conducted in compliance with the requirements of 21 CFR 312.7.[37]

If the trial does not have one of the four (4) automatically qualifying characteristics above, all seven (7) desirable characteristics in the 3rd level of the analysis should be met in order for the trial to qualify for the coverage of routine costs. A flow diagram is below to help you picture this.

*The THIRD level of the analysis*:

The seven (7) desirable characteristics in the third level of the analysis that should be met are:

1. The principal purpose of the trial is to test whether the intervention potentially improves the participants' health outcomes;
2. The trial is well supported by available scientific and medical information or it is intended to clarify or establish the health outcomes of interventions already in common clinical use;
3. The trial does not unjustifiably duplicate existing studies;
4. The trial design is appropriate to answer the research question being asked in the trial;
5. The trial is sponsored by a credible organization or individual capable of executing the proposed trial successfully;
6. The trial is in compliance with Federal regulations relating to the protection of human subjects; and
7. All aspects of the trial are conducted according to the appropriate standards of scientific integrity.

A flow diagram is shown in Fig. 2.2 to help.

**This Flow Diagram can also be downloaded from Appendix 38.**

The National Coverage Determination is based upon the authority found in §1862(a)(1)(E) of the Social Security Act (Act). It is binding on all Medicare carriers, fiscal intermediaries, Peer Review Organizations, Health Maintenance Organizations, Competitive Medical Plans, Health Care Prepayment Plans, and Medicare+Choice organizations (§1852(a)(1)(A) of the Act).[38]

Local Coverage Determinations (LCDs)

LCDs affirm whether a particular CPT code is reimbursable by Medicare or whether it is not reimbursable. You will need the CPT codes for the procedures in the study to look up whether they are covered or not. To find the current LCDs, use this url: https://www.cms.gov/medicare-coverage-database/downloads/downloadable-databases.aspx.

The CPT coders at your Institution should be able to perform the Local Coverage Determinations. Check with your Revenue Cycle Department or Hospital Billing Department.

*IDE Medicare Coverage Information and Steps to Request Coverage*

**Regulations:**

- The Medicare Prescription Drug, Improvement, and Modernization Act of 2003 (MMA)
- 42 CFR § 405 Subpart B

The FDA categorizes IDE-approved devices based on whether available data demonstrate that initial questions of safety and effectiveness have been resolved. IDE-approved devices are assigned to one of two categories:

- Category A—Experimental
- Category B—Non-Experimental/Investigational

https://www.fda.gov/MedicalDevices/DeviceRegulationandGuidance/HowtoMarketYourDevice/InvestigationalDeviceExemptionIDE/ucm051480.htm#labeling

**What is a Category A device?**

**Experimental Device**

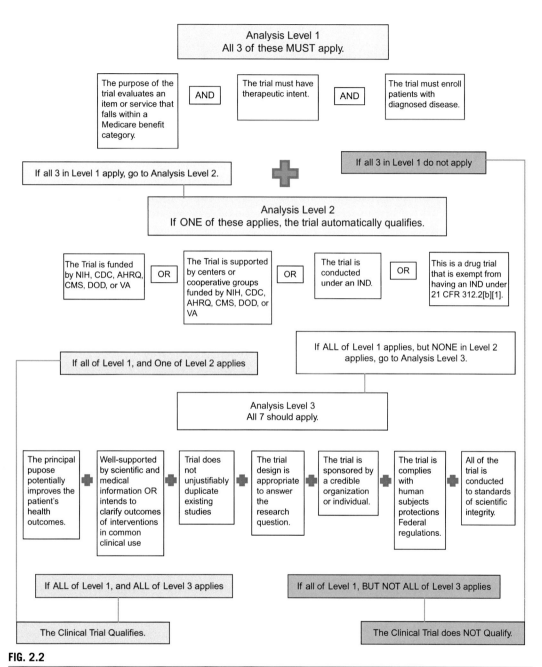

**FIG. 2.2**

Medicare Coverage Analysis flow diagram.

42 CFR 405.201(b): "…a device for which 'absolute risk' of the device types has not been established (that is, initial questions of safety and effectiveness have not been resolved) and the FDA is unsure whether the device type can be safe and effective."

Category A if one or more of the following criteria are met:

- No PMA (Premarketing Approval), 510(k) clearance or *de novo* request has been granted for the proposed device or similar devices, and non-clinical and/or clinical data on the proposed device do not resolve initial questions of safety and effectiveness.
- The proposed device has different characteristics compared to a legally marketed device; and information related to the marketed device does not resolve initial questions of safety and effectiveness for the proposed device. Available non-clinical and/or clinical data on the proposed device also do not resolve these questions.
- The proposed device is being studied for a new indication (a health problem or disease for which the device has not been FDA approved) or new intended use for which information from the proposed or similar device related to the previous indication does not resolve initial questions of safety and effectiveness. Available non-clinical and/or clinical data on the proposed device relative to the new indication or intended use also do not resolve these questions.[39]

📝 Coverage: A Category A IDE trial will allow coverage by a health insurance company or Medicare of routine healthcare items and services performed in the trial per the regulation. However, you must request coverage. (See the process for requesting coverage below.) The Category A device, itself, is not covered.

### What is a Category B device?
### Non-Experimental/Investigational Device

42 CFR 405.201(b). "…a device for which the incremental risk is the primary risk in question (that is, initial questions of safety and effectiveness of that device type have been resolved), or it is known that the device type can be safe and effective because, for example, other manufacturers have obtained FDA premarket approval or clearance for that device type."

Category B if one or more of the following criteria are met:

- No PMA (Premarket approval), 510(k) clearance or *de novo* request has been granted for the proposed device or similar devices; however, available clinical data (e.g., feasibility study data) and/or non-clinical data for the proposed device or a similar device resolve the initial questions of safety and effectiveness.
- The proposed device has similar characteristics compared to a legally marketed device, and information related to the marketed device resolves the initial questions of safety and effectiveness for the proposed device. Additional non-clinical and/or clinical data on the proposed device may have been used in conjunction with the leveraged information to resolve these questions.
- The proposed device is being studied for a new indication or new intended use; however, information from the proposed or similar device related to the previous indication resolves the initial questions of safety and effectiveness. Additional non-clinical and/or clinical data on the proposed device may have been used in conjunction with the leveraged information to resolve these questions.[40]

📝 Coverage: A Category B IDE trial will allow Medicare or health insurance coverage of the Category B device and the routine healthcare items and services performed in the trial per the regulation. However, you must request coverage.

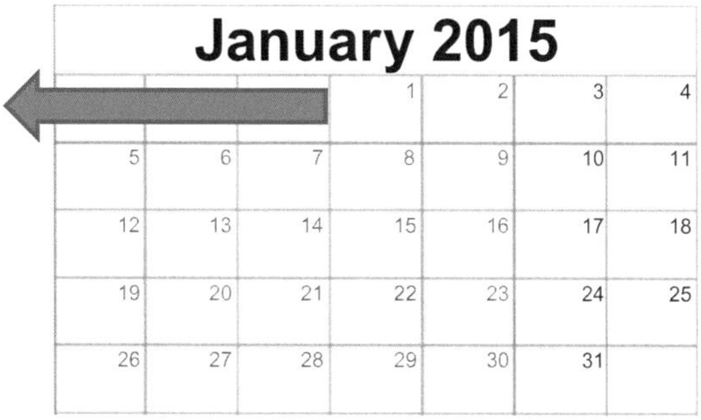

**FIG. 2.3**

Calendar prior to 1/01/15.

⚠ Without going through the process to request coverage as outlined below, your IDE studies will run the risk of being denied payment. With that said, each health insurance company has its own policies. Some will reimburse for an IDE study, some will not, but you will not be allowed to submit a health insurance claim for payment if you do not request coverage and then receive approval from a MAC (Medicare Administrative Contractor) or CMS.

Requesting coverage process:

**If the IDE was FDA approved PRIOR to 1/01/15** (see Fig. 2.3)

Contact your local Medicare Administrative Contractor (MAC). The MACs are designated by the State you live in. To find your MAC for your State, go to:

https://www.cms.gov/Medicare/Medicare-Contracting/Medicare-Administrative-Contractors/Downloads/MACs-by-State-July-2016.pdf or see Appendix 8 for the MACs by State List as of July 2016.

You will need to follow along with the documents and process required by your MAC as you navigate to their website. (The MAC list does not provide urls, so you will have to use a search engine to look them up.)

As an example, the State of Maryland uses the MAC Novitas Solutions. Novitas Solutions is assigned to several States, namely:

Arkansas, Colorado, New Mexico, Oklahoma, Texas, Louisiana, Mississippi, Delaware, DC, Maryland, New Jersey, and Pennsylvania

Novitas requires a Submission Checklist (known as Form FP172 (R8-15), which includes identifying information, contact information, and the following documents:

- The completed and signed Submission Checklist: See Appendix 9.
- FDA IDE Approval Letter with a date of approval prior to 1/01/15
- IRB Approval Letter
  - The letter must not be expired.
- Informed consent form
- Study Protocol or Summary, which includes "Therapeutic Intent"

This information must be faxed. (The fax number is on the form.)

Form FP172 (R8-15) can be found here: http://www.novitas-solutions.com/webcenter/content/conn/UCM_Repository/uuid/dDocName:00008268

For more information, see Novitas Solutions, Inc. website: http://www.novitas-solutions.com

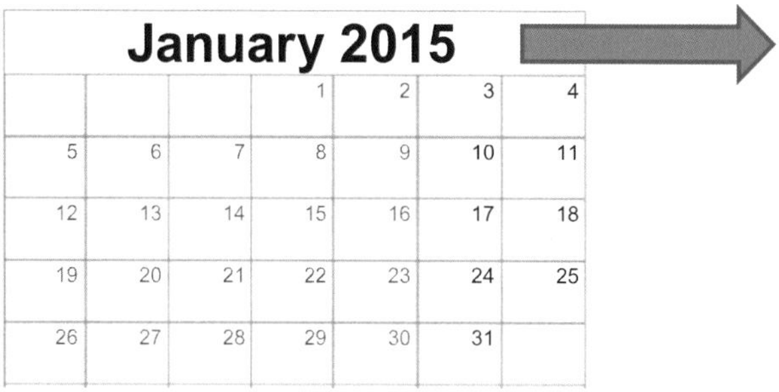

**FIG. 2.4**

Calendar after 1/01/15.

Click on your Jurisdiction.

**If the IDE was FDA approved on or after 1/01/15, the following steps apply** (see Fig. 2.4).

1. Submit a request packet to CMS.
   a. Use the IDE Study Criteria Checklist and Crosswalk Table in Appendix 10.
   b. Contents of the request packet include:
      i. FDA approval letter of the IDE.
      ii. IDE study protocol.
      iii. IRB approval letter
      iv. NCT number (from ClinicalTrials.gov)
      v. Medicare Coverage IDE Study Criteria located in your study materials
      vi. Supporting materials, as appropriate
      vii. Request Letter that describes the scope and nature of the IDE study, discussing how the IDE study meets each of the Medicare Coverage IDE Study Criteria. See the IDE Study Criteria Checklist and Crosswalk Table, Appendix 10, to know what the Medicare Coverage IDE Study Criteria are.
         1. The Request Letter should focus on how the IDE study meets each of the regulatory Medicare coverage IDE study criteria, which are:
1. The principal purpose of the study is to test whether the device improves health outcomes of appropriately selected patients.
2. The rationale for the study is well supported by available scientific and medical information, or it is intended to clarify or establish the health outcomes of interventions already in common clinical use.
3. The study results are not anticipated to unjustifiably duplicate existing knowledge.
4. The study design is methodologically appropriate and the anticipated number of enrolled subjects is adequate to confidently answer the research question(s) being asked in the study.
5. The study is sponsored by an organization or individual capable of successfully completing the study.
6. The study is in compliance with all applicable Federal regulations concerning the protection of human subjects found at 21 CFR parts 50, 56, and 812, and 45 CFR part 46.

7. Where appropriate, the study is not designed to exclusively test toxicity or disease pathophysiology in healthy individuals. Studies of all medical technologies measuring therapeutic outcomes as one of the objectives may be exempt from this criterion only if the disease or condition being studied is life threatening and the patient has no other viable treatment options.
8. The study is registered with the National Institutes of Health (NIH) National Library of Medicine's (NLM) ClinicalTrials.gov.
9. The study protocol describes the method and timing of release of results on all prespecified outcomes, including release of negative outcomes and that the release should be hastened if the study is terminated early.
10. The study protocol must describe how Medicare beneficiaries may be affected by the device under investigation, and how the study results are or are not expected to be generalizable to the Medicare beneficiary population. Generalizability to populations eligible for Medicare due to age, disability, or other eligibility status must be explicitly described.

Requests may be submitted via e-mail to: clinicalstudynotification@cms.hhs.gov
E-mails are preferred over hard copies.

**For Email Submissions**

- In Subject line, please use the following format: [IDE#]-[NCT#]-[Company Name]-[Device Name]-[FDA Category]:
  E.g., "A112233-NCT12345678-Acme Co-Device X-B"
- For attached files, please use the following conventions:
  - File names should clearly indicate the document type (e.g., "Request Letter," "IRB Approval Letter").
  - Each document type should be a separate file (i.e., the Request Letter should be separate from the IDE Study Protocol).
  - Word, PDF, and Excel file types are preferred.

**For Hard Copy Submissions**
Mail to:
Centers for Medicare and Medicaid Services
Center for Clinical Standards and Quality
Director, Coverage and Analysis Group
ATTN: Clinical Study Certification
Mail Stop: S3-02-01
7500 Security Blvd.
Baltimore, MD 21244
Source: https://www.cms.gov/medicare/coverage/ide/

There is an online site where you can check to see if your IDE trial has met CMS' standards for coverage. It is: https://www.cms.gov/Medicare/Coverage/IDE/Approved-IDE-Studies.html.

Of note, if approved by CMS, studies with the Category A are approved for coverage of routine services only. Studies with the Category B are approved for coverage of the Category B device and related services, and routine services.

## 2.9 HOW TO REGISTER A CLINICAL TRIAL AT WWW.CLINICALTRIALS.GOV

*Purpose of section*:

- Explains what ClinicalTrials.gov is and why it is important
- Explains how to register your trial through ClinicalTrials.gov
- Explains how to manage and update the registration
- Explains mandatory steps to add trial results to ClinicalTrials.gov
- Provides the language regarding ClinicalTrials.gov that is required in consent forms

ClinicalTrials.gov is a registry and results database of publicly and privately supported clinical studies of human participants conducted around the world. The regulations for ClinicalTrials.gov registration were updated on 9/21/2016 with an effective date of 1/18/2017. The regulations can be found at 42 CFR 11.[41]

This section will describe the key elements in registering your trial through ClinicalTrials.gov.

STEP 1

Only "applicable clinical trials" must be registered through ClinicalTrials.gov. See the ClinicalTrials.gov NIH Applicable Clinical Trial Checklist in Appendix 11 to determine whether your trial is an "applicable clinical trial" and must be registered.

The longer version to evaluating whether your trial is an applicable clinical trial can be found in the Code of Federal Regulations as described below:

42 CFR 11.22

The study is a pediatric postmarket surveillance of a device product as required by FDA under section 522 of the Federal Food, Drug, and Cosmetic Act (21 U.S.C. 3601).

OR

The study is an applicable device clinical trial with one or more arms that meets all of the following criteria:

(A) Study Type is interventional;

(B) Primary Purpose of the clinical trial is other than a feasibility study;

(C) The clinical trial studies a U.S. FDA-regulated Device Product; and

(D) One or more of the following applies:

**(1)** At least one Facility Location is within the United States or one of its territories,

**(2)** A device product under investigation is a Product Manufactured in and Exported from the U.S. or one of its territories for study in another country, or

**(3)** The clinical trial has a U.S. Food and Drug Administration IDE Number.

OR

(2) *Applicable drug clinical trial.* A clinical trial with one or more arms that meets the following conditions is an applicable drug clinical trial:

**(i)** Study Type is interventional;

**(ii)** Study Phase is other than phase 1;

**(iii)** The clinical trial studies a U.S. FDA-regulated Drug Product; and

**(iv)** One or more of the following applies:

**(A)** At least one Facility Location for the clinical trial is within the United States or one of its territories,

(B) A drug product (including a biological product) under investigation is a Product Manufactured in and Exported from the U.S. or one of its territories for study in another country, or

(C) The clinical trial has a U.S. Food and Drug Administration IND Number.

STEP 2

Determine who the Responsible Party is who is required to submit study information in ClinicalTrials.gov.

The updated regulation specifies that there must be one (and only one) responsible party for purposes of submitting information about an applicable clinical trial. The <u>sponsor</u> of an applicable clinical trial will be considered the responsible party, unless and until the sponsor <u>designates</u> a qualified <u>principal investigator</u> as the responsible party.[42]

Review your contract/award to see if the "Responsible Party" is specified. If not, call your Sponsor and ask! If your study is Investigator Initiated and qualifies for submission, the Principal Investigator is the Responsible Party.

STEP 3

Each institution has what is called a "PRS account," which stands for "Protocol Registration and Results System account." Every organization is given ONE PRS account only. All investigators who conduct trials at your organization are typically designated as users of this one PRS account. In tandem, each organization assigns one person (or more) to be the Administrator(s) of the PRS account.

Check your organization's ClinicalTrials.gov policy and procedure, to learn who the PRS Account Administrator is.

If your medical center does not have a PRS account, you must apply to obtain the account. Go to https://www.clinicaltrials.gov/ct2/manage-recs/how-apply and scroll down to the "Obtaining a PRS Account" section to learn what you need to do.

Once you know the PRS Account Administrator, the Responsible Party will need to ask him or her for a user login for ClinicalTrials.gov.

STEP 4

Know your deadlines. (See Fig. 2.5.)

The responsible party must register an applicable clinical trial within **21 calendar days** of enrolling the first subject.

Compliance with the updated regulation:

Effective date: January 18, 2017

Responsible parties had 90 calendar days after the effective date (1/18/17) to come into compliance with the requirements of this rule.[43]

STEP 5

Once you have your login and you have confirmed that you are the Responsible Party and that your trial is an applicable clinical trial, navigate to www.clinicaltrials.gov to start your trial registration process.

Contents of a ClinicalTrials.gov registration can be found at 42 CFR 11.28 along with "descriptive information" to define what is being requested.

Fill in the content of your applicable clinical trial registration. Follow along with the headings and prompts.

If you have a question about registering or need help, e-mail register@clinicaltrials.gov for support.

| MONTH | | | | | | |
|---|---|---|---|---|---|---|
| M | T | W | Th | F | Sa | Su |
| | | 1 | 2 | 3 | 4 | 5 |
| 6 | 7 | 8 | 9 | 10 | 11 | 12 |
| 13 | 14 | 15 | 16 | 17 | 18 | 19 |
| | 21 | 22 | 23 | 24 | 25 | 26 |
| 27 | 28 | 29 | 30 | | | |

**FIG. 2.5**

21 calendar days.

Release/Submit your registration. (You will see the prompt to do so.)

STEP 6

Two responses to your submission will happen next. There is no action on your part in this step. Responses:

1. The NIH Director will post a clinical trial registration within 30 calendar days of a registration submission. See the exception for devices that have not been approved or cleared. (42 CFR 11.35)
2. You will receive a ClinicalTrials.gov identifying number, called an "NCT number."
   a. This stands for "National Clinical Trial number." The format for the ClinicalTrials.gov identifier is "NCT" followed by an 8-digit number, e.g., NCT00000672.
   b. The NCT number will be sent to you by e-mail first. In 2-5 business days after the e-mail, you will see it on the first page of your registration in ClinicalTrials.gov.
   c. Reference this number if you contact ClinicalTrials.gov support for any questions in the future.

Your registration is complete!

**Updates & Results**

The Responsible Party is required by the regulations to update the ClinicalTrials.gov submission over time and to provide results at the end.

Here are two definitions you will need to know in order to proceed:

Primary Completion Date—The date that the last participant in a clinical study was examined or received an intervention and that data for the primary outcome measure were collected. Whether the clinical study ended according to the protocol or was terminated does not affect this date. National Institutes of Health Clinical Trial Glossary

Study Completion Date—The date that the final data for a clinical study were collected because the last study participant has made the final visit to the study location (that is, "last subject, last visit") National Institutes of Health Clinical Trial Glossary

**Requirements for Updating Your ClinicalTrials.gov submission:**
The reference for updating your ClinicalTrials.gov submission is found at 42 CFR 11.64.
If the clinical trial was initiated before January 18, 2017:

1. In general: for the updates of any information that was in your initial submission: once per year;
2. Recruitment status: within 30 (calendar) days after any change in overall recruitment status; and,
3. Primary completion date: Update this date within 30 (calendar) days after the clinical trial reaches its actual primary completion date.

If the clinical trial was initiated on or after January 18, 2017:

1. In general: for the updates of any information that was in your initial submission: once per year
2. Study start date: If the first human subject was not enrolled in the clinical trial at the time of registration (ClinicalTrials.gov registration submission), the Study Start Date... must be updated (within) 30 calendar days (of) the first human subject (enrollment).
3. Recruitment status: within 30 (calendar) days after any change in overall recruitment status
4. Individual site status: within 30 (calendar) days of a change in status for any individual site
5. Human Subjects Protection Review Board Status: update within 30 (calendar) days after a change in status
6. Primary completion date: Update this date within 30 (calendar) days after the clinical trial reaches its actual primary completion date.
7. Study completion date: within 30 (calendar days) after the clinical trial reaches its actual study completion date
   a. Definition: study completion date—the date that the final data for a clinical study were collected because the last study participant has made the final visit to the study location (that is, "last subject, last visit") National Institutes of Health Clinical Trial Glossary
8. Responsible Party: within 30 (calendar) days of a change in the Responsible Party
9. Device Product Not Approved or Cleared by U.S. FDA: within 15 (calendar) days after a change in approval or clearance status
10. Protocol amendment requiring communication to human subjects in the trial: within 30 (calendar) days of the protocol amendment being approved by a human subjects' protection review board
11. Clinical trial results: Update any registration submission information at the time you submit your clinical trial results and continue to update your results once every 12 months if changes occur.

**Requirements for adding Results to your ClinicalTrials.gov submission:**
Results must be submitted no later than 1 year after the primary completion date of the applicable clinical trial. See exceptions at 42 CFR 11.44.
See the clinical trial results information that must be submitted into ClinicalTrials.gov at 42 CFR 11.48.[44]

Of note, you are required to submit Adverse Event information in your results. The final rule that went into effect 1/18/17 "requires the responsible party to submit information summarizing the number and frequency of adverse events experienced by participants enrolled in a clinical trial, by arm or comparison group, as well as a brief description of each arm or group as a component of clinical trial results information. It also requires submission of three tables of adverse event information: One summarizing all serious adverse events; another one summarizing other adverse events that occurred with a frequency of 5 percent or more in any arm of the clinical trial; and finally, one summarizing all-cause mortality data by arm or group. This final rule clarifies that these adverse event tables must include information about events that occurred, regardless of whether or not they were anticipated or unanticipated. In addition, this rule requires responsible parties to provide the time frame for adverse event data collection and specify whether the collection approach for adverse events was systematic or non-systematic."[45]

NIH will post your clinical trial results information within 30 days of your submission of the results.

**Additional Information**

Regulation 42 CFR 11 Subpart D (which is 42 CFR 11.60) outlines the requirements for voluntary submission of clinical trial information for studies that are not applicable clinical trials if you wish to do so.

**Consequences of Non-Compliance With ClinicalTrials.gov registrations:**

⚠ Civil or criminal judicial actions can incur for failure to comply with 42 CFR 11.

⚠ Also, "if an applicable clinical trial is funded in whole or part by the Department of Health and Human Services, any required grant or progress report forms must include a certification that the responsible party has made all required registration and results submissions" within ClinicalTrials.gov. "If it is not verified that the required registration and results clinical trial information for each applicable clinical trial for which a grantee is the responsible party has been submitted, any remaining funding for a grant or funding for a future grant to such grantee will not be released." 42 CFR 11.66(c)

Consent Language

📝 **The following exact statement must be included in the informed consent documents of "applicable clinical trials":**

"A description of this clinical trial will be available on http://www.ClinicalTrials.gov, as required by U.S. Law. This Web site will not include information that can identify you. At most, the Web site will include a summary of the results. You can search this Web site at any time."

https://www.fda.gov/ScienceResearch/SpecialTopics/RunningClinicalTrials/FDAsRoleClinicalTrials.govInformation/default.htm

For the European community, there is an International Clinical Trials Registry Platform (ICTRP) through the World Health Organization (WHO).

"The International Clinical Trials Registry Platform (ICTRP) is a global initiative that aims to make information about all clinical trials involving human beings publicly available. It was established in 2006 in response to demand from countries through the World Health Assembly for: a voluntary platform to link clinical trials registers in order to ensure a single point of access and the unambiguous identification of trials with a view to enhancing access to information by patients, families, patient groups and others. {World Health Assembly, 2005 16 /id}"

More information can be found here: http://www.who.int/ictrp/en/.

There is a publication called the "International Standards for Clinical Trial Registries" by the World Health Organization, and can be found here: http://apps.who.int/iris/bitstream/10665/76705/1/9789241504294_eng.pdf?ua=1&ua=1.

Additionally, the **European** Medicines Agency has a clinical trial registry called the "**European Clinical Trials Database** (EudraCT)". It is currently in Version 10, "EudraCT V10."

This new version marks the final step of a process through which summary clinical trial results will be made publicly available through the EU Clinical Trials Register (EU CTR).

**https://eudract.ema.europa.eu/**

The *EU Clinical Trials* Register provides a free and accurate search of *clinical trials* in *European* Union member states and the *European* Economic Area.

The European Union Clinical Trials Register allows you to search for protocol and results information on: interventional clinical trials that are conducted in the European Union (EU) and the European Economic Area (EEA), which started after 1 May 2004; clinical trials conducted outside the EU/EEA that are linked to European pediatric-medicine development.[46]

The EU clinical trials register has been a primary registry in the World Health Organization (WHO)'s Registry Network since September 2011 and is a WHO Registry Network data provider. It is also available on the WHO ICTRP.

## 2.10 FLOWCHART FOR SEQUENCE/TIMING OF ALL TASKS IN THIS CHAPTER

See Fig. 2.6.

**Workflow for industry sponsored clinical trials' significant documents at study start-up**

This is a Best Practice. Your Institution's sequence of events and Department assignments may differ.

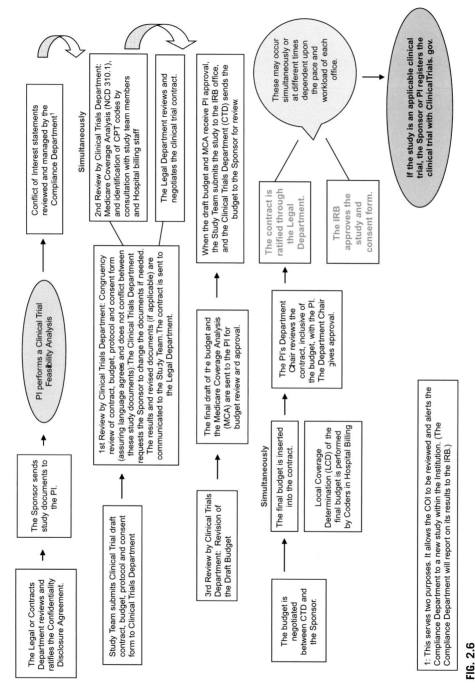

The flowchart contains the following text boxes:

The Legal or Contracts Department reviews and ratifies the Confidentiality Disclosure Agreement.

The Sponsor sends study documents to the PI.

PI performs a Clinical Trial Feasibility Analysis

Conflict of Interest statements reviewed and managed by the Compliance Department[1]

**Simultaneously**

Study Team submits Clinical Trial draft contract, budget, protocol and consent form to Clinical Trials Department

1st Review by Clinical Trials Department: Congruency review of contract, budget, protocol and consent form (assuring language agrees and does not conflict between these study documents). The Clinical Trials Department requests the Sponsor to change the documents if needed. The results and revised documents (if applicable) are communicated to the Study Team. The contract is sent to the Legal Department.

2nd Review by Clinical Trials Department: Medicare Coverage Analysis (NCD 310.1), and identification of CPT codes by consultation with study team members and Hospital billing staff

The Legal Department reviews and negotiates the clinical trial contract.

3rd Review by Clinical Trials Department: Revision of the Draft Budget

The final draft of the budget and the Medicare Coverage Analysis (MCA) are sent to the PI for budget review and approval.

When the draft budget and MCA receive PI approval, the Study Team submits the study to the IRB office, and the Clinical Trials Department (CTD) sends the budget to the Sponsor for review.

**Simultaneously**

The budget is negotiated between CTD and the Sponsor.

The final budget is inserted into the contract.

Local Coverage Determination (LCD) of the final budget is performed by Coders in Hospital Billing

The PI's Department Chair reviews the contract, inclusive of the budget, with the PI. The Department Chair gives approval.

These may occur simultaneously or at different times dependent upon the pace and workload of each office.

The contract is ratified through the Legal Department.

The IRB approves the study and consent form.

**If the study is an applicable clinical trial, the Sponsor or PI registers the clinical trial with ClinicalTrials. gov.**

1: This serves two purposes. It allows the COI to be reviewed and alerts the Compliance Department to a new study within the Institution. (The Compliance Department will report on its results to the IRB.)

**FIG. 2.6**

Flowchart for sequence of start-up tasks.

# ENDNOTES

[1] Full information on the ICH GCP (International Conference on Harmonisation Good Clinical Practices) can be found here: http://ichgcp.net/ [accessed 28.03.18].

[2] 21 CFR 54—Financial Disclosure by Clinical Investigators https://www.gpo.gov/fdsys/granule/CFR-2011-title21-vol1/CFR-2011-title21-vol1-part54 [accessed 28.03.18].

[3] Guidance for Clinical Investigators, Industry, and FDA Staff Financial Disclosure by Clinical Investigators, February 2013. https://www.fda.gov/downloads/regulatoryinformation/guidances/ucm341008.pdf [accessed 28.03.18].

[4] Ibid.

[5] Ibid.

[6] Text of 42 CFR Part 50 Subpart F: https://grants.nih.gov/grants/compliance/42_cfr_50_subpart_f.htm [accessed 28.03.18].

[7] Ibid.

[8] 42 CFR 50.603, https://www.gpo.gov/fdsys/granule/CFR-2007-title42-vol1/CFR-2007-title42-vol1-sec50-603 [accessed 28.03.18].

[9] NIH Financial Conflict of Interest, https://grants.nih.gov/grants/policy/coi/index.htm [accessed 28.03.18].

[10] https://admin.share.aahrpp.org/Website%20Documents/AAHRPP_Accreditation_Standards.PDF [accessed 28.03.18].

[11] Please see: http://ichgcp.net/58-compensation-to-subjects-and-investigators [accessed 28.03.18].

[12] Please see: http://ichgcp.net/5-sponsor [accessed 28.03.18].

[13] https://www.accessdata.fda.gov/scripts/cdrh/cfdocs/cfcfr/CFRSearch.cfm?CFRPart=50.

[14] Ibid.

[15] Protection of Human Subjects, FDA, https://www.accessdata.fda.gov/scripts/cdrh/cfdocs/cfcfr/CFRSearch.cfm?fr=50.25 [accessed 28.03.18].

[16] National Institutes of Health, https://humansubjects.nih.gov/coc/index [accessed 28.03.18].

[17] The Genetic Information Nondiscrimination Act of 2008 (Pub.L. 110–233, 122 Stat. 881, https://www.gpo.gov/fdsys/pkg/PLAW-110publ233/content-detail.html [accessed 28.03.18].

[18] Further information on the Genetic Nondiscrimination Act of 2008, https://www.hhs.gov/ohrp/regulations-and-policy/guidance/guidance-on-genetic-information-nondiscrimination-act/index.html [accessed 28.03.18].

[19] Ibid.

[20] U.S. Equal Employment Opportunity Commission, Genetic Information Discrimination. http://www.eeoc.gov/laws/types/genetic.cfm [accessed 28.03.18].

[21] NIH on Genetic Discrimination, Fact Sheet, https://report.nih.gov/nihfactsheets/ViewFactSheet.aspx?csid=81 [accessed 28.03.18].

[22] Please see: https://grants.nih.gov/grants/guide/rfa-files/RFA-RM-10-001.html, Part II, Research Objectives [accessed 28.03.18].

[23] 45 CFR 46.116 (c ) and (d), https://www.hhs.gov/ohrp/regulations-and-policy/regulations/45-cfr-46/index.html [accessed 28.03.18].

[24] Ibid.

[25] 21 CFR 50.27(b) (2) and 45 CFR 46.117 (b) (2) https://www.accessdata.fda.gov/scripts/cdrh/cfdocs/cfcfr/CFRSearch.cfm?fr=50.27 [accessed 28.03.18].

[26] 45 CFR 46.402 (b)) https://www.hhs.gov/ohrp/sites/default/files/ohrp/policy/ohrpregulations.pdf [accessed 28.03.18].

[27] Ibid.

[28] Ibid.

[29] 45 CFR 46.408 (e)). https://www.hhs.gov/ohrp/regulations-and-policy/regulations/45-cfr-46/index.html [accessed 28.03.18].

[30] Ibid.

[31] NIH Source for *Regulatory Requirements for Parent/Guardian Permission:* https://humansubjects.nih.gov/children1#Requirements_Child_Assent [accessed 28.03.18].

[32] U.S. Department of Health and Human Research, Research With Children FAQs https://www.hhs.gov/ohrp/regulations-and-policy/guidance/faq/children-research/index.html [accessed 28.03.18].

[33] ICH GCP, Financing p. 33, https://www.ich.org/fileadmin/Public_Web_Site/ICH_Products/Guidelines/Efficacy/E6/E6_R1_Guideline.pdf [accessed 28.03.18].

[34]Please see Section 8 in ICH GCP E6 R2, specifically Section 8.2 for the Essential Documents required for Good Clinical Practice, "Before the Clinical Phase of the Trial Commences", https://www.fda.gov/downloads/Drugs/Guidances/UCM464506.pdf [accessed 28.03.18].

[35]National Coverage Determination (NCD) for Routine Costs in Clinical Trials, https://www.cms.gov/medicare-coverage-database/details/ncd-details.aspx?NCAId=248&NcaName=Intensive+Behavioral+Therapy+for+Cardiovascular+Disease&ExpandComments=y&ver=2&NCDId=1&ncdver=2&bc=BEAAAAAAEEAAAA%3D%3D& [accessed 28.03.18].

[36]Centers for Medicare and Medicaid Services (CMS), Final National Coverage Determination, https://www.cms.gov/Medicare/Coverage/ClinicalTrialPolicies/downloads/finalnationalcoverage.pdf [accessed 28.03.18].

[37]The Investigational New Drug (IND) Exemption regulation at 21 CFR 312.2(b)(1), https://www.accessdata.fda.gov/scripts/cdrh/cfdocs/cfcfr/CFRSearch.cfm?fr=312.2 [accessed 28.03.18].

[38]CMS, Final National Coverage Determination, https://www.cms.gov/Medicare/Coverage/ClinicalTrialPolicies/downloads/finalnationalcoverage.pdf [accessed 28.03.18].

[39]FDA Categorization of Investigational Device Exemption (IDE) Devices to Assist the Centers for Medicare and Medicaid Services (CMS) with Coverage Decisions, Guidance for Sponsors, Clinical Investigators, Industry, Institutional Review Boards, and Food and Drug Administration Staff, Document issued on December 5, 2017. https://www.fda.gov/downloads/MedicalDevices/DeviceRegulationandGuidance/GuidanceDocuments/ucm504091.pdf [accessed 29.03.18].

[40]Ibid.

[41]42 CFR 11. https://www.gpo.gov/fdsys/granule/CFR-2010-title42-vol3/CFR-2010-title42-vol3-sec424-11/content-detail.html [accessed 28.03.18].

[42]Note: This final rule details the requirements for submitting registration and summary results information, including adverse event information, for specified clinical trials of drug products (including biological products) and device products and for pediatric postmarket surveillances of a device product to ClinicalTrials.gov, the clinical trial registry and results data bank operated by the National Library of Medicine (NLM) of the National Institutes of Health (NIH). https://www.federalregister.gov/documents/2016/09/21/2016-22129/clinical-trials-registration-and-results-information-submission#sectno-reference-11.8%20 [accessed 28.03.18].

[43]Ibid.

[44]Further information on results submitted to ClinicalTrials.gov https://www.gpo.gov/fdsys/pkg/CFR-2016-title42-vol1/pdf/CFR-2016-title42-vol1-part11.pdf [accessed 28.03.18].

[45]https://www.federalregister.gov/documents/2016/09/21/2016-22129/clinical-trials-registration-and-results-information-submission#sectno-reference-11.8%20 [accessed 28.03.18].

[46]European Union Clinical Trials Register, https://www.clinicaltrialsregister.eu/ctr-search/search [accessed 28.03.18].

# RECRUITING CLINICAL RESEARCH SUBJECTS

# 3

*Purpose of chapter*:

- Explains Activities Preparatory to Research
- Provides Internal patient recruitment strategies, including Physician Outreach, Medical Center Patient Databases, patient chart reviews and billing code reviews, and Grand Rounds
- Provides External patient recruitment strategies, including Professional associations, clinical trial listing services, call centers, and community outreach, and print, broadcast, and digital advertising and outreach

## 3.1 ACTIVITIES PREPARATORY TO RESEARCH: IDENTIFYING AND/OR CONTACTING SUBJECTS FOR STUDY RECRUITMENT

*Purpose of section*:

- How to identify subjects for your trial
- To know when you may contact potential subjects and when you cannot

A study team needs to become adept at the following tasks:

**(1)** reviewing medical records or a database during the feasibility analysis to see if there are enough potential subjects available to the team to accept the research study

**(2)** contacting potential subjects to see if they would be interested in consenting to and enrolling in a research study

These two tasks are considered "activities preparatory to research." Activities preparatory to research occur before consenting an individual, and therefore, before actual research occurs.

**For searching a database or patients' medical records**, the following applies:

Under 45 CFR 164.512(i)(1)(ii) ,the preparatory to research provision permits covered entities to use or disclose protected health information for purposes preparatory to research, such as to aid study recruitment. It does not permit the researcher to remove protected health information from the covered entity's site. As such, a researcher who is an employee or a member of the covered entity's workforce can use protected health information to <u>identify and contact</u> prospective research subjects.[1]

How this is practically carried out:

NO individual HIPAA authorization is required.
NO waiver of HIPAA authorization is required.
NO alteration of HIPAA Authorization is required<u>.</u>
NO data use agreement is required.

The Sourcebook for Clinical Research. https://doi.org/10.1016/B978-0-12-816242-2.00003-5

A REPRESENTATION IS REQUIRED:

The covered entity must obtain representations from a researcher that state:

**(1)** The use or disclosure is requested solely to review PHI as necessary to prepare a research protocol or for similar purposes preparatory to research,

**(2)** The PHI will not be removed from the covered entity in the course of review, and

**(3)** The PHI for which use or access is requested is necessary for the research.

The covered entity may permit the researcher to make these representations in written or oral form." You can find the source information here: https://privacyruleandresearch.nih.gov/pr_08.asp#8e (2/02/2007).[2]

**IRB** Check with your IRB regarding their procedure. Some institutions allow a letter to be written from the PI to the Chief Medical Officer of the PI's Department with the above information to cover the requirement.

Here is a table to succinctly express the requirement for representations:

See Appendix 12 for this same table, "Representations for Reviews Preparatory to Research" (see Table 3.1).

Human Subjects Protections Considerations:

Common Rule (45 CFR 46, part A)

A partial waiver of consent for recruitment, or a waiver of consent is required. (Which one depends upon the determination of your IRB).

New Common Rule (45 CFR 46, part A)

Consent or a waiver of consent is NOT required.

45 CFR 46.116(3)(g)

(g) Screening, recruiting, or determining eligibility. An IRB may approve a research proposal in which an investigator will obtain information or biospecimens for the purpose of screening, recruiting, or determining the eligibility of prospective subjects without the informed consent of the prospective subject or the subject's legally authorized representative, if either of the following conditions are met:

**(1)** The investigator will obtain information through oral or written communication with the prospective subject or legally authorized representative, or

**(2)** The investigator will obtain identifiable private information or identifiable biospecimens by accessing records or stored identifiable biospecimens.

# Table 3.1 Representations for Reviews Preparatory to Research

Activities Preparatory to Research
45 CFR 164.512(i)(1)(ii)
source: https://privacyruleandresearch.nih.gov/pr_08.asp

| GOAL | Regulation | Access | | Subjects | | HIPAA Requirement | | | | DUA | Notes |
|---|---|---|---|---|---|---|---|---|---|---|---|
| | | researcher within the covered entity | researcher outside the covered entity | Can the researcher identify potential subjects? | Can the researcher contact potential subjects? | HIPAA Authorization required | HIPAA partial waiver required | HIPAA alteration of authorization | HIPAA full waiver required | DUA required | |
| 1. Search a patient database to see if you will have enough potential, eligible participants for a research study<br>2. To identify prospective research participants for purposes of seeking their Authorization to use or disclose protected health information for a research study | Reviews Preparatory to Research<br>45 CFR 164.512(i)(1)(ii)<br><br>Proper representation must be received by the covered entity inclusive of:<br>1) the use or disclosure is requested solely to review PHI as necessary to prepare a research protocol or for similar purposes preparatory to research<br>2) the PHI will not be removed from the covered entity<br>3) The PHI for which use or access is requested is necessary for the research<br>These representations can be made in oral or written form. Check your IRB procedure. One implementation example of this is for the PI to provide the representations by writing a letter to the Chief Medical Officer of the PI's Department. | yes | no | yes | yes | no | no | no | no | no | See the Regulation to note that a "representation" must be provided. |

**For speaking with patients directly about the prospect of a research study,** the following apply:
**Treating Physician:**

**Option 1: The Treating Physician is also the PI of a Study:** A treating physician, who is also an Investigator in a Study, may speak to his or her patients about options for the care of the patient's condition including the prospect of enrolling in the physician's/PI's research study. No IRB review or authorizations are required for this conversation.

**Option 2: The Treating Physician is NOT the PI of a Study:** If a treating physician knows of a colleague's study, the treating physician may discuss the study with his/her patient and give the Study PI's contact information to the patient. The patient can contact the Study PI directly if he/she chooses to do so. (The treating physician cannot give the patient's PHI to the researcher.)

**Option 3: A treating physician may give a clinical summary to a researcher** to discuss whether his/her patient may meet recruitment criteria as long as the summary is deidentified. This can occur when a treating physician has a patient for which he/she is looking for alternatives to the standard of care. For example, the physician has tried various treatments without the outcomes he or she wishes and is looking for possible investigational methods to try.

No HIPAA authorization or waiver is required to hold these conversations.

**Call Centers:**

A Call Center receives phone calls from people about a research study advertisement they heard. The Call Center collects identifiable information and sends it to researchers or sends information about a study directly to a caller. A Call Center is a business outside of the covered entity, and therefore, is not required to comply with the Privacy Rule.

**For a study team OUTSIDE of the covered entity:**

A researcher who is not a part of the covered entity may not use the preparatory to research provision to contact prospective research subjects. Rather, the outside researcher could obtain contact information through a partial waiver of individual authorization by an IRB or Privacy Board as permitted at 45 CFR164.512(i)(1)(i). The IRB or Privacy Board waiver of authorization permits the partial waiver of authorization for the purposes of allowing a researcher to obtain protected health information as necessary to recruit potential research subjects. For example, even if an IRB does not waive informed consent and individual authorization for the study itself, it may waive such authorization to permit the disclosure of protected health information as necessary for the researcher to be able to contact and recruit individuals into the study.[3]

ICH GCP does not speak to identifying and contacting potential subjects.

---

## 3.2 INTRODUCTION TO RECRUITING SUBJECTS FOR A CLINICAL STUDY

*Purpose of section:*

- The importance of project management in recruiting
- Introduces the Subject Recruitment Tracking Log in the Appendix

Subject recruitment for a trial can be a true challenge. In fact, according to a clinical trial management firm, Forte Research, 48% of trials under-enroll study subjects, nine of out ten study sites reach enrollment goals if original timelines are doubled, and 11% of sites fail to enroll a single subject.[4] Hence, identifying, contacting, and finally, consenting, and enrolling the appropriate subjects in a trial require rigor and knowledge of regulatory requirements. Therefore, create a well-designed recruiting plan, weekly recruiting activities, and approvable advertising strategies.

This section will focus on the regulatory requirements for advertising and recruiting, and will equip you with successful recruiting strategies. To organize the recruitment strategies, we will look at:

- Internal strategies, using Institutional and Physician resources; and,
- External strategies, using outreach, external services, and direct advertising.

Recruiting subjects requires excellent project management, detailed planning, capable personnel, and persistent follow-through. *Do not be dismissive of these skills because they are administrative, not clinical.* Institutions that do not grant the proper respect, resources, and time to the <u>administration</u> of clinical trials will have frustrated physicians, poor team morale, research programs with consistent noncompliance, high staff turnover, and poor research outcomes. To aid recruitment project management, a "Subject Recruitment Tracking Log" can be found in Appendix 25.

Of note, the Federal regulations require IRB review and approval of all advertisements and recruiting strategies prior to any patient interaction with them; this occurs when the IRB initially reviews a protocol.[5]

## 3.2.1 METHODS FOR RECRUITING SUBJECTS INTERNALLY

*Purpose of section*:

- Provides suggestions for internal subject recruitment methods

Internal Recruiting Strategies:
**The most basic:**

1. **Medical Charts**: A Research Coordinator may review and flag patient charts for upcoming visits when the patients are **clinical** patients of the physician who is an Investigator on a study. This **ONLY** pertains when the patients are new or established patients of a physician who is an Investigator in a study.
2. **Posters**: IRB-approved and Sponsor-approved brochures and posters can be displayed within hospital common areas, including cafeterias, waiting rooms, elevators, and on message boards.
3. **TV Screens/Video**: Some Hospitals have TV screens in their Waiting Rooms for educational and advertisement purposes. Have your recruitment ad circulate through the video feed for the TV screens.
   a. An ad in the 60- to 90-second range is recommended and can be produced using basic video cameras and editing.
4. **Grand Rounds**: It can be useful for the PI to present studies at Hospital Grand Rounds and to ask for hospital physicians to mention the studies to their patients. Have a *Clinical Trial Overview Document* copied and ready to hand out.
5. **Database**: The RC can contact an institutional CPT and ICD-10 coder to request the relevant billing codes related to your trial. Then the Research Coordinator can search the in-house patient database for potential subjects. This database would be one that patients have consented to be a part of, including the consent to be contacted for future research studies.

**Physician Outreach and Medical Center Patient Databases:**

Investigators within a medical center or health system can provide study information to their fellow physicians internal to and external to the Investigator's medical center or health system via USPS mail, e-mail, or other communication channels. A physician-to-physician communication describes the trial and seeks to learn if the physician colleague may know of any patients from their own practice who would fit the inclusion and exclusion criteria of the trial.

For the physician-to-physician communication, we recommend composing a *Clinical Trial Overview Document*. The document provides basic trial information such as the title; purpose of the study; protocol summary; basic eligibility criteria; study site location(s); and, how to contact the site for further information. The *Overview* will serve as a handy and useful tool, which you can provide to the relevant individuals throughout the recruiting period. (Remember, the IRB and Sponsor must approve this document.)

From experience, having this document ready to go helps the PI speak to the salient aspects of a trial, without having to rely on memory, especially when he/she is conducting multiple trials.

And, another note from experience: Physicians are often concerned that the patients they refer to another physician for a trial will be taken from them and become the patients of another practice. Therefore, it is best that letters from the PI include the promise to **inform** a physician colleague if their patient enrolls in the trial and for the PI to be available to answer any questions and to provide updates on the status of a referred patient. A common mistake is that after a patient is referred, the referring physician hears nothing about the patient or trial and does not even receive a "Thank you."

Additionally, as a courtesy, the PI should refer to himself/herself as the "study doctor" only and encourage the referred patient to stay in communication with their clinical physician about their activity on the study.

When this physician-to-physician method is used, the colleague can inform their clinic patients about the study and provide them with the PI's contact information. However, the physician colleague MAY NOT give the PI the contact information of the patient. (See HIPAA information in Chapter 1, Section 1.8.)

## 3.3 METHODS FOR RECRUITING SUBJECTS EXTERNALLY

*Purpose of section*:

• Provides an overview of five (5) external Physician and institutional subject recruiting methods

**1.** Professional Associations

Clinical researchers can enlist the participation of relevant health care associations, local physician networking groups, advocacy groups, and online patient forums. Basic information on the proposed trial on websites and in newsletters can spur subject recruitment. The *Clinical Trial Overview Document* will be useful in concisely explaining the study to multiple groups.

**2.** Clinical Trials Listing Services

A Clinical Trials Listing Service (CTLS) is a database of available trials, providing information such as the study name, study design, purpose, eligibility, and contact information. Interested persons can look up trials for their diagnosis, then call the number on the Listing Service for more information. Please note: IRB approval is needed for most clinical trial listing sites.

Sites not requiring IRB approval include the AIDS Clinical Trials Information Service (ACTIS) at https://aidsinfo.nih.gov/clinical-trials and the National Cancer Institute's cancer clinical trial listing at https://www.cancer.gov/about-cancer/treatment/clinical-trials/search.[6]

In addition, there are websites that actively solicit volunteers for clinical trials. For example, https://www.researchmatch.org/ is run by NIH and allows a potential subject to review and gain more information about specific trials. Moreover, the site encourages researchers to register with the site, which NIH bills as "a free recruitment and feasibility analysis tool for researchers at participating institutions." Currently, the site has 558 studies ongoing, with 124,000 volunteers at 144 institutions.[7]

There is also a listing service called "ClinicalConnection," which can be found at https://clinicalconnection.com/Default.[8]

**3.** Call Centers

An Institution can hire the services of a paid, professional call center for clinical research recruiting for all of the studies occurring at its location. These centers are often open 24/7 and provide screening of eligible patients as well.

Alternatively, the institution can create an in-house call center; that is, hiring and training staff who answer dedicated recruiting phone lines and provide information on research studies ongoing in the medical center. Call center staff would prescreen interested individuals and then schedule screening visits for potential subjects who qualify for a particular trial. Varying shift times would allow for contact with potential patients, at times outside of typical work hours when they are free, such as 6 a.m. to 2 p.m. and 2 p.m. to 10 p.m.

Importantly, the IRB should have assurance that confidential information will be appropriately handled by a Call Center. For example, the following questions would need to be addressed:

**a.** What happens to personal information if the caller ends the interview or simply hangs up?

**b.** Are the data gathered by a marketing company? If so, are names and contact information sold to others?

**c.** Are names of non-eligible, potential candidates maintained in case they would qualify for another study?

**d.** Are paper copies of records shredded?

The acceptability of the procedures would depend on the sensitivity of the data gathered, including personal, medical, and financial.

**4.** Community Outreach

The following suggestions regarding Community Outreach take resources, time, and expertise; indeed, Institutions may have programs in place through which the PI/Study team can mention available studies. For example:

**Patient Support Groups**

These can be facilitated by regularly booking a room in the hospital and inviting patients who have the same diagnosis to meet and discuss their experience and provide emotional support to each other.

Study materials or/and *Clinical Trial Overview Documents* can be displayed for consideration.

**Patient-Networking Site**

The Medical Center web team could create a secure, password-protected, membership-only (for HIPAA reasons) Patient-Networking Site that patients voluntarily join. Trials and research studies can be advertised through this site.

**Educational Sessions**

Offer Educational Sessions about the diagnosis, coping mechanisms for it, and the latest research discoveries. These sessions can be in person or via WebEx. You will typically achieve higher attendance via WebEx due to convenience and anonymity. Advertise trials and research studies in these sessions.

**Mobile Clinic**

If your hospital has a mobile clinic to read blood pressure, check glucose levels, etc. in the community, have a research staff member on board to talk about studies for hypertension and diabetes – relevant to the services provided. (See Fig. 3.1.)

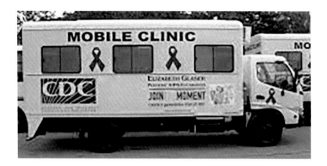

**FIG. 3.1**

Mobile Clinic photo.

## 3.4 EXTERNAL SUBJECT RECRUITING STRATEGIES INVOLVING DIRECT MEDIA

*Purpose of section*:

•   Provides an overview of external recruitment strategies involving direct media

External recruitment efforts involving direct media advertising cover a wide range of activities: Traditional media, defined as print and broadcast, and digital media, defined as Internet websites, e-mail marketing, and social media platforms such as Facebook, Twitter, YouTube, Instagram, and the range of instant messaging services.

First, and the least expensive is Print Ads.

**Print Ads:**

1. Advertise in a community paper that is distributed in the city or county where your Medical Center is. Choose the publication that targets readers in the demographic you need.

---

**AUTHOR'S CORNER**

For example, one of the authors worked in Ophthalmology. There was a study for cataracts that needed subjects. Cataracts are typically found in a senior demographic. Therefore, the author went to a Senior Center and an Assisted Living Facility near the Medical Center to see what people were reading. The author picked up a couple of free publications from these locations and placed an ad in one of them. A minimal fee was paid for the ad. The study enrolled several people from that ad.

---

2. Look for free or low-cost options. For example, advertising for subjects through the "volunteers" section under the "Community" heading of Craigslist. Try www.craigslist.org for the Craigslist in your area. The ad will post for one day only, so consider a Craigslist campaign in which you post on a periodic basis, e.g., weekly.

**Social Media** (see Figs. 3.2–3.5)

**FIG. 3.2**

Facebook icon.

**FIG. 3.3**

Twitter icon.

**FIG. 3.4**

YouTube icon.

**FIG. 3.5**

Snapchat icon.

Social Media is the new frontier for clinical trial recruitment. Effective use of social media requires skill, creativity, and patience, which is why such advertising is best left to the institution's Marketing and/or Communications department. With this in mind, the authors, one of whom has two decades of communications and marketing experience, offer these basic rules:

Create Personal Ads: The key for any media is to make the advertising personal and compelling. Human interest stories can be gripping with the use of words and images that evoke warmth and empathy, connecting with individuals who have a particular condition. Some examples of advertisements from the web that depicts well these principles are given in Figs. 3.6–3.8.

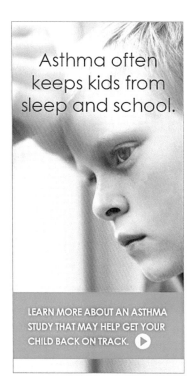

**FIG. 3.6**

Asthma ad.

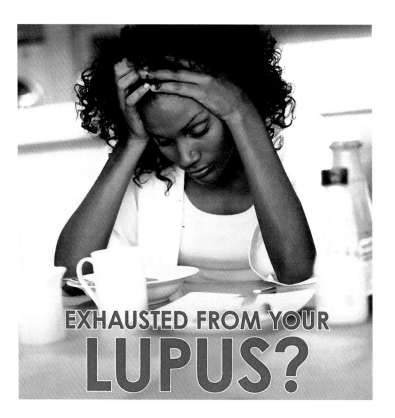

**FIG. 3.7**

Lupus ad.

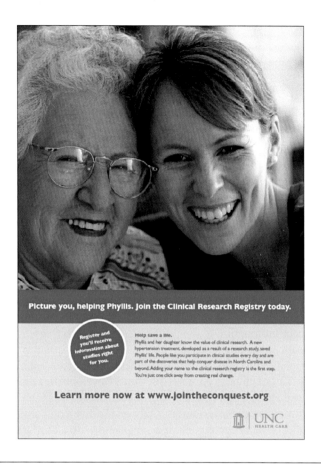

**FIG. 3.8**

Clinical Research Registry ad.

Facebook can serve as the foundation of a social media campaign for your research clinic. The page can feature your trials with evocative text and graphics and can even host your Clinical Trial Overview Document. In addition, the Facebook page leads to other forms of social media outreach, principally Twitter, but also such platforms as Instagram, YouTube, and Pinterest.

Of note, Google Analytics can provide your study team/your Marketing Department with return on investment (ROI) data from your advertising efforts by tracking and reporting on the traffic going to your website; you'll see which posts attract attention and which ones do not (https://analytics.google.com). And, currently, Google Analytics is free!

**a.** Your Institution will probably have branding standards, so check in with your branding office for anything that faces the public.

**b.** Keep it current and add content to it at least twice a month to keep traffic flowing to it. Write educational pieces, or what is of interest to your targeted demographic in the community, or an inspiring true story. Think of ways to gain the attention and interest of the people with whom you want to connect.

**c.** Don't forget to get IRB approval (and Sponsor approval if applicable).

A Note about Paid Recruitment Advertising Campaigns

It is uncommon that an institution has funding to run a media advertising campaign for study recruitment; however, sometimes an industry Sponsor is willing to financially support advertising. If so, there are firms that specialize in digital marketing for patient recruitment. Following are six such companies:

- https://www.bbkworldwide.com/referral-management/index.html
- https://www.forteresearch.com
- https://www.mdconnectinc.com/
- https://www.gopraxis.com/
- https://www.patientwise.com/
- http://www.viamark.com/patient-recruitment

Of note, the authors do not know the quality or reputations of these companies, only that they exist. Please perform your due diligence.

A Word About Digital Advertising Metrics

Virtually all patients are online as 80% of Internet users are actively seeking healthcare information. Even mature persons are online, with 71% of US adults aged 50–64 and 58% of those over 65 seeking medical information online.

According to a comprehensive, long-term poll undertaken by the Pew Internet & American Life Project, seeking health care information is the third-ranking online activity across all age groups. In addition, searching for health information, an activity that was once the primary domain of older adults, is now the third most popular online activity for all internet users 18 and older.[9]

And according to the Tufts University Center for Drug Development, drug sponsors are primarily using social media to distribute information (e.g., about drugs, diseases, and the company) and to listen to patient and professional conversations. Only one in five companies that use social media directly interacts with patients; most contract out their engagement to a third party or use more passive approaches, including placing banner ads on social media sites. Finally, social media is being used to recruit patients in about 11% of all trials.[10]

## 3.5 FDA GUIDANCE GOVERNING DIRECT ADVERTISING

*Purpose of section*:

- Provides overview of FDA Guidance Governing Direct Advertising

Both the FDA and Institutional Review Boards view advertising as the beginning of the informed consent process. The FDA has a *Guidance for Industry, Consumer-Directed Broadcast Advertisements* from August 1999 for Sponsors who want to advertise their drugs and products through TV, radio, and phone systems. The FDA also has an Information Sheet on *Recruiting Study Subjects,* which can be found here: https://www.fda.gov/RegulatoryInformation/Guidances/ucm126428.htm.

The FDA directs us in the following ways:

- Advertisements should be reviewed and approved by the IRB as part of the package for initial review.
- The following items may be included in advertisements:
  - the name and address of the clinical investigator and/or research facility;
  - the condition under study and/or the purpose of the research;

- in summary form, the criteria that will be used to determine eligibility for the study;
- a brief list of participation benefits, if any (e.g., a no-cost health examination);
- the time or other commitment required of the subjects; and
- the location of the research and the person or office to contact for further information;
- a note that subjects will receive compensation for their participation in a trial, but that payment cannot be emphasized or highlighted.[11]
- The following are items that cannot be included in advertisements:
  - Content cannot be "unduly coercive and does not promise a certainty of cure beyond what is outlined in the consent and the protocol." This is especially critical when a study may involve subjects who are likely to be vulnerable to undue influence.
  - As the FDA states, "No claims should be made, either explicitly or implicitly, that the drug, biologic or device is safe or effective for the purposes under investigation, or that the test article is known to be equivalent or superior to any other drug, biologic or device. Such representation would not only be misleading to subjects but would also be a violation of the Agency's regulations concerning the promotion of investigational drugs.
  - Advertisements cannot use terms such as "new treatment," "new medication," or "new drug" without explaining that the test article is investigational. "A phrase such as 'receive new treatments' leads study subjects to believe they will be receiving newly improved products of proven worth."
  - Advertisements cannot promise "free medical treatment," when the intent is only to say subjects will not be charged for taking part in the investigation. Advertisements may state that subjects will be paid, but should not emphasize the payment or the amount to be paid. Advertisements may note a "no-cost health examination" as a benefit for recruiting purposes.[12]

To summarize, recruiting subjects for a trial can be a formidable challenge but a well-designed, creative, and persistent campaign can yield the required subject pool.

# ENDNOTES

[1] Please see: Uses and disclosures for which an authorization or opportunity to agree or object is not required, 45 CFR 164.512, (i)(1)(ii) [accessed 28.03.18].
[2] https://privacyruleandresearch.nih.gov/pr_08.asp#8e [accessed 28.03.18].
[3] http://www.hhs.gov/hipaa/for-professionals/faq/317/can-the-prepatory-research-provision-be-used-to-recruit-individuals-to-a-research-study/index.html [accessed 28.03.18].
[4] https://forteresearch.com/news/infographic/patient-recruitment-enrollment-clinical-trials-infographic/ [accessed 28.03.18].
[5] https://www.fda.gov/regulatoryinformation/guidances/ucm126428.htm [accessed 28.03.18].
[6] https://www.cancer.gov/about-cancer/treatment/clinical-trials/search.
[7] See: www.researchmatch.org [accessed 03.28.18].
[8] https://clinicalconnection.com/Default [accessed 03.28.18].
[9] ABC "Health Online 2013", Pew Internet & American Life Project, AB—Pew Internet & American Life Project, 2010, http://www.pewinternet.org/2010/12/16/generations-2010 [accessed 28.03.18].
[10] "Drug Developers Circumspect about Using Social Media in Clinical Research," News release, March 16, 2014, Tufts Center for the Study of Drug Development [accessed 28.03.18].
[11] Please see: https://www.fda.gov/regulatoryinformation/guidances/ucm126428.htm [accessed 28.03.18].
[12] Ibid.

# CLINICAL TRIAL CONDUCT—A DAILY PERSPECTIVE

*Purpose of chapter*:

- Explains the role of HIPAA, De-Identification and Chart Reviews
- Explains Translation and Interpretation for study subjects
- Explains Blinding and Unblinding
- Explains Adverse Events (AE) and reporting
- Provides examples and descriptions of FDA forms, Sponsor forms and Study Team forms
- Explains the necessity of Project Management and offers Project Management ideas
- Describes Clinical Trial Coding for Claims
- Provides suggestions for Choosing a CTMS

## 4.1 HIPAA (HEALTH INSURANCE PORTABILITY AND ACCOUNTABILITY ACT) AND DE-IDENTIFIED CHART REVIEWS AND DATABASES

*Purpose of section*:

- Explains how to de-identify a subject's record correctly
- Provides information on what permissions are required to access records
- Describes when waivers apply
- Explains when the HIPAA Privacy Rule no longer applies

The HIPAA Privacy Rule and de-identifying medical record information or creating a de-identified database within your Institution:

"In the Privacy Rule, creating de-identified health information or a limited data set is a health care operation of the covered entity, and thus, does not require the covered entity to obtain an individual's Authorization, a waiver of the Authorization requirement, or representations for reviews preparatory to research..." https://privacyruleandresearch.nih.gov/research_repositories.asp

Once the data are de-identified, the data are not considered PHI, and therefore the Privacy Rule does not apply.

In tandem, de-identified data is considered non-human subjects research. This means it is EXEMPT from human subjects protections through the HHS federal regulations at 45 CFR 46. (The specific exemption for the collection or study of existing data is 45 CFR 46.101(4).) Therefore, consent or a waiver of consent is not necessary.

Check both Privacy Rule AND human subjects protections regulations when you question what authorization or consent is required, because "…the Privacy Rule does not override any requirements of 45 CFR part 46, and vice versa. In situations where both 45 CFR part 46 and the Privacy Rule apply, institutions must adhere to both sets of regulations." https://privacyruleandresearch.nih.gov/clin_research.asp

How to de-identify:

Here is what must be taken out of a medical record in order for a patient's data to be considered "de-identified":

---

The Privacy Rule allows a covered entity to de-identify data by removing all 18 elements that could be used to identify the individual or the individual's relatives, employers, or household members; these elements are enumerated in the Privacy Rule. The covered entity also must have no actual knowledge that the remaining information could be used alone or in combination with other information to identify the individual who is the subject of the information. Under this method, the identifiers that must be removed are the following:

1. Names.
2. All geographic subdivisions smaller than a state, including street address, city, county, precinct, ZIP Code, and their equivalent geographical codes, except for the initial three digits of a ZIP Code if, according to the current publicly available data from the Bureau of the Census:
   a. The geographic unit formed by combining all ZIP Codes with the same three initial digits contains more than 20,000 people.
   b. The initial three digits of a ZIP Code for all such geographic units containing 20,000 or fewer people are changed to 000.
3. All elements of dates (except year) for dates directly related to an individual, including birth date, admission date, discharge date, date of death; and all ages over 89 and all elements of dates (including year) indicative of such age, except that such ages and elements may be aggregated into a single category of age 90 or older.
4. Telephone numbers.
5. Facsimile numbers.
6. Electronic mail addresses.
7. Social security numbers.
8. Medical record numbers.
9. Health plan beneficiary numbers.
10. Account numbers.
11. Certificate/license numbers.
12. Vehicle identifiers and serial numbers, including license plate numbers.
13. Device identifiers and serial numbers.
14. Web universal resource locators (URLs).
15. Internet protocol (IP) address numbers.
16. Biometric identifiers, including fingerprints and voiceprints.
17. Full-face photographic images and any comparable images.
18. Any other unique identifying number, characteristic, or code, unless otherwise permitted by the Privacy Rule for re-identification.[1]

---

Covered entities may also use statistical methods to establish de-identification instead of removing all 18 identifiers. The covered entity may obtain certification by "a person with appropriate knowledge of and experience with generally accepted statistical and scientific principles and methods for rendering information not individually identifiable" that there is a "very small" risk that the information could be used by the recipient to identify the individual who is the subject of the information, alone or in combination with other reasonably available information.

📝 The person certifying statistical de-identification must document the methods used as well as the result of the analysis that justifies the determination. A covered entity is required to keep such certification, in written or electronic format, for at least **six** years from the date of its creation or the date when it was last in effect, whichever is later.

When you conduct a large retrospective chart review and obtain PHI, your IRB of record will need to approve a waiver of HIPAA authorization.

The CFR source regulation is:

**45 CFR 164.512**

(i) *Standard: Uses and disclosures for research purposes*—(1) *Permitted uses and disclosures.* A covered entity may use or disclose protected health information for research, regardless of the source of funding of the research, provided that:

(i) *Board approval of a waiver of authorization.* The covered entity obtains documentation that an alteration to or waiver, in whole or in part, of the individual authorization required by §164.508 for use or disclosure of protected health information has been approved by either:

1. An Institutional Review Board (IRB)
2. A privacy board that:
    **(1)** Has members with varying backgrounds and appropriate professional competency as necessary to review the effect of the research protocol on the individual's privacy rights and related interests;
    **(2)** Includes at least one member who is not affiliated with the covered entity, not affiliated with any entity conducting or sponsoring the research, and not related to any person who is affiliated with any of such entities; and
    **(3)** Does not have any member participating in a review of any project in which the member has a conflict of interest.

Below are the guidelines the IRB review when determining whether a HIPPA waiver should be approved. Pursuant to 21 CFR 56, the IRB must send a letter to the PI with the IRB's determination.

📝 Principal Investigators must be aware of the HIPPA waiver process so that they can provide the necessary information. The regulation is found at 45 CFR 164.512(i)(2).[2]

(2) *Documentation of waiver approval.* For a use or disclosure to be permitted based on documentation of approval of an alteration or waiver, under paragraph (i)(1)(i) of this section, the documentation must include all of the following:

(i) *Identification and date of action.* A statement identifying the IRB or privacy board and the date on which the alteration or waiver of authorization was approved;

(ii) *Waiver criteria.* A statement that the IRB or privacy board has determined that the alteration or waiver, in whole or in part, of authorization satisfies the following criteria:

(A) The use or disclosure of protected health information involves no more than a minimal risk to the privacy of individuals based on, at least, the presence of the following elements:

**(1)** An adequate plan to protect the identifiers from improper use and disclosure;
**(2)** An adequate plan to destroy the identifiers at the earliest opportunity consistent with conduct of the research, unless there is a health or research justification for retaining the identifiers or such retention is otherwise required by law; and
**(3)** Adequate written assurances that the protected health information will not be reused or disclosed to any other person or entity, except as required by law, for authorized oversight of the research study, or for other research for which the use or disclosure of protected health information would be permitted by this subpart;

(B) The research could not practicably be conducted without the waiver or alteration; and,

(C) The research could not practicably be conducted without access to and use of the protected health information.

## 4.2 TRANSLATION AND INTERPRETATION

*Purpose of section*:

- Defines the terms "translation" and "interpretation"
- Provides advice on translation services
- Provides regulatory and ICH GCP references on language requirements

Clinical trials increasingly have the opportunity to recruit non-English speaking subjects, partially because of the local and regional demographics of certain institutional sites. In this section, we discuss translation of study documents and interpretation for study visits for individuals who do not speak English, nor understand written English.

To clarify:

Translation is the <u>written</u> expression of one language into another language. (See Fig. 4.1.)

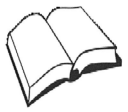

**FIG. 4.1**

Book icon.

Interpretation is the <u>spoken</u> expression of one language into another language. (See Fig. 4.2.)

**FIG. 4.2**

Speaking icon.

**A first and important note:** Your institution will only be able to invite persons speaking languages other than English into your research studies successfully IF AND ONLY IF your Institution has an interpretation call line with accessibility to multiple languages, or in-house interpreters available 24/7.

As noted in the Feasibility Analysis Checklist in Appendix 3, translating a consent form into another language to meet the demographic in your area is a first step only.

In addition, the study team must be able to speak with subjects at study visits, during the scheduling of phone calls, and have a plan in place for communication if a research subject calls outside of regular work hours with a question, or because they are experiencing an Adverse Event or Serious Adverse Event.

The study team needs to think through the various scenarios for communicating with study subjects who do not speak or read English.

The Code of Federal Regulations states the following about language:

---

**21 CFR 50.20:**

**Sec. 50.20 General requirements for informed consent**.
Except as provided in 50.23 and 50.24, no investigator may involve a human being as a subject in research covered by these regulations unless the investigator has obtained the legally effective informed consent of the subject or the subject's legally authorized representative. An investigator shall seek such consent only under circumstances that provide the prospective subject or the representative sufficient opportunity to consider whether or not to participate and that minimize the possibility of coercion or undue influence. **The information that is given to the subject or the representative shall be in language understandable to the subject or the representative.** No informed consent, whether oral or written, may include any exculpatory language through which the subject or the representative is made to waive or appear to waive any of the subject's legal rights, or releases or appears to release the investigator, the sponsor, the institution, or its agents from liability for negligence."

---

Moreover, there is additional guidance provided here:

**45 CFR 46.116**:

**§46.116 General requirements for informed consent.**

Except as provided elsewhere in this policy, no investigator may involve a human being as a subject in research covered by this policy unless the investigator has obtained the legally effective informed consent of the subject or the subject's legally authorized representative. An investigator shall seek such consent only under circumstances that provide the prospective subject or the representative sufficient opportunity to consider whether or not to participate and that minimize the possibility of coercion or undue influence. **The information that is given to the subject or the representative shall be in language understandable to the subject or the representative.** No informed consent, whether oral or written, may include any exculpatory language through which the subject or the representative is made to waive or appear to waive any of the subject's legal rights, or releases or appears to release the investigator, the sponsor, the institution or its agents from liability for negligence.[3]

---

**45 CFR 46.116 (a)(1)-(a)(6) General Requirements for Informed Consent New Common rule**
  (1) **Before involving a human subject in research covered by this policy, an investigator shall obtain the legally effective informed consent of the subject or the subject's legally authorized representative.**
  (2) **An investigator shall seek informed consent only under circumstances that provide the prospective subject or the legally authorized representative sufficient opportunity to discuss and consider whether or not to participate and that minimize the possibility of coercion or undue influence.**

(3)  **The information that is given to the subject or the legally authorized representative shall be in language understandable to the subject or the legally authorized representative.**

(4)  **The prospective subject or the legally authorized representative must be provided with the information that a reasonable person would want to have in order to make an informed decision about whether to participate, and an opportunity to discuss that information.**

(5)  **Except for broad consent obtained in accordance with paragraph (d) of this section:**

   (i)  **Informed consent must begin with a concise and focused presentation of the key information that is most likely to assist a prospective subject or legally authorized representative in understanding the reasons why one might or might not want to participate in the research. This part of the informed consent must be organized and presented in a way that facilitates comprehension.**

   (ii)  **Informed consent as a whole must present information in sufficient detail relating to the research, and must be organized and presented in a way that does not merely provide lists of isolated facts, but rather facilitates the prospective subject's or legally authorized representative's understanding of the reasons why one might or might not want to participate.**

(6)  **No informed consent may include any exculpatory language through which the subject or the legally authorized representative is made to waive or appear to waive any of the subject's legal rights, or releases or appears to release the investigator, the sponsor, the institution, or its agents from liability for negligence.**

𝒥𝑪ᴵᶜᴴ The ICH GCP E6 R2 states the following about language:

"4.8.6 **The language used in the oral and written information about the trial, including the written informed consent form**, should be as non-technical as practical and **should be understandable to the subject or the subject's legally acceptable representative and the impartial witness**, where applicable."[4]

For further information, see "Short Form Consent" in Chapter 2, Section 2.5.

**Acquiring Translation Services:**

There are a lot of translation services available through the internet, and the process of translating a document is as simple as uploading your document onto one of the company's websites. They take it from there!

Key "consent form translation" into an internet search engine. You will see at least a couple translation companies that cater to the translation of informed consent forms for human subjects research.

You can also key "document translation" into an internet search engine. There will be many more translation companies that can translate your research study documents.

Know your word count. These companies typically charge so many cents per word. Within Microsoft Word, the "Word Count" function can be found within the "Review" tab. Depending upon your version of Word, you may find the Word Count in the "Proofing" section of "Review" or in another section. Click on "Word Count" and a small window will appear with your word count; it is that easy!

Compare a few companies for cost and turnaround time. Choose the one that best suits your needs and budget. Some clinical trial sponsors are willing to pay for the cost of translation, so add it to your study budget for consideration.

IRB Check your IRB policy to see if they require:

1. A forward-and-back translation (explained below) or whether a forward translation will suffice;
2. A "Certificate of Accuracy" from the translating company.

What is a "back translation"?

The consent form or/and other research documents are translated into a language other than English. After this translation, a separate translator (from the same translation company) then translates the document(s) back into English. Each pair of documents is compared for language accuracy by yet another individual from the translation company.

What is a "Certificate of Accuracy"?

A "Certificate of Accuracy" guarantees that the translation complies with international translation standards, such as ISO 17100, or/and ASTM F2575.

A Certificate of Accuracy is recommended so that no subject can claim that the consent form was inadequate. It protects the Institution, and should provide each subject with a level of comfort that he or she is getting a solid representation of the research and its risks.

For international readers, the European Union has a translation-services standard called "European EN 15038." Canada goes by the "Canadian Standard for Translation Services CAN CGSB 131.10-2008."

## 4.3 BLINDING AND UNBLINDING IN A CLINICAL TRIAL

*Purpose of section*:

- Defines the terms "blinding" and "unblinding"
- Identifies different types of blinding
- Identifies administrative precautions for maintaining a blind

"Blinding" is defined as follows: Knowledge of the treatment intervention *is **hidden*** from the majority of individuals involved in a clinical trial. The majority members include the PI, study team members, clinical trial subjects, sponsor team members, and clinical staff providing care for a subject.

The reason for blinding is to remove bias. For example, if the PI and study team expect the investigational agent to be more effective than a placebo, their study documentation may reflect this expectation. In order to not be influenced, blinding is practiced.

Clinicaltrials.gov provides three definitions for "blinding":

**MASKING (or Blinding)**

A clinical trial design strategy in which one or more parties involved in the trial, such as the investigator or participants, do not know which participants have been assigned which interventions.

**SINGLE BLINDING (or Masking)**

A type of Masking in which one party involved in the clinical trial, either the investigator or participants, does not know which participants have been assigned which interventions.

An example of single blinding or masking is an IDE (Investigational Device Exemption) trial. The investigational device or comparison device (such as an FDA approved device) is masked to the subjects, while the Investigator and study team know the assignments.

**DOUBLE MASKING OR BLINDING**

A type of Masking in which two or more parties involved in the clinical trial do not know which participants have been assigned which interventions. Typically, the parties include the investigator and participants.

Double blinding is the most typical type of blinding in Industry sponsored drug clinical trials.

In double-blind trials, there will be appointed individuals who know the treatment assignments. All others involved with the trial will need to be blinded. These blinded individuals include:

**(a)** The Principal Investigator
**(b)** Any Sub-Investigators
**(c)** Co-Investigator if applicable
**(d)** Research Coordinator(s)
**(e)** Data Analysts

**(f)** Technicians performing tests or procedures on the subjects

**(g)** Research Nurse(s)

"Unblinding" is defined as follows: The treatment intervention *is **revealed*** by the breaking of a code, which identifies what intervention a subject was given. Unblinding can occur at the end of a trial, or when an individual subject experiences a serious adverse advent necessitating unblinding, or if a female subject becomes pregnant.

🧍‍ICH Guidance through ICH GCP E6 R2 is the following:

4.7 Randomization Procedures and Unblinding

The investigator should follow the trial's randomization procedures, if any, and should ensure that the code is broken only in accordance with the protocol. If the trial is blinded, the investigator should promptly document and explain to the sponsor any premature unblinding (e.g., accidental unblinding, unblinding due to a serious adverse event) of the investigational product(s).

5.13.4 Manufacturing, Packaging, Labeling, and Coding Investigational Product(s)

In blinded trials, the coding system for the investigational product(s) should include a mechanism that permits rapid identification of the product(s) in case of a medical emergency, but does not permit undetectable breaks of the blinding.

In Essential Documents:

8.2.17 Decoding Procedures for Blinded Trials

To document how, in case of an emergency, identity of blinded investigational product can be revealed without breaking the blind for the remaining subjects' treatment (referring to all other subjects in the trial).

The Code of Federal Regulations does not speak to blinding, unblinding, masking, or unmasking.

👍 In order to maintain the blind in clinical trials, the following administrative precautions need to be taken:

**(1)** The investigational agent needs to look like the placebo so that those blinded cannot tell which is which. For example:
  **a.** Liquids need to have the same viscosity and color.
  **b.** Pills or capsules need to be the same size and color.
  **c.** If there is any smell emanating from the investigational agent, it will need to be replicated in the placebo.

**(2)** Labeling needs to be the same for the investigational agent and the placebo.

**(3)** Coding/numbering needs to be similar enough that those blinded cannot figure out the difference between the investigational agent and the placebo.

**(4)** Packaging, including tamper seals, need to be identical.

**(5)** Shipping documentation needs to conceal the actual substance.

**(6)** Clearly define the access/permissions on any electronic database or web portal or CTMS or other software program used for the study so that those who are blinded are kept separate from the research pharmacy or other party(ies) who know which product is being given to whom. (Permissions for those who are blinded are kept separate from those who are unblinded.)

**(7)** Make sure radiology images are labeled in such a way to keep the blind.
  **a.** Of note, this matter of labeling has been a cause of a break in the blind in some trials. A member of the study team will need to notify the Radiology Department of the trial and the need for a change in their usual labeling. (See the sponsor's protocol for details. De-identification may be needed or the use of the Subject ID instead of the subject's name, etc.)

i. The Radiology Department will need to create and enforce a process for the changed labeling so that <u>all shifts</u> will be aware.

---

## AUTHOR'S NOTE

An important note is that the research subject's safety ALWAYS takes precedence. If the subject has a serious adverse event or unanticipated problem or medical emergency or becomes pregnant, the Principal Investigator may decide that unblinding is warranted.

**NOTE: The PI has the ultimate authority to request unblinding.**

---

PIs should follow the study protocol for the proper unblinding procedure created by the Sponsor. This procedure should be known prior to an emergency so that action can occur quickly.

Typically, study team members and Sponsor personnel responsible for the management of the trial remain blinded. See the sponsor's protocol for details.

Once a subject's blind is broken, that subject must be withdrawn from the study. Follow the protocol's direction for follow-up care.

---

## 4.4 ADVERSE EVENTS AND REPORTING IN A CLINICAL TRIAL

*Purpose of section*:

- Defines the various terms found in the Federal regulations for all types of adverse events experienced in clinical trials
- Outlines the requirements for managing, documenting, and reporting these events to the relevant stakeholders

Below is a chart defining "Adverse Events", "Serious Adverse Events", and related terms (Table 4.1):

**Table 4.1 Adverse Events Terms**

| Term | Reference |
|---|---|
| **Adverse Event**: Any untoward medical occurrence associated with the use of a drug in humans, whether or not considered drug related | 21 CFR 312.32 (a) Title 21, Volume 5, Revised 4/1/15 |
| *Adverse event*: Any untoward medical occurrence in a patient or clinical investigation subject administered a pharmaceutical product and which does not necessarily have a causal relationship with this treatment. An adverse event (AE) can therefore be any unfavorable and unintended sign (including an abnormal laboratory finding), symptom, or disease temporally associated with the use of a medicinal (investigational) product, whether or not related to the medicinal (investigational) product | ICH GCP E6 R2 Glossary 1.2 |
| *External adverse event*: Those adverse events experienced by subjects at institutions other than yours in a multicenter clinical trial in which your center participates<br><br>Also: An Adverse Event in a multicenter study that occurs at a site external to an Investigator's local site | **Guidance on Reviewing and Reporting Unanticipated Problems Involving Risks to Subjects or Others and Adverse Events**, www.hhs.gov, **January 15, 2007**<br>Martien |

**Table 4.1 Adverse Events Terms—cont'd**

| Term | Reference |
|---|---|
| *Internal adverse event*: Those adverse events experienced by subjects at your own institution in a multicenter clinical trial in which your center participates<br>Also: An Adverse Event that occurs within a multicenter study at an Investigator's local site | **Guidance on Reviewing and Reporting Unanticipated Problems Involving Risks to Subjects or Others and Adverse Events**, www.hhs.gov, **January 15, 2007**<br>Martien |
| Adverse effect: | (Not defined but mentioned in 21 CFR 312.55 and 312.150 and 312.310) |
| Adverse experience: | Not defined, but found in 21 CFR 312.33, 21 CFR 312.44, 21 CFR 312.53 |
| **Adverse Drug Reaction (ADR)**: In the pre-approval clinical experience with a new medicinal product or its new usages, particularly as the therapeutic dose(s) may not be established: all noxious and unintended responses to a medicinal product related to any dose should be considered adverse drug reactions. The phrase "responses to a medicinal product" means that a causal relationship between a medicinal product and an adverse event is at least a reasonable possibility, i.e., the relationship cannot be ruled out. Regarding marketed medicinal products: a response to a drug which is noxious and unintended and which occurs at doses normally used in man for prophylaxis, diagnosis, or therapy of diseases or for modification of physiological function | ICH GCP E6 R2 Glossary 1.1 |
| **Serious Adverse Event or Serious Suspected Adverse Reaction**: An adverse event…is serious…if it results in any of the following outcomes:<br>• Death<br>• A life-threatening adverse event<br>• Inpatient hospitalization<br>• Prolongation of existing hospitalization<br>• A persistent or significant incapacity or substantial disruption of the ability to conduct normal life functions<br>• Or a congenital anomaly/birth defect (in a fetus or newborn of the research subject's) | 21 CFR 312.32 (a) Title 21, Volume 5, Revised 4/1/15 |
| **Suspected Adverse Reaction**: Any adverse event for which there is a reasonable possibility that the drug caused the adverse event | 21 CFR 312.32 (a) Title 21, Volume 5, Revised 4/1/15 |
| **Reasonable possibility**: Evidence to suggest a causal relationship between the drug and the adverse event | 21 CFR 312.32 (a) Title 21, Volume 5, Revised 4/1/15 |
| **Adverse Reaction**: Any adverse event caused by a drug | 21 CFR 312.32 (a) Title 21, Volume 5, Revised 4/1/15 |
| **Unexpected**: An adverse event or suspected adverse reaction that is not listed in the Investigator Brochure (IB) | 21 CFR 312.32 (a) Title 21, Volume 5, Revised 4/1/15 |
| **Unanticipated Problems**:<br>• A single occurrence of a serious, unexpected event that is uncommon and strongly associated with drug exposure•<br>  A single occurrence, or more often a small number of occurrences, of a serious, unexpected event that is not commonly associated with drug exposure, but uncommon in the study population | Guidance for Clinical Investigators, Sponsors and IRBs: Adverse Event Reporting to IRBs—Improving Human Subject Protection, January 2009, by HHS, FDA, OC, CDER, CBER, CDRH, GCPP |

| Table 4.1 Adverse Events Terms—cont'd | |
| --- | --- |
| **Term** | **Reference** |
| • Multiple occurrences of an AE that, based on aggregate analysis, is determined to be an unanticipated problem<br>• An AE that is described or addressed in the Investigator's Brochure, protocol or consent, but occurs at a specificity or severity that is inconsistent with prior observations<br>• An AE that is described or addressed in the Investigator's Brochure, protocol or consent, but for which the rate of occurrence in the study represents a clinically significant increase in the expected rate of occurrence<br>• Any other AE or safety finding that would cause the sponsor to modify the Investigator's Brochure, study protocol or consent | |
| Unanticipated Adverse Device Effect(s) (UADE) | 21 CFR 812 |

HHS regulations at 45 CFR 46.103(a) and (b)(5) require that institutions have written procedures to ensure that the following incidents related to research conducted or supported by a federal department or agency are promptly reported to OHRP:

**a. Any unanticipated problems involving risks to subjects or others;**
**b. Any serious or continuing non-compliance with this policy or the requirements or determinations of the IRB; and**
**c. Any suspension or termination of IRB approval.**[5]

"Adverse event," "adverse effect," "adverse experience," "serious adverse event" are not found AT ALL in 45 CFR 46, including the New Common Rule. Only "Unanticipated problem" is found in 45 CFR 46 & ONLY in 45 CFR 46.103 within the Common Rule. In the New Common Rule, "unanticipated problem" is mentioned once only in 45 CFR 46.108(a)(4)(i). Within the Common Rule and the New Common Rule, both reference establishing "written procedures for ensuring prompt reporting" in relation to "unanticipated problems."

21 CFR 812 only uses "unanticipated adverse device effect(s)" and "adverse device effects"

ᴊᴄ︎ᴵᶜᴴ **ICH GCP E6 R2**

4.11 Safety Reporting

4.11.1 All serious adverse events (SAEs) should be reported immediately to the sponsor except for those SAEs that the protocol or other document (e.g., Investigator's Brochure) identifies as not needing immediate reporting. The immediate reports should be followed promptly by detailed, written reports.

The immediate and follow-up reports should identify subjects by unique code numbers assigned to the trial subjects rather than by the subjects' names, personal identification numbers, and/or addresses. The investigator should also comply with the applicable regulatory requirement(s) related to the reporting of unexpected serious adverse drug reactions to the regulatory authority(ies) and the IRB/IEC.

4.11.2 Adverse events and/or laboratory abnormalities identified in the protocol as critical to safety evaluations should be reported to the sponsor according to the reporting requirements and within the time periods specified by the sponsor in the protocol.

4.11.3 For reported deaths, the investigator should supply the sponsor and the IRB/IEC with any additional requested information (e.g., autopsy reports and terminal medical reports).

21 CFR 312.32 IND safety reporting definitions

(a) *Definitions*. The following definitions of terms apply to this section:

*Adverse event* means any untoward medical occurrence associated with the use of a drug in humans, whether or not considered drug related.

*Life-threatening adverse event* or *life-threatening suspected adverse reaction*. An adverse event or suspected adverse reaction is considered "life-threatening" if, in the view of either the investigator or sponsor, its occurrence places the patient or subject at immediate risk of death. It does not include an adverse event or suspected adverse reaction that, had it occurred in a more severe form, might have caused death.

*Serious adverse event* or *serious suspected adverse reaction*. An adverse event or suspected adverse reaction is considered "serious" if, in the view of either the investigator or sponsor, it results in any of the following outcomes: Death, a life-threatening adverse event, inpatient hospitalization or prolongation of existing hospitalization, a persistent or significant incapacity or substantial disruption of the ability to conduct normal life functions, or a congenital anomaly/birth defect. Important medical events that may not result in death, be life-threatening, or require hospitalization may be considered serious when, based upon appropriate medical judgment, they may jeopardize the patient or subject and may require medical or surgical intervention to prevent one of the outcomes listed in this definition. Examples of such medical events include allergic bronchospasm requiring intensive treatment in an emergency room or at home, blood dyscrasias or convulsions that do not result in inpatient hospitalization, or the development of drug dependency or drug abuse.

*Suspected adverse reaction* means any adverse event for which there is a reasonable possibility that the drug caused the adverse event. For the purposes of IND safety reporting, "reasonable possibility" means there is evidence to suggest a causal relationship between the drug and the adverse event. Suspected adverse reaction implies a lesser degree of certainty about causality than adverse reaction, which means any adverse event caused by a drug.

✒ *Unexpected adverse event* or *unexpected suspected adverse reaction*. An adverse event or suspected adverse reaction is considered "unexpected" if it is not listed in the investigator brochure or is not listed at the specificity or severity that has been observed; or, if an investigator brochure is not required or available, is not consistent with the risk information described in the general investigational plan or elsewhere in the current application, as amended. For example, under this definition, hepatic necrosis would be unexpected (by virtue of greater severity) if the investigator brochure referred only to elevated hepatic enzymes or hepatitis. Similarly, cerebral thromboembolism and cerebral vasculitis would be unexpected (by virtue of greater specificity) if the investigator brochure listed only cerebral vascular accidents. "Unexpected," as used in this definition, also refers to adverse events or suspected adverse reactions that are mentioned in the investigator brochure as occurring with a class of drugs or as anticipated from the pharmacological properties of the drug, but are not specifically mentioned as occurring with the particular drug under investigation.

**See the "Adverse Events Plus Reporting Table" for when and to whom to report in Appendix 1. To aid your Adverse Event reporting, reference the**

Common Terminology Criteria for Adverse Events (CTCAE) Version 4.0

Published: May 28, 2009 (v4.03: June 14, 2010)

U.S. DEPARTMENT OF HEALTH AND HUMAN SERVICES

National Institutes of Health

National Cancer Institute

Here is the link: https://evs.nci.nih.gov/ftp1/CTCAE/CTCAE_4.03_2010-06-14_QuickReference_5x7.pdf.

The CTCAE will provide terminology definitions and a grading scale for AEs. Here is the opening summary page. (See Fig. 4.3.)

## Common Terminology Criteria for Adverse Events v4.0 (CTCAE)
### Publish date: May 28, 2009

**Quick Reference**

The NCI Common Terminology Criteria for Adverse Events is a descriptive terminology which can be utilized for Adverse Event (AE) reporting. A grading (severity) scale is provided for each AE term.

**Components and Organization**

**SOC**

System Organ Class, the highest level of the MedDRA hierarchy, is identified by anatomical or physiological system, etiology, or purpose (e.g., SOC Investigations for laboratory test results). CTCAE terms are grouped by MedDRA Primary SOCs. Within each SOC, AEs are listed and accompanied by descriptions of severity (Grade).

**CTCAE Terms**

An Adverse Event (AE) is any unfavorable and unintended sign (including an abnormal loboratory finding), symptom, or disease temporally associated with the use of a medical treatment or procedure that may or may _not_ be considered related to the medical treatment or procedure. An AE is a term that is a unique representation of a specific event used for medical documentation and scientific analyses. Each CTCAE v4.0 term is a MedDRA LLT (Lowest Level Term).

**Definitions**

A brief definition is provided to clarify the meaning of each AE term.

**Grades**

Grade refers to the severity of the AE. The CTCAE displays Grades 1 through 5 with unique clinical descriptions fo severity for each AE based on this general guideline:

| | |
|---|---|
| Grade 1 | Mild; asymptomatic or mild symptoms; clinical or diagnostic observations only; intervention not indicated. |
| Grade 2 | Moderate; minimal, local or noninvasive intervention indicated; limiting age-appropriate instrumental ADL*. |
| Grade 3 | Severe or medically significant but not immediately life-threatening; hospitalization or prolongation of hospitalization indicated; disabling; limiting self care ADL**. |
| Grade 4 | Life-threatening consequences; urgent intervention indicated. |
| Grade 5 | Death related to AE. |

A Semi-colon indicates 'or' within the description of the grade.

A single dash (-) indicates a grade is not available.

Not all Grades are appropriate for all AEs. Therefore, some AEs are listed with fewer than five options for Grade selection.

**Grade 5**

Grade 5 (Death) is not appropriate for some AEs and therefore is not an option.

**Activities of Daily Living (ADL)**

*Instrumental ADL refer to preparing meals, shopping for groceries or clothes, using the telephone, managing money, etc.

**Self care ADL refer to bathing, dressing and undressing, feeding self, using the toilet, taking medications, and not bedridden.

† CTCAE v4.0 incorporates certain elements of the MedDRA terminology. For further details on MedDRA refer to the MedDRA MSSO web site (http://www.meddramsso.com).

**FIG. 4.3**

CTCAE.

# 4.5 THE VARIOUS FORMS USED IN A CLINICAL TRIAL

*Purpose of section*:

- Introduces the FDA forms, Sponsor forms, and self-developed study team forms used in a clinical trial
- Provides key information on procedures for the submission of FDA forms by clinical trials sites and sponsors
- Explains details of electronic and hard copy submission requirements

Before, during, and after a clinical trial, there are a number of key forms and documents requiring submission to the U.S. Food and Drug Administration (FDA). Submissions can be made two ways:

1. Electronically, through portals maintained by FDA.
2. By mailing hard copies through surface mail, through delivery services, such as the U.S. Postal Service, United Parcel Service, Federal Express, and DHL.

**Below is a list of the commonly required FDA Forms, accompanied by a brief description of form content and purpose.**

To get the current FDA forms for INDs: https://www.fda.gov/Drugs/DevelopmentApprovalProcess/HowDrugsareDevelopedandApproved/ApprovalApplications/InvestigationalNewDrugINDApplication/ucm071073.htm.

**Form FDA 1571 Investigational New Drug Application (IND)**

Purpose: The 1571 requests the FDA to authorize the use of an investigational drug in humans. It serves as a summary page for the actual submission. (See Fig. 4.4.)

Next page | Export data | Import data | Reset form

DEPARTMENT OF HEALTH AND HUMAN SERVICES
Food and Drug Administration
INVESTIGATIONAL NEW DRUG APPLICATION (IND)
*(Title 21, Code of Federal Regulations (CFR) Part 312)*

Form Approved: OMB No. 0910-0014
Expiration Date: February 28, 2019
*See PRA Statement on page 3.*

NOTE: No drug/biologic may be shipped or clinical investigation begun until an IND for that investigation is in effect (21 CFR 312.40)

1. Name of Sponsor
2. Date of Submission *(mm/dd/yyyy)*
3. Sponsor Address
Address 1 *(Street address, P.O. box, company name c/o)*
Address 2 *(Apartment, suite, unit, building, floor, etc.)*
City
State/Province/Region
Country
ZIP or Postal Code
4. Telephone Number *(Include country code if applicable and area code)*
5. Name(s) of Drug *(Include all available names: Trade, Generic, Chemical, or Code)*
Continuation page for #5
6. IND Number *(If previously assigned)*
7. (Proposed) Indication for Use
Is this indication for a rare disease (prevalence <200,000 in U.S.)? ☐ Yes ☐ No
Does this product have an FDA Orphan Designation for this indication? ☐ Yes ☐ No
If yes, provide the Orphan Designation number for this indication:
Continuation page for #7
8. Phase(s) of Clinical Investigation to be conducted ☐ Phase 1 ☐ Phase 2 ☐ Phase 3 ☐ Other *(Specify)*:
9. List numbers of all Investigational New Drug Applications (21 CFR Part 312), New Drug Applications (21 CFR Part 314), Drug Master Files (21 CFR Part 314.420), and Biologics License Applications (21 CFR Part 601) referred to in this application.

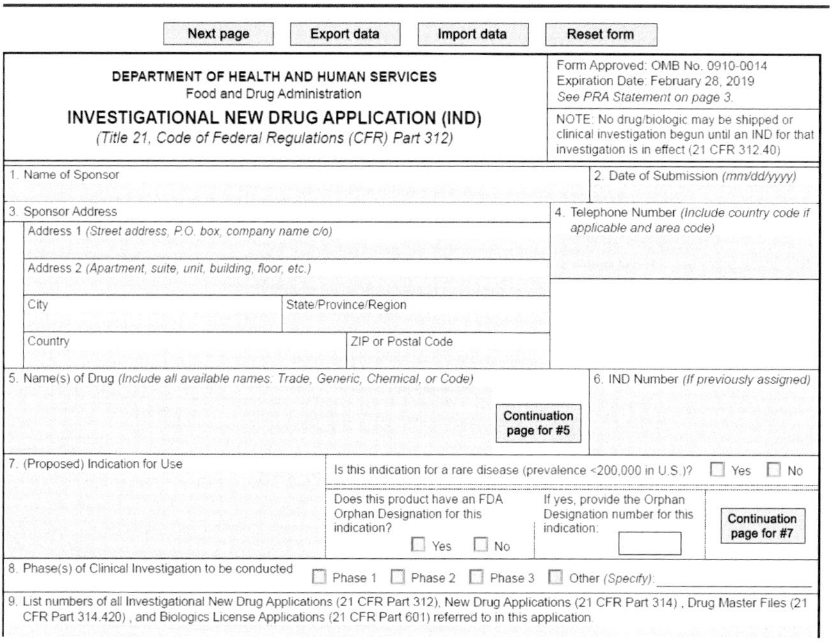

**FIG. 4.4**

FDA 1571 form sample.

Who fills it out: the Sponsor—whether a Sponsor Investigator or an Industry Sponsor

Where it is sent: the FDA

**Website Link:**

Form https://www.fda.gov/downloads/AboutFDA/ReportsManualsForms/Forms/UCM083533.pdf

Instructions https://www.fda.gov/downloads/aboutfda/reportsmanualsforms/forms/ucm182850.pdf

**Form FDA 1572 Statement of Investigator (Site)**

Purpose: The 1572 has two purposes:

**(1)** to provide the sponsor with information about the investigator's qualifications and the clinical site that will enable the sponsor to establish and document that the investigator is qualified and the site is an appropriate location at which to conduct the clinical investigation, and

**(2)** to inform the investigator of his/her obligations and obtain the investigator's commitment to follow pertinent FDA regulations.

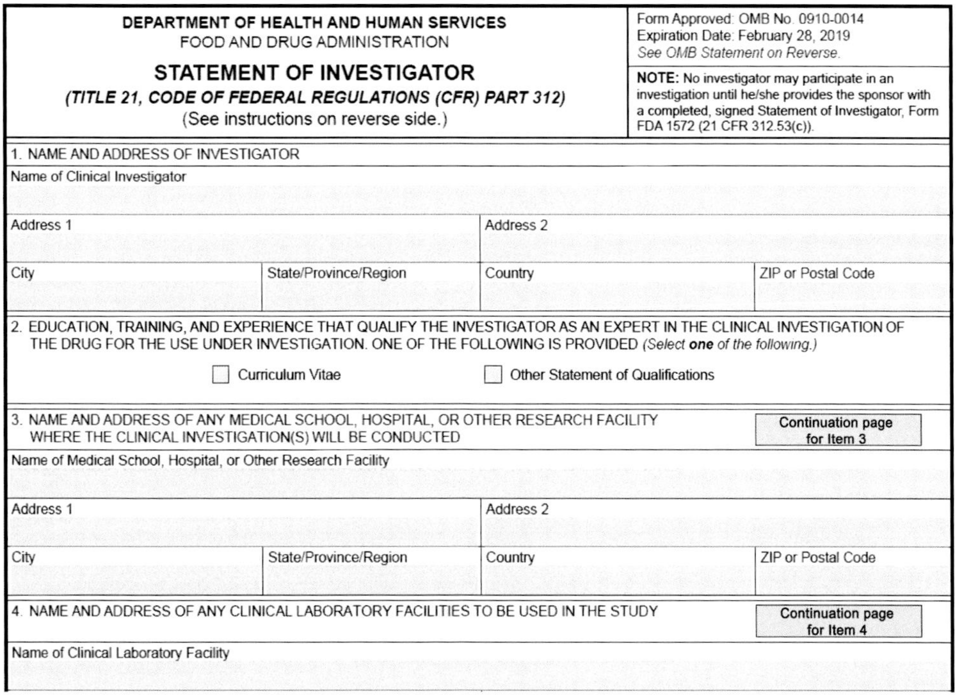

https://www.fda.gov/downloads/regulatoryinformation/guidances/ucm214282.pdf.

**DEPARTMENT OF HEALTH AND HUMAN SERVICES**
FOOD AND DRUG ADMINISTRATION

**STATEMENT OF INVESTIGATOR**
***(TITLE 21, CODE OF FEDERAL REGULATIONS (CFR) PART 312)***
(See instructions on reverse side.)

Form Approved: OMB No. 0910-0014
Expiration Date: February 28, 2019
*See OMB Statement on Reverse.*

**NOTE:** No investigator may participate in an investigation until he/she provides the sponsor with a completed, signed Statement of Investigator, Form FDA 1572 (21 CFR 312.53(c)).

1. NAME AND ADDRESS OF INVESTIGATOR
Name of Clinical Investigator
Address 1 | Address 2
City | State/Province/Region | Country | ZIP or Postal Code

2. EDUCATION, TRAINING, AND EXPERIENCE THAT QUALIFY THE INVESTIGATOR AS AN EXPERT IN THE CLINICAL INVESTIGATION OF THE DRUG FOR THE USE UNDER INVESTIGATION. ONE OF THE FOLLOWING IS PROVIDED *(Select **one** of the following.)*
☐ Curriculum Vitae ☐ Other Statement of Qualifications

3. NAME AND ADDRESS OF ANY MEDICAL SCHOOL, HOSPITAL, OR OTHER RESEARCH FACILITY WHERE THE CLINICAL INVESTIGATION(S) WILL BE CONDUCTED — **Continuation page for Item 3**
Name of Medical School, Hospital, or Other Research Facility
Address 1 | Address 2
City | State/Province/Region | Country | ZIP or Postal Code

4. NAME AND ADDRESS OF ANY CLINICAL LABORATORY FACILITIES TO BE USED IN THE STUDY — **Continuation page for Item 4**
Name of Clinical Laboratory Facility

**FIG. 4.5**

FDA 1572 statement of investigator sample.

Who fills it out: Typically, a Research Coordinator fills it out. The PI reviews it and reads the Commitments in Section 9 and signs then dates it.

Where it is sent: the Sponsor (The Sponsor will include it with their IND Application to the FDA.) (See Fig. 4.5.)

**Website Links:**

Form https://www.fda.gov/downloads/AboutFDA/ReportsManualsForms/Forms/UCM074728.pdf

Instructions https://www.fda.gov/downloads/AboutFDA/ReportsManualsForms/Forms/UCM223432.pdf

Guidance https://www.fda.gov/downloads/regulatoryinformation/guidances/ucm214282.pdf

**Form FDA 3454 Certification: Financial Interests and Arrangements of Clinical Investigators**

Purpose: FORM FDA 3454 certifies:

1. That a clinical investigator has no disclosable financial interests in or arrangements with any sponsor of the covered clinical study (21 CFR § 54.4(a)(1)); or
2. That the applicant acted with due diligence but was unable to obtain financial interests' information (option 3 on the form)

| DEPARTMENT OF HEALTH AND HUMAN SERVICES<br>Food and Drug Administration<br>**CERTIFICATION: FINANCIAL INTERESTS AND ARRANGEMENTS OF CLINICAL INVESTIGATORS** | Form Approved: OMB No. 0910-0396<br>Expiration Date: March 31, 2019 |
|---|---|

*TO BE COMPLETED BY APPLICANT*

With respect to all covered clinical studies (or specific clinical studies listed below (if appropriate)) submitted in support of this application, I certify to one of the statements below as appropriate. I understand that this certification is made in compliance with 21 CFR part 54 and that for the purposes of this statement, a clinical investigator includes the spouse and each dependent child of the investigator as defined in 21 CFR 54.2(d).

*Please mark the applicable check box.*

☐ (1) As the sponsor of the submitted studies, I certify that I have not entered into any financial arrangement with the listed clinical investigators (enter names of clinical investigators below or attach list of names to this form) whereby the value of compensation to the investigator could be affected by the outcome of the study as defined in 21 CFR 54.2(a). I also certify that each listed clinical investigator required to disclose to the sponsor whether the investigator had a proprietary interest in this product or a significant equity in the sponsor as defined in 21 CFR 54.2(b) did not disclose any such interests. I further certify that no listed investigator was the recipient of significant payments of other sorts as defined in 21 CFR 54.2(f).

Clinical Investigators

☐ (2) As the applicant who is submitting a study or studies sponsored by a firm or party other than the applicant, I certify that based on information obtained from the sponsor or from participating clinical investigators, the listed clinical investigators (attach list of names to this form) did not participate in any

**FIG. 4.6**

FDA 3454 sample.

Who fills it out: applicants who submit a marketing application for a drug, biological product or device.

Where it is sent: to the FDA (The Sponsor will include it with their IND Application to the FDA.) (See Fig. 4.6.)

**Website Links:**

Form https://www.fda.gov/downloads/AboutFDA/ReportsManualsForms/Forms/UCM048304.pdf

Guidance https://www.fda.gov/downloads/regulatoryinformation/guidances/ucm341008.pdf

**Form FDA 3455 Disclosure: Financial Interests and Arrangements of Clinical Investigators**

Purpose: Form FDA 3455 discloses financial interests in and/or arrangements with any sponsor of the covered clinical study by each clinical investigator, or the investigator's spouse or dependent child(ren).

| DEPARTMENT OF HEALTH AND HUMAN SERVICES<br>Food and Drug Administration<br><br>**DISCLOSURE: FINANCIAL INTERESTS AND<br>ARRANGEMENTS OF CLINICAL INVESTIGATORS** | Form Approved: OMB No. 0910-0396<br>Expiration Date: March 31, 2019 |
| --- | --- |

*TO BE COMPLETED BY APPLICANT*

The following information concerning _____ , who participated
Name of clinical investigator

as a clinical investigator in the submitted study_____
Name of

_____ is submitted in accordance with 21 CFR part 54. The
*clinical study*

named individual has participated in financial arrangements or holds financial interests that are required to be disclosed as follows:

*Please mark the applicable check boxes.*

☐ any financial arrangement entered into between the sponsor of the covered study and the clinical investigator involved in the conduct of the covered study, whereby the value of the compensation to the clinical investigator for conducting the study could be influenced by the outcome of the study;

☐ any significant payments of other sorts made on or after February 2, 1999, from the sponsor of the covered study, such as a grant to fund ongoing research, compensation in the form of equipment, retainer for ongoing consultation, or honoraria;

☐ any proprietary interest in the product tested in the covered study held by the clinical investigator;

**FIG. 4.7**

FDA 3455 Disclosure form sample.

Who fills it out: applicants who submit a marketing application for a drug, biological product or device.

Where it is sent: to the FDA (The Sponsor will include it with their IND Application to the FDA.) (See Fig. 4.7.)

**Website Links:**

Form https://www.fda.gov/downloads/AboutFDA/ReportsManualsForms/Forms/UCM048310.pdf

Guidance https://www.fda.gov/downloads/regulatoryinformation/guidances/ucm341008.pdf

**Form FDA 3500A—MedWatch MANDATORY reporting of adverse events and product problems by manufacturers, importers, distributors, and user facilities.**

Purpose: mandatory reporting of Adverse Events

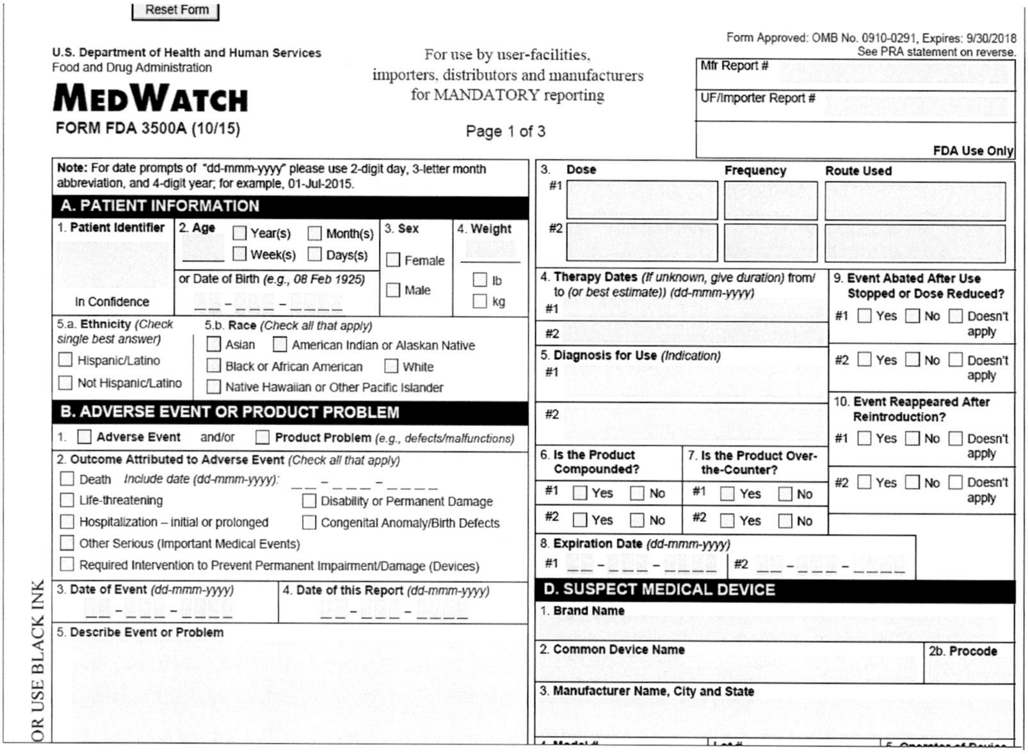

Reset Form

U.S. Department of Health and Human Services
Food and Drug Administration

**MEDWATCH**

FORM FDA 3500A (10/15)

For use by user-facilities, importers, distributors and manufacturers for MANDATORY reporting

Page 1 of 3

Form Approved: OMB No. 0910-0291, Expires: 9/30/2018
See PRA statement on reverse.

Mfr Report #

UF/Importer Report #

FDA Use Only

**Note:** For date prompts of "dd-mmm-yyyy" please use 2-digit day, 3-letter month abbreviation, and 4-digit year; for example, 01-Jul-2015.

**A. PATIENT INFORMATION**

1. Patient Identifier — In Confidence
2. Age — Year(s) / Month(s) / Week(s) / Days(s); or Date of Birth (e.g., 08 Feb 1925)
3. Sex — Female / Male
4. Weight — lb / kg

5.a. Ethnicity (Check single best answer) — Hispanic/Latino / Not Hispanic/Latino

5.b. Race (Check all that apply) — Asian / American Indian or Alaskan Native / Black or African American / White / Native Hawaiian or Other Pacific Islander

**B. ADVERSE EVENT OR PRODUCT PROBLEM**

1. Adverse Event and/or Product Problem (e.g., defects/malfunctions)
2. Outcome Attributed to Adverse Event (Check all that apply)
   - Death Include date (dd-mmm-yyyy):
   - Life-threatening
   - Disability or Permanent Damage
   - Hospitalization – initial or prolonged
   - Congenital Anomaly/Birth Defects
   - Other Serious (Important Medical Events)
   - Required Intervention to Prevent Permanent Impairment/Damage (Devices)
3. Date of Event (dd-mmm-yyyy)
4. Date of this Report (dd-mmm-yyyy)
5. Describe Event or Problem

3. Dose / Frequency / Route Used — #1, #2

4. Therapy Dates (If unknown, give duration) from/to (or best estimate)) (dd-mmm-yyyy) — #1, #2

5. Diagnosis for Use (Indication) — #1, #2

6. Is the Product Compounded? — #1 Yes No; #2 Yes No

7. Is the Product Over-the-Counter? — #1 Yes No; #2 Yes No

8. Expiration Date (dd-mmm-yyyy) — #1, #2

9. Event Abated After Use Stopped or Dose Reduced? — #1 Yes No Doesn't apply; #2 Yes No Doesn't apply

10. Event Reappeared After Reintroduction? — #1 Yes No Doesn't apply; #2 Yes No Doesn't apply

**D. SUSPECT MEDICAL DEVICE**

1. Brand Name
2. Common Device Name
2b. Procode
3. Manufacturer Name, City and State

OR USE BLACK INK

**FIG. 4.8**

MedWatch form sample.

For the purpose of the form, the FDA defines "Adverse event" this way: Any incident where the use of a product (drug or biologic, including human cell, tissue, or cellular or tissue-based product (HCT/P)), at any dose, or a medical device (including in vitro diagnostic products) is suspected to have resulted in an adverse outcome in a patient.

Who fills it out: The Sponsor or the CRO (for the Sponsor), importers, distributors, manufacturers, or user facilities

Definition: user facility—A user facility is a federally sponsored research facility available for external use to advance scientific or technical knowledge. https://science.energy.gov/user-facilities/ which allow scientific users from universities, national laboratories, and industry to carry out experiments and pursue groundbreaking discoveries that would otherwise not be possible due to the cost. https://www.anl.gov/user-facilities

Where it is sent: the FDA and the manufacturer (see Fig. 4.8).

**Website Links:**

Form https://www.fda.gov/downloads/AboutFDA/ReportsManualsForms/Forms/UCM048334.pdf

Instructions https://www.fda.gov/downloads/aboutfda/reportsmanualsforms/forms/ucm295636.pdf

**Form FDA 3674 Certificate of Compliance**

Purpose: To certify compliance with ClinicalTrials.gov requirements, FDA requires that applicants complete and submit Form FDA 3674 with certain human drug, biological product, and device applications and submissions. In general, FDA recommends that a Form FDA 3674 accompany the following applications and submissions to FDA:

- Investigational New Drug Application (IND)
- New Clinical Protocol Submitted to an IND
- New Drug Application (NDA)
- Efficacy Supplement to an Approved NDA
- Biologics License Application (BLA)
- Efficacy Supplement to an Approved BLA
- Abbreviated New Drug Application (ANDA)
- Premarket Approval Application (PMA)
- PMA Panel Track Supplement
- Humanitarian Device Exemption (HDE)
- 510(k) submissions that refer to, relate to, or include information on a clinical trial

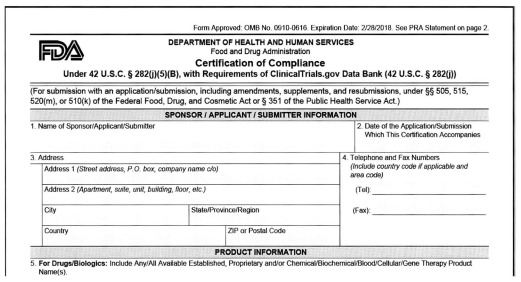

**FIG. 4.9**

FDA 3674 form sample.

Note—FDA does not require the submission of a Form FDA 3674 with an Investigational Device Exemption (IDE) application, as this was not required by FDAAA. https://www.fda.gov/scienceresearch/specialtopics/runningclinicaltrials/fdasroleclinicaltrials. govinformation/default.htm

Who fills it out: applicants submitting the above-mentioned applications, which would be a Sponsor or Manufacturer

Where it is sent: the FDA (see Fig. 4.9).

**Website Links:**

Form https://www.fda.gov/downloads/AboutFDA/ReportsManualsForms/Forms/UCM048364.pdf

Instructions https://www.fda.gov/downloads/aboutfda/reportsmanualsforms/forms/ucm354618.pdf
**Form FDA 3926 Individual Patient Expanded Access Applications** (Physician at Site)
Purpose: Expanded Access (Compassionate Use) of an IND. See Chapter 6, Section 6.1.

| DEPARTMENT OF HEALTH AND HUMAN SERVICES<br>Food and Drug Administration<br>**Individual Patient Expanded Access<br>Investigational New Drug  Application (IND)**<br>*(Title 21, Code of Federal Regulations (CFR) Part 312)* | Form Approved: OMB No. 0910-0814<br>Expiration Date: April 30, 2019<br>*See PRA Statement on last page.* |
|---|---|

| **1. Patient's Initials** | **2. Date of Submission** *(mm/dd/yyyy)* |
|---|---|

| **3.a. Initial Submission**<br>☐ Select this box if this form is an initial submission for an individual patient expanded access IND, and complete only fields 4 through 8, and fields 10 and 11. | **3.b. Follow-Up Submission**<br>☐ Select this box if this form accompanies a follow-up submission to an existing individual patient expanded access IND, and complete the items to the right in this section, and fields 8 through 11. | Investigational Drug Name<br><br>Physician's IND Number |
|---|---|---|

**4. Clinical Information**
Indication

Brief Clinical History *(Patient's age, gender, weight, allergies, diagnosis, prior therapy, response to prior therapy, reason for request, including an explanation of why the patient lacks other therapeutic options)*

**5. Treatment Information**
Investigational Drug Name

Name of the entity that will supply the drug *(generally the manufacturer)*

**FIG. 4.10**

FDA 3926 form sample.

Who fills it out: a Physician at a medical institution
Where it is sent: the FDA (see Fig. 4.10).
**Website Links:**
Form https://www.fda.gov/downloads/AboutFDA/ReportsManualsForms/Forms/UCM504572.pdf
Instructions https://www.fda.gov/downloads/aboutfda/reportsmanualsforms/forms/ucm504574.pdf
**Form FDA 356h Application to Market a New or Abbreviated New Drug or Biologic for Human Use**
Purpose:

- Accompanies regulatory submissions to new drug applications (NDAs), biologic license applications (BLAs), abbreviated new drug applications (ANDAs), and supplements
- Describes the reason for, and content of, the submission
- Captures information used to populate FDA system

| DEPARTMENT OF HEALTH AND HUMAN SERVICES Food and Drug Administration **APPLICATION TO MARKET A NEW OR ABBREVIATED NEW DRUG OR BIOLOGIC FOR HUMAN USE** (Title 21, Code of Federal Regulations, Parts 314 & 601) | Form Approved: OMB No. 0910-0338 Expiration Date: March 31, 2020 *See PRA Statement on page 3.* |
|---|---|
| | 1. Date of Submission *(mm/dd/yyyy)* |

| **APPLICANT INFORMATION** | 2. Name of Applicant | |
|---|---|---|
| 3. Telephone Number *(Include country code if applicable and area code)* | 4. Facsimile (FAX) Number *(Include country code if applicable and area code)* | |
| 5. Applicant Address | | |

| Address 1 *(Street address, P.O. box, company name c/o)* | Email Address |
|---|---|
| Address 2 *(Apartment, suite, unit, building, floor, etc.)* | Applicant DUNS |
| City / State/Province/Region | |
| Country / ZIP or Postal Code | U.S. License Number if previously issued |

6. Authorized U.S. Agent *(Required for non-U.S. applicants)*

| Authorized U.S. Agent Name | Telephone Number *(Include area code)* |
|---|---|
| Address 1 *(Street address, P.O. box, company name c/o)* | FAX Number *(Include area code)* |
| Address 2 *(Apartment, suite, unit, building, floor, etc.)* | Email Address |
| City / State | |
| ZIP Code | U.S. Agent DUNS |

| **PRODUCT DESCRIPTION** | 7. NDA, ANDA, or BLA Application Number | 8. Supplement Number *(If applicable)* |
|---|---|---|
| 9. Established Name *(e.g., proper name, USP/USAN name)* | | |
| 10. Proprietary Name *(Trade Name) (If any)* | | |
| 11. Chemical/Biochemical/Blood Product Name *(If any)* | | |
| 12. Dosage Form | 13. Strengths | 14. Route of Administration |

**FIG. 4.11**

FDA 356h form sample.

Who fills it out: applicants submitting an NDA, BLA, or ANDA, which would be a Sponsor or Manufacturer

Where it is sent: the FDA (see Fig. 4.11).

**Website Links:**

**Form FDA 356h Application to Market a New or Abbreviated New Drug or Biologic for Human Use**

Form https://www.fda.gov/downloads/AboutFDA/ReportsManualsForms/Forms/UCM082348.pdf

Instructions https://www.fda.gov/downloads/AboutFDA/ReportsManualsForms/Forms/UCM321897.pdf

**Please Note: Do not confuse the MedWatch 3500A form with the MedWatch 3500. The MedWatch 3500 form is strictly for general public use.**

**Form FDA 3500 MedWatch The FDA Safety Information and Adverse Event Reporting Program—Voluntary**

Purpose: For VOLUNTARY reporting of adverse events, product problems and product use errors

Form FDA 3500 may be used by health professionals or consumers for **VOLUNTARY** reporting of adverse events, product use errors, product quality problems, and therapeutic failures for:

- drugs (prescription and over-the-counter)
- biologics (including blood components, blood derivatives, allergenics, human cells, tissues, and cellular and tissue-based products (HCT/Ps))
- medical devices (including in vitro diagnostic products)
- combination products
- special nutritional products (dietary supplements, infant formulas, medical foods)
- cosmetics (such as moisturizers, makeup, shampoos and conditioners, face and body washes, deodorants, nail care products, hair dyes and relaxers, and tattoos)
- foods/beverages (including reports of serious allergic reactions)

Adverse events involving **investigational (study) drugs, such as those relating to Investigational New Drug (IND) applications, including those for cellular products administered under IND,** should be reported as required in the study protocol and sent to the address and contact person listed in the study protocol. They should generally not be submitted to FDA MedWatch as voluntary reports.

Form https://www.fda.gov/downloads/AboutFDA/ReportsManualsForms/Forms/UCM163919.pdf
Instructions https://www.fda.gov/Safety/MedWatch/HowToReport/DownloadForms/ucm149236.htm

### How to Submit FDA Forms
**Background on Electronic Submissions to the FDA**

The FDA's Electronic Submissions Gateway (ESG) is the Agency system for accepting electronic regulatory submissions. ESG serves as an exchange point for FDA and its partners to transact a variety of documents and submissions.

The FDA ESG enables the FDA to process regulatory information automatically, functioning as a single point of entry for receiving and processing all electronic submissions within a secure environment. The FDA ESG complies with the secure Hypertext Transfer Protocol (HTTP) messaging standards and uses digital certificates for secure communication. The electronic submission process encompasses the receipt, acknowledgment of receipt (to the sender), routing and notification (to the relevant receiving Center or Office) of the delivery of an electronic submission.

The FDA ESG is a conduit, or "highway," along which submissions travel to reach their final destination. The FDA ESG does not open or review submissions, but automatically routes them to the proper FDA Center or Office. Clinical trial sites, and/or sponsors, can send and receive documents from the Gateway via a web interface or server-to-server communications.

**How To Register for an Electronic Submissions' Account With FDA**

Registering to use the FDA ESG involves a sequence of steps to be conducted for all submitters and types of submissions. It is best to register well in advance of when you plan to make a submission. The account creation process includes a testing phase designed to ensure that the FDA ESG can successfully receive your electronic submission and that the electronic submission is prepared according to published guidelines.

The testing phase is done through the FDA ESG test system. Once the submitter's test submission has passed the testing phase, an account will be set up to allow submissions through the FDA ESG production system. All relevant information, including detailed descriptions of the steps and contact information for requests and assistance, can be found on the FDA ESG website at the following link: https://www.fda.gov/ForIndustry/ElectronicSubmissionsGateway/ucm2005551.htm.

**FDA's Electronic Submission Platforms**

FDA ESG provides two methods—WebTrader (WT) and AS2—for making electronic submissions to FDA.

1. **WebTrader**: WebTrader is a web-based interface used to send documents and receive receipts and acknowledgments from the FDA. The WebTrader application makes communication with the FDA simple and cost effective. WebTrader requires each user from a Submitter (trial site and/or sponsor) to register for their own unique WebTrader account. To view the steps needed to setup a WebTrader account, please click on the following link: https://www.fda.gov/ForIndustry/ElectronicSubmissionsGateway/CreateanESGAccount/ucm114831.htm.

2. **AS2 (System-to-System)**: Submitting parties have the option to access the Electronic Submissions Gateway via system-to-system communication. System-to-system communication (often referred to as an AS2 Account) provides an automated connection to the FDA for submissions, receipts, and acknowledgments. The system-to-system communication requires server and software procurement and configuration from trial sites and/or sponsors. System-to-system communication requires one user from an organization to register for the organizational account. Submissions can be sent automatically or manually and receipts and acknowledgments may be received asynchronously or synchronously. To see the steps needed to setup an AS2 account, please click here: https://www.fda.gov/ForIndustry/ElectronicSubmissionsGateway/CreateanESGAccount/ucm425405.htm.

Plan and prepare early for electronic submission and obtain clarification from the appropriate FDA Review Division in advance.

**For submission-related questions, email: esub@fda.hhs.gov**

**For study data-related questions, email: edata@fda.hhs.gov**

The Proper Format for Electronic Submissions

After Registering with FDA's Electronic Submission Gateway, the next step is ensuring your submissions are in the proper format.

The Electronic Common Technical Document (eCTD) is the standard format for submitting applications, amendments, supplements, and reports to FDA's Center for Drug Evaluation and Research (CDER) and Center for Biologics Evaluation and Research (CBER). An eCTD submission has five modules: region-specific information, summary documents, quality-related information, non-clinical study reports, and clinical study reports. The forms requiring eCTD submission include the following:

- New Drug Application (NDA)
- Abbreviated New Drug Application (ANDA)
- Investigational New Drug Application (IND)
- Master files: Drug Master File (DMF) and Biologics Master File (BMF)
- Emergency Use Authorization (EUA)

When submissions arrive in eCTD format, reviewers can easily find and access the information they need to review, whether it was part of the original submission or added later by the product sponsor. Using eCTD also simplifies the process for submitters, because it is the same format used by drug regulatory agencies in other countries.

Since January 2017, the eCTD format has been required for certain submissions to CBER and CDER. Beginning on **May 5, 2018,** Commercial Investigational New Drug Applications (INDs) and Master Files must be submitted using eCTD format.

Here is the link for an introduction to eCTD: https://www.fda.gov/Drugs/DevelopmentApprovalProcess/FormsSubmissionRequirements/ElectronicSubmissions/ucm330116.htm#learn.

A useful, downloadable PDF on eCTD can be found here: https://www.fda.gov/downloads/Drugs/GuidanceComplianceRegulatoryInformation/Guidances/UCM333969.pdf.

### Mandatory Steps Prior to Requesting an NDA, ANDA, and IND Application Number

There are two mandatory steps for a sponsor to complete prior to requesting an Application Number:

1. You must apply for a secure e-mail account with the FDA by contacting secureemail@fda.hhs.gov. If using a U.S. Agent to request the number, please be sure that the agent has established a secure e-mail account.
2. Before you can submit an application to FDA, you must have a pre-assigned application number.

Following is the link providing the details for applying for a Pre-Assigned Application Number from the Center for Drug Evaluation and Research: https://www.fda.gov/Drugs/DevelopmentApprovalProcess/FormsSubmissionRequirements/ElectronicSubmissions/ucm114027.htm.

**Following is the link providing details for applying for a Pre-Assigned Application Number from the Center for Biological Evaluation and Research:** https://www.fda.gov/BiologicsBloodVaccines/GuidanceComplianceRegulatoryInformation/ProceduresSOPPs/ucm109641.htm.

---

Plan accordingly and avoid rushing when submitting to help avoid mistakes. What may seem like a small error can have big implications—such as a wrong digit in your application number.

---

### Hard Copy Submissions

An ever-increasing amount of regulatory filing and data transfer is carried out over the Internet, as exemplified by the detailed procedures developed by the FDA with respect to clinical trials. There are some institutions and study teams that prefer hard copy delivery and filing of the relevant documentation.

To that end, below are a range of FDA addresses to which forms and documentation can be sent by surface mail carriers.

### Form FDA 3500A MANDATORY Reporting Form

For Pre-Marketing IND Safety Reports: Adverse events involving investigational drugs under Investigational New Drug (IND) applications should be reported as required in the study protocol and sent to the address and contact person listed in the study protocol.

Sponsors and Sponsor-Investigators must submit Mandatory serious adverse event (SAE) reports under the IND to the following addresses:

**Center for Drug Evaluation and Research (CDER) INDs:**
U.S. Food and Drug Administration
Center for Drug Evaluation and Research
5901-B Ammendale Road
Beltsville, MD 20705-1266

**CDER-only Biologic INDs:**
U.S. Food and Drug Administration
Center for Drug Evaluation and Research
Therapeutic Biologic Products Document Room
5901-B Ammendale Road
Beltsville, MD 20705-1266

**Center for Biologics Evaluation and Research (CBER) INDs:**
U.S. Food and Drug Administration
Center for Biologics Evaluation and Research
Document Control Center
10903 New Hampshire Avenue
WO71, G112
Silver Spring, MD 20993-0002
**For Physicians/Emergency Requests**

If there is an emergency that requires the patient to be treated before a written submission can be made, FDA may allow the treatment use to proceed without a written submission, provided the applicable criteria are met. In an emergency situation, the request to use the drug may be made via telephone, fax, or other means of electronic communication, and authorization to ship and use the drug may be given by the FDA official over the telephone during normal business hours (8 am to 4:30 pm EST weekdays). Note: See the Emergency Use of a Test Article, Chapter 6, Section 6.3.

**Drugs:** For questions about expanded access for emergency use for investigational drugs, contact CDER's Division of Drug Information (DDI) at phone: 855-543-3784 or 301-796-3400.

**Biologics:** For questions about expanded access for emergency use for investigational biologics, contact CBER's Office of Communication, Outreach, and Development at phone: 240-402-7800 or 800-835-4709; or e-mail:industry.biologics@fda.hhs.gov.

**Devices:** For questions about expanded access for emergency use for medical devices, contact CDRH at phone: 301-796-5640; or fax 301-847-8120.

**After hours (after 4:30 pm EST weekdays and all day on weekends)—All questions about and requests for expanded access for emergency use for drugs, biologics, and medical devices should be directed to the FDA Emergency Call Center, telephone: 866-300-4374.**

**For Expanded Access Requests**

In a non-emergency situation, a written request (IND) for individual patient use of an investigational drug must be received by the FDA before shipment of and treatment with the drug may begin.

For general questions about non-emergency individual patient expanded access for drugs, contact the Office of Health and Constituent Affairs' Expanded Access Team at 301-796-8460 or PatientNetwork@fda.hhs.gov.

**Drugs:** For questions about expanded access for a specific investigational drug, contact CDER's Division of Drug Information at 855-543-3784.

**Biologics:** For questions about non-emergency individual expanded access for biologics, contact CBER at 240-402-8010 or 800-835-4709.

**Devices:** For questions about non-emergency individual expanded access for medical devices, contact CDRH at 301-796-5640 or 301-847-8120.

**Here is a link to Contact Information at All FDA Centers**: https://www.fda.gov/NewsEvents/PublicHealthFocus/ExpandedAccessCompassionateUse/ucm429610.htm#CBER-chart_info.

**Additional Resources**

Below are links to useful, important, and up-to-date FDA Fact Sheets:

Fact Sheet—eCTD Submission Requirements: What You Need to Know (PDF—224KB) https://www.fda.gov/downloads/Drugs/DevelopmentApprovalProcess/FormsSubmissionRequirements/ElectronicSubmissions/UCM511230.pdf.

Fact Sheet—FDA Electronic Submissions Gateway (PDF—208KB) https://www.fda.gov/downloads/Drugs/DevelopmentApprovalProcess/FormsSubmissionRequi  rements/ElectronicSubmissions/UCM511233.pdf.

Fact Sheet—Getting Started: Creating an ESG Account (PDF—210KB) https://www.fda.gov/downloads/Drugs/DevelopmentApprovalProcess/FormsSubmissionRequirements/ElectronicSubmissions/UCM511234.pdf.

Fact Sheet—New Requirements for Electronic Submissions of DMFs (PDF—208KB) https://www.fda.gov/downloads/Drugs/DevelopmentApprovalProcess/FormsSubmissionRequirements/ElectronicSubmissions/UCM511231.pdf.

Following are key tips on self-explanatory forms that a Sponsor will provide or that the Study Team will need to create.

While the FDA forms are required for submissions, requests, and reporting, the forms to follow are needed or required for the day-to-day conduct of trials.

**Delegation of Responsibility/Delegation of Authority** See Section 4.5.1 and Appendix 15 for two sample forms.

**Financial Disclosure Form** (internal to your Institution) See Conflict of Interest, Chapter 2, Section 2.2.

**Screening and Enrollment Log** See Appendix 13 for a template form. This Log serves to document every person screened or screened and enrolled for your study. It is **CRITICAL** that this Log exists in every type of study, whether it is Industry Sponsored, Investigator initiated, or a non-profit consortium study, and so on. The study team must **always know** who has undergone any research procedure or activity and who has been enrolled. This is a matter of human subjects protection.

**Subject Identification Code List** (this includes subject names and their study ID).

**Visitor Log**—Anyone, such as a monitor, or auditor, who reviews study documents (Binder, eCRFs, etc.) must sign the visitor log.

**Maintenance/Calibration Log**—For any equipment needing periodic calibration, a log is kept to manifest that maintenance was performed and to document the settings/proper calibration of the instruments.

**Protocol Deviation Log** (what was the deviation, when did it occur, comments)

**SAE Tracking Log**—for monitor/Sponsor/CRO

**Safety Report Tracking Log** (note that Safety Reports were received, the date received, and that they were signed off/acknowledged)

**Drug Accountability Log or Device Accountability Log**
Date received
Identifying information, i.e., Lot #, bottle # or Device #
Packing slip
For Drug: Date of return from Subject, amount remaining (volume, number of pills, etc.)

**Dispensation information (AKA Subject Drug Log or Subject Device Log)**
Drug: name of drug or blinded code, what amount, to whom (subject ID)
Device: Which device was given or blinded code, to whom (subject ID)

**Note to File** Notes to File are for administrative notations that are significant. For example, "the IRB meeting intended to provide Continuing Review on 7/29/18 was cancelled. The new IRB meeting date will be 8/17/18."

These forms can be found in your Regulatory Binder or in the eCRF/database. If you are conducting an Investigator Initiated trial without formal structure from an external Sponsor, keep these logs in mind and create simple Excel spreadsheets or Access databases that will suffice to track what is needed.

**Regulatory Binder Checklist** See Appendix 14 for an NIH Regulatory Binder Checklist

The Regulatory Binder maintains all essential documents and significant correspondence in hard copy form. The documents are literally placed in a 3-ring binder. Monitors review it in Industry-

Sponsored trials. It can be created by study teams for Investigator-Initiated trials, and other trials for which it is not provided by a Sponsor or CRO.

## 4.5.1 DELEGATION OF AUTHORITY (DOA)/DELEGATION OF RESPONSIBILITY

*Purpose of section*:

- Provides a definition of the term "Delegation of Authority"
- Identifies what study team member should be on the DOA log
- Outlines the training requirements for the study team members on the log
- Introduces two Delegation of Authority/Responsibility Logs in the Appendix

The "Delegation of Authority" is also known as the "Delegation of Responsibility". It is a log created to record the <u>significant</u> study-related duties and which member of the study team will be performing these duties.

Who is considered a study team member that needs to be on this log?

Study team members typically are the following:

- Principal Investigator
- Co-Investigator
- Sub-Investigators
- Research Coordinator
- Research Nurse
- Data Manager/Analyst
  - If there is funding to hire a Data Manager/Analyst, he or she will be considered a study team member. Otherwise, the Research Coordinator takes on this role by entering and managing the study data.

Per the NIH National Cancer Institute, Research (Study) Team Members are:

- Principal Investigator
- Research Nurse
- Data Manager
- Staff physician or nurse who treat patients according to the clinical trial protocol (not Standard of Care)[6]

Note that the log is for SIGNIFICANT study-related duties (not for every task in the protocol). It is up to the PI, or the PI in consultation with the Sponsor, to determine which protocol duties are considered "significant."

If a significant task is assigned to an individual outside of the study team members listed above and the task is written on the Delegation of Authority, the assigned person becomes a member of the study team, and is required to be trained in the protocol, regulations, and ICH GCP just like the core study team members are.

**Regulatory Guidance on assigning protocol tasks:**

The investigator is responsible for conducting studies in accordance with the protocol (see 21 CFR 312.60, Form FDA-1572, 21 CFR 812.43 and 812.100). In some cases, a protocol may specify the qualifications of the individuals who are to perform certain protocol-required tasks (e.g., physician, registered nurse), in which case the protocol must be followed even if state law permits individuals with different qualifications to perform the task (see 21 CFR 312.23(a)(6) and 312.40(a)(1)). For example, if the state in which the study site is located permits a nurse practitioner or physician's assistant to perform physical examinations under the supervision of a physician, but the protocol specifies that physical examinations must be done by a physician, a physician must perform such exams.[7]

The Investigator must ensure that every study team member listed on the Delegation of Authority is adequately trained.

<u>What Is Adequate Training?</u>

The investigator should ensure that there is adequate training for all staff participating in the **conduct** of the study, including any new staff hired after the study has begun in order to meet an unanticipated workload or to replace staff who have left. The investigator should ensure that staff:

- Are familiar with the purpose of the study and the protocol
- Have an adequate understanding of the specific details of the protocol and attributes of the investigational product needed to perform their assigned tasks
- Are aware of regulatory requirements and acceptable standards for the conduct of clinical trials and the protection of human subjects
- Are competent to perform or have been trained to perform the tasks they are delegated; and
- Are informed of any pertinent changes during the conduct of the trial and receive additional training as appropriate.

When the sponsor provides training for the conduct of the study, the investigator should ensure that staff receive the sponsor's training and/or any information (e.g., training materials) from that training that is pertinent to the staff's role in the study.[8]

ICH **ICH GCP sections that pertain to the Delegation of Authority:**

4.1.5: The investigator should maintain a list of appropriately qualified persons to whom the investigator has delegated significant trial-related duties.

4.2.5: The investigator is responsible for supervising any individual or party to whom the investigator delegates study tasks conducted at the trial site.

2.8: Each individual involved in conducting a trial should be qualified by education, training, and experience to perform his or her respective task(s).

For drug studies, the following regulation applies to the training requirement:

NOTE: (Read all bullets. You will see the relevance when you reach the last bullet.)

21 CFR 312.53

(vi) A commitment by the investigator that he or she:

- **(a)** Will conduct the study(ies) in accordance with the relevant, current protocol(s) and will only make changes in a protocol after notifying the sponsor, except when necessary to protect the safety, the rights, or welfare of subjects;
- **(b)** Will comply with all requirements regarding the obligations of clinical investigators and all other pertinent requirements in this part;
- **(c)** Will personally conduct or supervise the described investigation(s);
- **(d)** Will inform any potential subjects that the drugs are being used for investigational purposes and will ensure that the requirements relating to obtaining informed consent (21 CFR part 50) and institutional review board review and approval (21 CFR part 56) are met;
- **(e)** Will report to the sponsor adverse experiences that occur in the course of the investigation(s) in accordance with 312.64;
- **(f)** Has read and understands the information in the investigator's brochure, including the potential risks and side effects of the drug; and

**(g)** Will ensure that all associates, colleagues, and employees assisting in the conduct of the study(ies) are informed about their obligations in meeting the above commitments.

**See Appendix 15 for 2 sample Delegation of Authority logs.**

## 4.6 PROJECT MANAGEMENT FOR CLINICAL TRIALS

*Purpose of section*:

- Emphasizes that beyond the clinical focus of trials, solid administrative management is important to successful clinical trial conduct
- Provides suggestions and describes real case scenarios of institutional breakdowns in trial administration—and how they can be resolved

Below is a graph detailing Real Case Scenarios that the authors have experienced in their careers. Every scenario could have been avoided. If your site/you experience a single—or several—of these breakdowns, you should immediately create a project management improvement plan. *Such breakdowns can place your institution and your research in jeopardy* (Fig. 4.12 and Table 4.2).

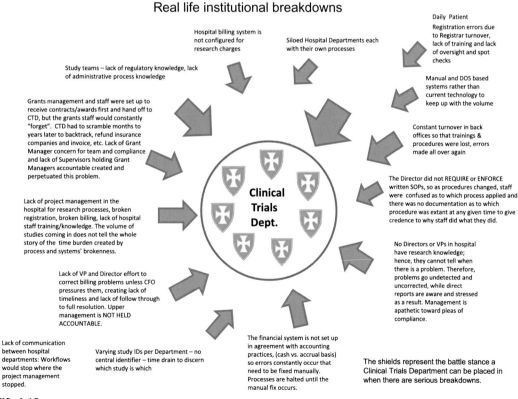

**FIG. 4.12**

Real-life institutional breakdowns.

**Table 4.2 What To DO**

| | | Project Management<br>Using the Observed Institutional Breakdowns as a guide… | |
|---|---|---|---|
| | | **What NOT To Do** | **What to DO** |
| | 1 | Allow each Department to have their own IDs for each study. This creates inefficient time use as no one knows which study a Department is referencing without researching it to figure it out each time | Create ONE ID that is used throughout your medical center to identify a study. If needed, ADD it as a field into each Department so that Departments can keep their unique IDs and add the universal ID for reference for all. |
| | 2 | Allow Directors and VPs to be unaware of problems, unwilling to fix problems and apathetic to the needs and pressures on employees. Allow Directors and VPs to have a disregard for regulatory compliance | Supervisors of Directors and VPs need to physically visit Departments, unannounced, and speak candidly with a range of staff about Department operations. Look at their computer screens. See what they see. Go through an SOP with them. See if it is current and if anyone knows it. Supervisors cannot rely on reports from the Directors and VPs, who may not be forthcoming or aware of problems. The Supervisors of Directors and VPs need to hold their direct reports accountable for the culture, condition, and regulatory compliance of their Departments. |
| | 3 | Allow poor or lack of project management | Require sound project management by Six Sigma experts or people who have proven to create, organize, and manage workflows well. |
| | 4 | Do not set up one Department to provide work to another Department whose personnel continuously fail to follow through and show no concern for the receiving Department | Test workflows. If they are not working, if handoffs are not being done, CHANGE the process. Give the responsibility to managers and staff who are engaged and prove they can follow through. |
| | 5 | Allow PIs and RCs to disregard or be ignorant to the Code of Federal Regulations, ICH GCP, HIPAA law, and/or medical center policies and procedures | Train your PIs and RCs in federal regulations, ICH GCP, HIPAA law, and medical center policies and procedures. Hold them accountable to follow through. Set up QA programs to test whether PIs and RCs are complying and have knowledge. |
| | 6 | Refuse to purchase or upgrade a hospital billing system that cannot perform for research charges (separating Standard of Care from research sponsor payments) | Purchase or upgrade your hospital billing system to handle research charges as well as clinical charges. |
| | 7 | Allow Medical Center Departments to have their own processes regarding research, fostering siloes | Centralize research processes so that every Department in the medical center is in unison and able to talk the same language and have efficient workflows. |
| | 8 | Allow Registrars to be inadequately trained in research registration. Allow Supervisors of Registrars to not hold Registrars accountable and to not spot check their registrations | Train Registrars in research registrations. Hold Supervisors accountable to train new Registrars and to provide ongoing training if Registrars are not registering correctly. Supervisors must spot check/audit Registrars' work on a periodic basis to make sure registrations are being done correctly. Billing and claims flow from registration. If errors are not spotted and corrected at registration, they will cause greater problems in billing. |

| Table 4.2 | What To DO—cont'd | |
|---|---|---|
| | **Project Management** | |
| | **Using the Observed Institutional Breakdowns as a guide...** | |
| | **What NOT To Do** | **What to DO** |
| 9 | Keep old systems that can't keep up with volume and research complexity | Get rid of old technology that cannot keep pace with the volume of work and complexities of research. Upgrade or acquire new systems. |
| 10 | Allow high turnover to continue. Allow a Director or Manager of a Department with high turnover to provide all reports, reasons, and solutions | Assess high turnover. Do not allow excuses from the Director/Manager over a high turnover Department. The Director/Manager may well be hiding a problem they do not want exposed. The Supervisor of the Department Manager/Director with high turnover needs to become closely involved with the Department, speaking candidly to the staff, in order to understand the problem. In the real-life institutional breakdown, one scenario involved a Director with poor project management skills, who created confusing and multilayer procedures that left the staff confused and unable to understand processes. In addition, changes were made frequently that left staff confused, and which also left records in disarray. The Department was too disorganized to function well and managers were not held accountable to make certain staff were doing their jobs correctly. |
| 11 | Allow SOPs to be spoken, rather than documented. Allow SOPs to not be dated to provide clarity as to what process was extant at any given time | **Document, document, document, and date.** All SOPs should be written and accessible to all staff. Every stakeholder should be a part of creating an SOP so that all voices are heard, there is buy in, and the SOP works for all aspects of a process. |
| 12 | Allow your upper management and executives to have clinical expertise only in a research institution | Hire upper management and executives who are certified in the Code of Federal Regulations, ICH GCP, and have practical experience in clinical research. Clinical management cannot properly manage research (without knowledge of research). |
| 13 | Purchase or retain financial systems that do not work with your form of accounting—whether accrual or cash basis. Allow manual workarounds consistently and at a growing pace | Purchase or upgrade financial systems that work with your accounting methodology. Avoid manual workarounds. |

## Project Management

1. Set up workflows with all Departments that provide services for research protocols. You will need to have a plan and clear communication for:
   a. Notifying Departments that their services are needed
   b. Registering subjects
   c. Billing subjects
   d. Paying Departments for their services for research protocols
      All individuals involved in research, from administrative support to the clinics where research visits are being conducted, need to be a part of the documented workflow so that as subject visits are being performed, Accounting, Billing, and the individual departments that need to fulfill procedures within a protocol are aware of the study and have scheduling and billing processes in place.

Therefore, the Institutional research policy must be inclusive of all departments that interface with a research study. Here are the Departments to include. (This list is not all-inclusive):

a. Anesthesiology
b. Laboratory
c. Cardiology
d. Radiology
e. Investigative Drug Services (IDS)/ Research Pharmacy
f. Any Specialty Units providing research nurses or space in which to hold research subject visits
g. Pulmonary
h. Physical Therapy/Occupational Therapy

---

## AUTHOR'S CORNER

AN ACTUAL OCCURRENCE:

At one hospital, the Physical Therapy Department (PT) was left out of the research workflow. PT was not informed when a new study, requiring PT procedures, was approved at the hospital. Research Coordinators would show up at the PT Department with research subjects at the time of their visits with no scheduling or forewarning to PT. PT had not been given the protocol to review prior and the therapy required took three hours per subject! PT did not have the opportunity to staff for these visits, so a lot of pressure was placed on the department. Additionally, because PT was not recognized, the PT procedures were not factored into the study budget prior to approval. Consequently, they were not paid for their work. An Amendment had to be created, which was met with great reluctance by the Sponsor (because their total budget for this multicenter trial had already been set) and took months to resolve. Avoid such scenarios by ensuring every Department whose services are needed for the study are included in your research workflow.

---

Below is a brief list of seemingly pedestrian but actually, problematic administrative challenges the authors have encountered, and, the resulting project management corrections. These fixes will be useful if you find yourself in a similar situation:

1. Make sure you have a naming convention for all electronic files and folders.
   In the office the author joined, no naming conventions were created. Whatever was on a file was saved. We had files such as N263-7. What was that? (Was it a contract, a budget, a protocol, a note to file and to which study did it belong?) Imagine hundreds of these. We had to open each file to discover what it was and to rename it.
   1. Naming convention example:
      a. Last Name of PI_Sponsor Name_protocol #_type of document_date
   2. Sample:
      a. Williams_ABC Pharmaceutical Co_M3652-897_CTA_2-22-17
2. All Institutions/Departments involved in research studies must know which studies are active and which studies have closed.
3. Make sure each active study has a ratified contract/award/grant and budget.
4. Create your unique medical center ID (a universal ID that all Departments share) for each study / so that it is identifiable when the study moves through various Departments and systems.
5. Depending upon how an Institution is set up, there needs to be a Department, which creates registration forms or a process to identify patients that are research subjects whose procedural costs are being paid by a sponsor or funder and not the patient's medical insurance.

6. Make sure there are separate payment streams through your software systems and medical center processes.
7. Document, document, document. Keep records. Know where they are. Make study records accessible to all stakeholders.
8. Perform a Medicare Coverage Analysis.
9. Follow and have a process for ALL regulations through your IRB or Compliance Department; it is essential that study team members know the regulations.

🕮 ICH  ICH GCP has the following to say regarding trial management:

5.5.1 The sponsor should utilize appropriately qualified individuals to supervise the overall conduct of the trial, to handle the data, to verify the data, to conduct the statistical analyses, and to prepare the trial reports.

In the Introduction to Essential Elements…

8.1 …Filing essential documents at the investigator/institution and sponsor sites in a timely manner can greatly assist in the successful management of a trial by the investigator, sponsor, and monitor.

In the Introduction to the Investigator's Brochure (IB)…

7.1 …The IB also provides insight to support the clinical management of the study subjects during the course of the clinical trial.

In the Monitoring Report Addendum…

5.18.6(e) …Reports of on-site and/or centralized monitoring should be provided to the sponsor (including appropriate management and staff responsible for trial and site oversight)

In the Manufacturing, Packaging, Labeling, and Coding Investigational Product(s)…

5.13.2 The sponsor should determine, for the investigational product(s), acceptable storage temperatures, storage conditions (e.g., protection from light), storage times, reconstitution fluids and procedures, and devices for product infusion, if any. The sponsor should inform all involved parties (e.g., monitors, investigators, pharmacists, storage managers) of these determinations.

## 4.7 CODING FOR CLINICAL TRIAL CLAIMS

*Purpose of section*:

- Explains what ICD-10 codes, CPT codes, and HCPCS modifiers must be used to identify clinical trials on claims
- Introduces the Medicare Claims Processing Manual

### Clinical Trial Coding

All of the information in this section comes from the *Medicare Claims Processing Manual: Chapter 32—Billing Requirements for Special Services, Revision 3556, 7-01-2016*, Section 69, and can be found at: https://www.cms.gov/Regulations-and-Guidance/Guidance/Manuals/downloads/clm104c32.pdf.

**A.** Clinical Trial Number on Claims
Effective for claims with dates of service on or after January 1, 2014, it is **mandatory** to report a clinical trial number on claims for items/services provided in clinical trials/studies/registries. The clinical trial number used is the 8-digit NCT number from ClinicalTrials.gov, i.e. NCT00000654.

i. Providers report the 8-digit number on the following claims locators:
- 837 professional claim format-Loop 2300 REF02 (REF01=P4) (do not use 'CT' on the electronic claim); or
- CMS-1500 paper form-place in Field 19 (preceded by 'CT').

**B.** Diagnosis Code

In addition to the clinical trial number, Routine Costs Submitted by Practitioners/Suppliers on Claims with dates of service on or after January 1, 2008 should include:

- If ICD-9-CM is applicable, ICD-9 diagnosis code V70.7
- If ICD-10-CM is applicable, ICD-10 diagnosis code Z00.6 (in either the primary/secondary positions)

**C.** HCPCS Modifier

i. • HCPCS modifier Q0 or Q1 as appropriate
   **a.** Q0: Investigational clinical service provided in a clinical research study that is in an approved research study
   **b.** Q1: Routine clinical service provided in a clinical research study that is in an approved clinical research study
   **NOTE:** The Q1 modifier is line item specific and must be used to identify items and services that constitute <u>medically necessary routine patient care or treatment of complications</u> arising from a Medicare beneficiary's participation in a Medicare-covered clinical trial. Items and services that are provided solely to satisfy data collection and analysis needs and that are not used in the clinical management of the patient are not covered and may not be billed using the Q1 modifier. Items and services that are not covered by Medicare by virtue of a statutory exclusion or lack of a benefit category also may not be billed using the Q1 modifier. When billed in conjunction with the V70.7/Z00.6 diagnosis code, the Q1 modifier will serve as the provider's attestation that the service meets the Medicare coverage criteria (i.e., was furnished to a beneficiary who is participating in a Medicare qualifying clinical trial and represents routine patient care, including complications associated with qualifying trial participation).
   **1.** Effective for claims processed after September 28, 2009, with dates of service on or after January 1, 2008, claims submitted with modifier Q1 shall be returned as unprocessable if ICD-9-CM code V70.7 (if ICD-9 is applicable) or ICD-10-CM code Z00.6 (if ICD-10-CM is applicable) is not submitted on the claim.

**D.** Inpatient Clinical Trial Claims
   **a.** Institutional providers billing clinical trial service(s) must report ICD-9 diagnosis code <u>V70.7</u> if ICD-9 is applicable or, if ICD-10-CM is applicable, ICD-10 diagnosis code <u>Z00.6</u> in either the primary or secondary position and a <u>condition code 30</u> regardless of whether all services are related to the clinical trial or not.
   **b.** HCPCS codes are not reported on inpatient claims. Therefore, the HCPCS modifier requirements (i.e., Q0/Q1) as outlined in the outpatient clinical trial section immediately below, are not applicable to inpatient clinical trial claims.

**E.** Outpatient Clinical Trial Claims

On all outpatient clinical trial claims, providers need to do the following:

**a.** Report condition code 30,

**b.** Report ICD-9 diagnosis code V70.7, if ICD-9-CM is applicable, in the primary or secondary position;

**c.** Report ICD-10 diagnosis code Z00.6, if ICD-10-CM is applicable, in the primary or secondary position; and

**d.** Identify all lines that contain an investigational item/service with a HCPCS modifier of:
  **i.** Q0 for dates of service on or after 1/1/08

**e.** Identify all lines that contain a routine service with a HCPCS modifier of
  **i.** Q1 for dates of service on or after 1/1/08

**Billing and Processing Fee for Service Claims for Covered Clinical Trial Services Furnished to Managed Care Enrollees**

For dates of service on or after September 19, 2000, and until notified otherwise by CMS, Medicare contractors will pay for covered clinical trial services furnished to beneficiaries enrolled in managed care plans. Providers who furnish covered clinical trial services to managed care beneficiaries must be enrolled with Medicare in order to bill on a fee-for-service basis. Providers that wish to bill fee for service but have not enrolled with Medicare must contact their local carrier, intermediary, regional home health intermediary or National Supplier Clearinghouse, as appropriate, to obtain an enrollment application.

Determine payment for covered clinical trial services furnished to beneficiaries enrolled in managed care plans in accordance with applicable fee for service rules, except that beneficiaries are not responsible for the Part A or Part B deductibles (i.e., assume the Part A or Part B deductible has been met). Managed care enrollees are liable for the coinsurance amounts applicable to services paid under Medicare fee for service rules.

The clinical trial coding requirements for managed care enrollee claims are the same as those for regular Medicare fee for service claims. However, for beneficiaries enrolled in a managed care plan, institutional providers must not bill outpatient clinical trial services and non-clinical trial services on the same claim. If covered outpatient services unrelated to the clinical trial are rendered during the same day/stay, the provider must split bill so that ONLY the clinical trial services are contained on a single claim and billed as fee-for-service (this allows the Medicare claims processing system to not apply deductible when the patient is found to be in a managed care plan). Any outpatient services unrelated to the clinical trial should be billed to the managed care plan.

**IDE (Investigational Device Exemption)**

For IDEs, see section 68 of the *Medicare Claims Processing Manual: Chapter 32—Billing Requirements for Special Services, Revision 3556, 7-01-2016*

https://www.cms.gov/Regulations-and-Guidance/Guidance/Manuals/downloads/clm104c32.pdf

Section 68—Investigational Device Exemption (IDE) Studies

68.1—Billing Requirements for Providers Billing for Routine Care Items and Services in Category A IDE Studies

68.2—Billing Requirements for Providers Billing for Category B IDE Devices and Routine Care Items and Services in Category B IDE Studies

68.4—Billing Requirements for Providers Billing Routine Costs of Clinical Trials Involving a Category B IDE

## 4.8 CHOOSING A CTMS

*Purpose of section*:

- Provides pointers on CTMS selection
- Introduces the CTMS Decision Worksheet in the Appendix

A Clinical Trials Management System (CTMS) purposes to provide an administrative hub for operational tasks within a clinical trial. It is a software solution.

A CTMS will organize and provide operational task solutions such as: subject visit scheduling; study status (e.g., open, closed, in data analysis); tracking (e.g., for the completion of each study start up activity); flags for milestones such as subject accrual being met; billing; financial management; and, provision for dashboards, metrics, and reporting.

You will want to choose wisely the tasks your CTMS is configured to accomplish. The goal is to ease administrative burden. You do not want yet another data entry system. Depending on how much your Institution is willing to spend, you can get a CTMS with standard features or you can customize it.

Be careful to avoid redundancy with your EMR, eCRFs/EDCs, and IRB submissions. You will want a system that can integrate with the software systems your Institution has in place and that can download from one system into another. You do not want to manually enter the same data points into multiple systems!

For example, in the authors' experience, one Medical Center captured the list of Inclusion and Exclusion Criteria in their CTMS. The Study Coordinator had to check off that each criterion was met in the CTMS system. This was iterative. The Study Coordinator will already be doing the exact same task in the Case Report Form/EDC, and it does not serve an administrative purpose for the CTMS. (You can easily note that a subject was enrolled through a CTMS with a simple check mark in a box. This is needed administratively. The detail leading up to it is not. Do not make your CTMS a Case Report Form when you have separate Case Report Forms to fill out. Do not make your CTMS a burden.)

**THINK**. What administrative tasks, if centralized and taken from a manual process to an electronic system, will REDUCE the administrative burden, create greater efficiency, and provide quickly accessed reports? This is what you want your CTMS to accomplish.

There is a CTMS Decision Worksheet in Appendix 16 that will allow you to compare vendors side by side for the various features you want a CTMS to accomplish.

You will be able to quickly exclude particular vendors by asking what software systems (EMRs, EDCs, billing systems, scheduling systems, IRB solutions) they are compatible with. If their CTMS cannot integrate with the systems your Institution has, you will be wise to find other vendors that can integrate.

Ask your physicians and administrative staff what operational pain points they have when conducting clinical research. The answers received from your colleagues across multiple hospital departments will shed light on what you will need your CTMS to accomplish.

Be aware of how much the end user/Medical Center personnel can add, delete, or revise fields and how much the vendor has to intervene in this process. The more independence you can have without going to the vendor for changes, the more efficient and less costly a system will be for your center.

Many CTMSs have a subject payment solution within them. Be aware of what is included in the CTMS package before you contract with a separate vendor.

Create your team infrastructure of managers, data entry specialists, subject matter experts and IT specialists who can see your CTMS purchase through a typical 12 month or more implementation and integration process.

# ENDNOTES

[1]Additional information can be found here: https://privacyruleandresearch.nih.gov/pr_08.asp [accessed 28.03.18].

[2]Additional Information can be found here: https://www.hhs.gov/hipaa/for-professionals/privacy/guidance/disclosures-public-health-activities/index.html [accessed 28.03.18].

[3]Additional information can be found here: https://www.hhs.gov/ohrp/regulations-and-policy/regulations/45-cfr-46/index.html [accessed 28.03.18].

[4]Office for Human Research Protections (OHRP), Guidance on Reporting Incidents to OHRP, https://www.hhs.gov/ohrp/compliance-and-reporting/guidance-on-reporting-incident/index.html [accessed 28.03.18].

[5]Additional Information can be found here: https://evs.nci.nih.gov/ [accessed 28.03.18].

[6]Additional information can be found here: https://www.cancer.gov/about-cancer/treatment/clinical-trials/what-are-trials/team [accessed 28.03.18].

[7]Guidance for Industry, Investigator Responsibilities—Protecting the Rights, Safety, and Welfare of Study Subjects, https://www.fda.gov/downloads/Drugs/.../Guidances/UCM187772.pdf [accessed 28.03.18].

[8]Ibid.

# ORGANIZATIONS WITH OVERSIGHT RESPONSIBILITY IN CLINICAL RESEARCH

## 5

*Purpose of chapter*:
   Provides definitions and roles for the following organizations:

- Institutional Review Board (IRB)
- Central Institutional Review Board (Central IRB)
- Data-Safety-Monitoring Board (DSMB), also known as the Data-Monitoring Committee (DMC)
- Clinical Endpoint Committee (CEC)
- Association for the Accreditation of Human Research Protection Programs (AAHRPP)
- U.S. Food and Drug Administration (FDA)—Oversight Function

   The complexity and sensitivity of clinical research necessarily requires guidance, monitoring, and oversight, all of which are overseen by several institutional, non-profit, and government organizations. We begin with the most familiar—the IRB.

## 5.1 THE INSTITUTIONAL REVIEW BOARD

*Purpose of section*:

- Describes the Institutional Review Board (IRB)

   Following is the FDA's definition of the IRB:
   "Under FDA regulations, an IRB is an appropriately constituted group that has been formally designated to review and monitor biomedical research involving human subjects. In accordance with FDA regulations, an IRB has the authority to approve, require modifications in (to secure approval), or disapprove research. This group review serves an important role in the protection of the rights and welfare of human research subjects."

   "The purpose of IRB review is to assure, both in advance and by periodic review, that appropriate steps are taken to protect the rights and welfare of humans participating as subjects in the research. To accomplish this purpose, IRBs use a group process to review research protocols and related materials (e.g., informed consent documents and investigator brochures) to ensure protection of the rights and welfare of human subjects of research."[1]

   🏃ICH According to the ICH GCP E6 R2 Glossary, an IRB and Institutional Ethics Committee (IEC) are two names for the same functional group. The term IRB is predominantly used in the United States while the term IEC is predominantly used internationally.

**Here are the ICH GCP E6 R2 definitions:**

**Institutional Review Board**

1.31 IRB An independent body constituted of medical, scientific, and non-scientific members, whose responsibility is to ensure the protection of the rights, safety, and well-being of human subjects involved in a trial by, among other things, reviewing, approving, and providing continuing review of trial protocol and amendments and of the methods and material to be used in obtaining and documenting informed consent of the trial subjects.

**Independent Ethics Committee (IEC)**

1.27 Independent Ethics Committee (IEC) An independent body (a review board or a committee, institutional, regional, national, or supranational), constituted of medical professionals and non-medical members, whose responsibility it is to ensure the protection of the rights, safety, and well-being of human subjects involved in a trial and to provide public assurance of that protection, by, among other things, reviewing and approving/providing favorable opinion on, the trial protocol, the suitability of the investigator(s), facilities, and the methods and material to be used in obtaining and documenting informed consent of the trial subjects.[2]

Composition of an IRB

According to 21 CFR 56.107, each IRB Committee is composed of at least five (5) members with the following characteristics:

1. Varying backgrounds;
2. Diversity;
3. Professional competence;
4. Knowledge in:
   a. Regulations;
   b. Applicable law;
   c. Standards of professional conduct and practice; and
   d. Institutional commitments.
5. Representation from both genders;
6. At least one member whose primary concerns are in the scientific area;
7. At least one member whose primary concerns are in nonscientific areas; and,
8. One member who is not affiliated with the institution and is also not a part of the immediate family of a person affiliated with the institution.

Additionally, consultants with particular expertise may be asked to join IRB meetings in order to review protocols as needed.[3]

## 5.2 THE CENTRAL INSTITUTIONAL REVIEW BOARD

*Purpose of section*:

• Describes the Central IRB

The FDA defines the Central IRB as follows:

"A centralized IRB review process involves an agreement under which multiple study sites in a multicenter trial rely in whole or in part on the review of an IRB other than the IRB affiliated with the research site. Because the goal of the centralized process is to increase efficiency and decrease duplicative efforts that do not contribute to meaningful human subject protection, it will usually be preferable that a central IRB take responsibility for all aspects of IRB review at each site participating in the centralized review process. Other approaches may be appropriate as well. For example, an institution may permit a central IRB to be entirely responsible for initial and continuing review of a study, or apportion IRB review responsibilities between the central IRB and its own IRB."

This definition came from, and more information can be gained from, the *Guidance for Industry: Using a Centralized IRB Review Process in Multicenter Clinical Trials* at: https://www.fda.gov/downloads/RegulatoryInformation/Guidances/ucm127013.pdf.[4]

**What is the difference between a central IRB and a single IRB?**

Both are designed to help streamline IRB review, and the terms are sometimes used interchangeably. As the NIH notes, in general:

*A Central IRB* is the IRB of record that provides the ethical review for all sites participating in more than one multi-site study. The sites are usually in a network, consortium, or particular program.

*A Single IRB* is the IRB of record, selected on a study-by-study basis, which provides the ethical review for all sites participating in a multi-site study.[5]

See Chapter 8, Section 8.1 for more information on the Single IRB.

---

## 5.3  DATA SAFETY MONITORING BOARD, ALSO KNOWN AS THE DATA MONITORING COMMITTEE

*Purpose of section*:

- Describes the Data Safety Monitoring Board (DSMB), also known as the Data Monitoring Committee (DMC)

The DSMB and DMC are terms that are used interchangeably. The National Institutes of Health (NIH) refers to these Committees as "Safety Monitoring Committees."

The FDA notes: "A clinical trial DMC is a group of individuals with pertinent expertise that reviews on a regular basis accumulating data from one or more ongoing clinical trials. The DMC advises the sponsor regarding the continuing safety of trial subjects and those yet to be recruited to the trial, as well as the continuing validity and scientific merit of the trial."

Sponsors of INDs, IDEs, and new biologics are required to monitor their studies per Federal Regulations. For example: 21 CFR 312.56 *(c) The sponsor shall review and evaluate the evidence relating to the safety and effectiveness of the drug as it is obtained from the investigator.*

Other references include 21 CFR 312.50 and 312.56 for drugs and biologics, and 21 CFR 812.40 and 21 CFR 812.46 for devices.[6]

DMCs are generally recommended for any controlled trial of any size that will compare rates of mortality or major morbidity, but a DMC is not required or recommended for most clinical studies. DMCs are generally not needed, for example, for trials at early stages of product development. They are also generally not needed for trials addressing lesser outcomes, such as relief of symptoms, unless the trial population is at elevated risk of more severe outcomes..."

There is a Guidance available online, named Guid*ance for Clinical Trial Sponsors: Establishment and Operation of Clinical Trial Data Monitoring Committees,* at: https://www.fda.gov/downloads/RegulatoryInformation/Guidances/ucm127073.pdf.[7]

ℐᶜ⁺ᴴ The ICH GCP E6 R2 Glossary defines a Data Monitoring Committee this way:
1.25 Independent Data Monitoring Committee (IDMC) (DSMB, Monitoring Committee, DMC)
An IDMC that may be established by the sponsor to assess at intervals the progress of a clinical trial, the safety data, and the critical efficacy endpoints, and to recommend to the sponsor whether to continue, modify, or stop a trial.[8]

## 5.4 CLINICAL ENDPOINT COMMITTEE

*Purpose of section*:

• Describes the CEC

The CEC is a centralized committee formed independent of a study in order to review and classify safety and/or efficacy endpoints without bias. CECs are often utilized to standardize assessment and statistical analysis. CECs are particularly useful when endpoints are subjective, or complexity is involved, or there are cultural differences that can impact data in a multi-site international trial, or when studies cannot be blinded.

A clinical trial sponsor will contract with a company that provides CEC review and reporting, who will provide independent assessment.

## 5.5 ASSOCIATION FOR THE ACCREDITATION OF HUMAN RESEARCH PROTECTION PROGRAMS, INC.

*Purpose of section*:

• Describes the AAHRPP

AAHRPP is an independent, non-profit accrediting agency for human research protection programs (HRPPs).

Human Research Protection Programs (HRPP) are the offices that support IRBs. Studies are submitted to the IRB through the HRPP within an Institution. Studies are analyzed and requests are sent to study teams to correct or revise aspects of their research study submissions in order to be compliant with regulations, laws, and ICH GCP before the submission goes to the IRB for review.

AAHRPP evaluates the individual HRPPs. If an HRPP is accredited by AAHRPP, it means the program has achieved an approved, high level of quality in human subjects protections within scientifically and ethically sound research. To learn whether a medical center's HRPP has been accredited, and for further information, you can navigate to the AAHRPP website at: www.aahrpp.org.[9]

Of note, the offices that support IRBs can be called by other names as well, such as HRPO, or Human Research Protections Office and other similar variations.

## 5.6 WHAT YOU NEED TO KNOW ABOUT FDA INSPECTIONS, COMPLIANCE, & ENFORCEMENT

*Purpose of section*:

• Provides an overview of FDA inspections of clinical trial sites

- Provides FDA tips for clinical investigators on proper regulatory conduct of a trial
- Provides an overview of FDA enforcement mechanisms when trials are found operationally deficient
- Introduces the FDA Audit Documentation Checklist in Appendix 38.

<u>FDA Clinical Trial Site Inspections</u>

Study teams should be ready for the day when an individual from the FDA calls your site to schedule an inspection. This introduction means that there is the potential for virtually every aspect of your trial to be scrutinized for adherence to relevant federal regulations. Don't panic! If you have followed the regulations, been attentive to the tips in this book, and have used the forms and templates in the Appendix, you will be ready.

As a backdrop, following are some relevant statistics on FDA clinical inspections:

In Fiscal Year 2017, the FDA conducted 700 clinical research inspections—512 of Clinical Investigators, 73 of Sponsors for Good Clinical Practice, and 101 of IRBs/Radioactive Drug Research Committees (RDRC). Thirty-two percent of the Clinical Investigator inspections resulted in findings for which follow-up action by the inspected site was either suggested or required. Eighteen percent of IRB/RDRC inspections resulted in suggested follow-up action. Put more frankly: More than one-fourth of all investigations by the FDA into clinical trial environments resulted in voluntary or official action required.

Viewed more closely, for those clinical investigator inspections performed for FDA's Center for Drug Evaluation and Research (CDER), the post-inspection correspondence issued on clinical investigator deficiencies was in these categories:

Protocol deficiencies—26%

Records deficiencies—14%

Drug accountability—3%

Consent—2%

IRB communication—2%

Adverse Events—1%

https://www.fda.gov/downloads/aboutfda/centersoffices/officeofmedicalproductsandtobacco/cder/ucm438250.pdf.[10]

Highly trained professionals from FDA's Office of Regulatory Affairs (ORA) conduct the investigations and the results are reviewed by both ORA and the Office of Scientific Investigations (OSI) within the FDA's Center for Drug Evaluation and Research (CDER). As the authors know firsthand, both ORA and CDER are top-notch, nationally and internationally recognized entities.

FDA inspections of clinical trials sites are typically performed under the following circumstances:

- During ongoing clinical trials to provide real-time assessment of the investigator's conduct of the trial and protection of human subjects;
- To verify the accuracy and reliability of data that has been submitted to the FDA;
- As a result of a complaint to the FDA about the conduct of the study at a particular investigational site;
- In response to sponsor concerns;
- Upon termination of the clinical site;
- At the request of an FDA review division; and,
- In the event of trials related to certain classes of investigational products that FDA has identified as products of special interest in its current work plan (i.e., targeted inspections based on current public health concerns). https://www.fda.gov/downloads/RegulatoryInformation/Guidances/UCM126553.pdf.[11]

General FDA Guidance on Clinical Trial Sites

FDA's regulatory Guidances and the Code of Federal Regulations amount to hundreds of pages and provide in detail the rules under which a clinical trial should operate.

A more general and more useful articulation of the rules of efficient and proper operation of a regulatory compliant clinical trial is offered by FDA's OSI executives. The information below comes directly from these officials and hence should be given attention:

1. A PI should assemble a well-trained, responsible clinical trial team with proven skills in documentation. *Documentation, in all aspects of a trial, is vital.* Indeed, OSI executives emphasize that all trial staff should be experts in what the agency calls "ALCOA." This stands for Accurate, Legible, Contemporaneous, Original, and Attributable documentation.

2. To underscore the importance of documentation, FDA executives use the following example:

---

"In one of your trial source documents, there is the notation `BP 110/70.' But within the New Drug Application listing, the item is referred to as 'BP 110/*80*'." The question becomes: Was this error **a transcription error** within the Case Report Form [CRF]—the result of a data entry error—or a "data hiccup" at the sponsor's end? It is critical that the RC [Research Coordinator] check the CRF to determine whether this error is a site or sponsor issue. The RC then must determine: Was this error an isolated case or systemic? In either case, this minor error can have ramifications. The OSI executive, who noted she was speaking for many of her colleagues in FDA, emphasized: "A study is only as good as the data. And if your data is not useable, it will be thrown out."

---

3. The following are of keen importance to FDA executives:
- An accurate, continually updated Delegation log;
- Complete documentation of staff training;
- Documentation of the timely correction of problems;
- Detailed and documented plans for supervision and oversight of site personnel and activities;
- Written and well-known SOPs for site processes and procedures; and,
- Project management and quality control.

---

A lack of precision in data entry—which is a key focus of FDA executives—is easily discernable to FDA investigators and can impede your trial.

---

FDA officials have told the authors that the linchpin term for clinical trial operations is *Quality*. This shouldn't be viewed as an amorphous term but should guide the actions of every team member. The PI, say FDA officials, should build a culture of excellence, with no room for staff who cut corners, hide mistakes, and ignore details.

### What to Expect Before, During, and After an FDA Inspection

Let's say that phone call from an FDA investigator occurs and a site visit is scheduled. Please note you will have between five to 14 days' notice prior to the inspector's arrival.

Here's what you should have on hand prior to the inspection:

- Protocol
- Investigator Brochure and IND Safety Reports
- FDA Form 1572 with accompanying CVs
- IRB-approved Informed Consent Form
- IRB-Approved advertising
- Study-related correspondence excluding investigator agreement and financial information
- Monitor sign-in log
- Laboratory certification documents
- Drug accountability records
- Each subject's signed informed consent

In addition, you should have your site physically prepared; that is, you should review the support areas (pharmacy, lab) to be sure they are in good order, because the inspector often will visit various areas of the facility.

Most important, be prepared to answer the following questions related to the study, i.e., who assisted in performing the study, what were each person's specific duties, how did the sponsor monitor the study, what about drug accountability, i.e., drugs received, dispensed to/ returned from subjects; was drug returned to sponsor.

You also need to coach your staff on how to interact with the FDA—professional, but not effusive. One FDA Guidance notes that "In an attempt to impress the FDA inspector, some investigators have made the unfortunate mistake of providing unsolicited information and even offering up records from other studies only to be later cited for deficiencies in areas that were not part of the original inspection plan."

There is an FDA Audit Documentation Checklist in Appendix 38 you can use to prepare for your audit and to note corrections needed throughout the audit as well as FDA inspector comments.

**The Inspection**

Next, an FDA investigator arrives at your site and presents his/her credentials. The inspection takes place normally during a span of two to seven days. During this time, there is an examination of the facility and interviews of staff. There is a close review of study records, including the protocol, consent documents, CRFs, safety reporting, human subjects' protection, IRB reviews, and the data submitted to FDA.

Following are some of the matters that are routinely examined and ascertained by the FDA Investigator:

- Who performed various aspects of the protocol for the study (e.g., who verified inclusion and exclusion criteria, who obtained informed consent, who collected adverse event data);
- Whether the IRB approved the protocol, informed consent form, and any amendments to the protocol prior to implementation;
- Whether the clinical investigator and study staff adhered to the sponsor's protocol and investigational plan and whether protocol deviations were documented and reported appropriately;
- Whether informed consent documents were signed by the subject or the subjects' legally authorized representative prior to entry in the study (i.e., before the performance of any study-related procedures);

- Whether authority to conduct aspects of the study were delegated, and if so, how the conduct of the study was supervised by the clinical investigator;
- Where specific aspects of the investigation were performed;
- How the study data were obtained and where the study data were recorded;
- Accountability for the investigational product, including shipping records and disposition of unused investigational product;
- Whether the clinical investigator disclosed information regarding his financial interests to the sponsor and/or interests of any subinvestigator(s), spouse(s) and dependent children;
- The monitor's communications with the clinical investigator;
- The monitor's evaluations of the progress of the investigation; and,
- Corrective actions in response to previous FDA inspections, if any, and regulatory correspondence or sponsor and/or monitor correspondence. https://www.fda.gov/downloads/RegulatoryInformation/Guidances/UCM126553.pdf.[12]

In addition, "The FDA investigator also may audit the study data by comparing the data filed with the agency or the sponsor, if available, with records related to the clinical investigation. Such records may include the case report forms and supporting source documentation including signed and dated consent forms and medical records including, for example, progress notes of the physician, the subject's medical chart(s), and the nurses' notes. These records may be in hard copy and/or an electronic format. For electronic records and/or electronic signatures, the FDA investigator may gather information to determine whether 21 CFR part 11 requirements have been met."[13]

Moreover, "FDA may also examine subjects' medical records that are part of the clinical investigation and look prior to study start date for the diagnosis to verify whether the condition under study was in fact diagnosed, the study eligibility criteria were met, and whether the subject received any potentially interfering medication prohibited by the protocol. The FDA investigator may also review subjects' records covering a period after completion of study-related activities to determine if there was proper follow-up as outlined in the protocol, and if the clinical investigator submitted all reportable adverse events, including all clinical signs and symptoms."[14]

In addition to the review of documentation, following are some of the questions your team must be prepared to answer:

- How were subjects recruited, enrolled, and randomized?
- Did the study involve blinded and unblinded staff?
- Who had access to the treatment assignments and in what situations? Study staff, pharmacists, CRO, sponsor, or other third party?

Moreover, in addition to the record reviews and interviews, trial personnel are required to permit FDA investigators to access, copy, and verify any records or reports associated with the trial.[15]

*What does the FDA normally discover in an inspection?*

Some of the common deficiencies that have been observed by FDA investigators during a study inspection include:

- Failure to follow the investigational plan and signed investigator statement/agreement, which amounts to a failure to conduct or supervise the study in accordance with the current protocol(s);
- Protocol deviations, that is failure to appropriately document and report any medically necessary protocol deviations; inadequate record keeping[16];

- Inadequate accountability for the investigational product; Inappropriate delegation of medical tasks that contravene the protocol, including: Screening evaluations, obtaining medical histories and assessment of inclusion/exclusion criteria conducted by individuals with inadequate medical training (e.g., a medical assistant); physical examinations performed by unqualified personnel; evaluation of adverse events by individuals lacking appropriate medical training, knowledge of the clinical protocol; knowledge of the investigational product;, familiarity with the investigational product needed to be able to discuss the risks and benefits of a clinical trial with prospective subjects; and, inadequate subject protection, including informed consent issues.[17]

**What happens after an Inspection?**

At the end of an inspection, the FDA investigator conducts an exit interview with the clinical investigator or his/her representative. At this interview, the FDA investigator reviews and discusses the findings from the inspection. If there are concerns, the FDA inspector fills out an FDA Form 483 (Inspectional Observations) and gives a copy to the Investigator. (Please see Appendix 18 for an example of an FDA Form 483.)

Some common deficiencies:

- Failure to follow the investigational plan (protocol) and signed investigator statement/agreement (e.g., failure to conduct or supervise the study in accordance with the relevant, current protocol). See 21 CFR 312.60 and 812.110(b).
- Protocol deviations (e.g., failure to appropriately document and report any medically necessary protocol deviations). See 21 CFR 312.66 and 812.150(a)(4).
- Inadequate recordkeeping. See 21 CFR 312.62 and 812.140(a).
- Inadequate accountability for the investigational product. See 21 CFR 312.62(a) and 812.140(a)(2).
- Inadequate subject protection, including informed consent issues. See 21 CFR part 50, 312.60, and 812.100.

**FDA Form 483**

As noted above, if deficiencies were found, the Inspector issues a written FDA Form 483 to the clinical investigator. The Form 483 describes any inspectional observations that, in the opinion of the FDA investigator conducting the inspection, represent deviations from applicable statutes and regulations.

The clinical investigator may respond to the Form 483 observation orally during the exit interview or respond in writing after the inspection. Indeed, the FDA encourages facilities to respond in writing with their corrective action plan and then implement that corrective action plan expeditiously. FDA Form 483 FAQ: https://www.fda.gov/ICECI/Inspections/ucm256377.htm.

In addition, the inspector fills out an Establishment Inspection Report (EIR), which is an overview of the inspection itself, listing for example, the individuals interviewed, the trial site documents examined, and notes on the inspectional findings. The EIR will contain the following findings:

1. **No Action Indicated (NAI).** No objectionable conditions or practices were found during an inspection (or the objectionable conditions found do not justify further regulatory action). An example of a finding that would not justify further action is a slight deviation from the protocol, but one that was not placing subjects in jeopardy, nor significant enough to halt the trial. Approximately 20% of investigations end in the NAI category.
2. **Voluntary Action Indicated (VAI).** Objectionable conditions or practices were found, but the agency is not prepared to take or recommend any administrative or regulatory action. An example

of this type of finding is that certain assessments of patients were not completed in appropriate fashion, and this should be corrected but does not warrant enforcement action by the FDA. Approximately 70% end in the VAI category.

3. **Official Action Indicated (OAI)**. Regulatory and/or administrative actions will be recommended by the FDA. Examples of these findings are: Subject assessments were not conducted at all; trial records have been falsified to cover up these actions, and there are other, repeated, and deliberate failures to comply with the regulations. Approximately 10% end in the OAI category.[18] Further info here: https://www.fda.gov/downloads/ICECI/Inspections/FieldManagementDirectives/UCM382035.pdf.

Following the inspection, the FDA investigator sends the EIR, the FDA Form 483 (if one was issued) and any other materials collected during the inspection to the relevant FDA Center, i.e., Center for Drug Evaluation and Research (CDER), Center for Biologics Evaluation and Research (CBER), or the Center for Devices and Radiological Health (CDRH). The Center reviews the documents and one of the following letters is sent to the investigator:

---

It is important to note that the Form 483 does not constitute a final FDA determination of whether any condition is in violation of the Food, Drug and Cosmetic Act or any of its regulations. The relevant FDA Center (CDER, CBER, CDRH) reviews the Form 483 and the EIR and then will take into account any responses made by the company. The FDA considers all of this information and then determines what further action, if any, is appropriate to protect public health.[19]

---

### At the end of an inspection

After the FDA Investigator forwards his/her report to the relevant FDA Center, the report is analyzed and the Center issues one of the following deliberations:

1. A letter that generally states that FDA observed basic compliance with pertinent regulations. Note that a letter is not always sent when FDA observes no significant deviations.
2. An *Informational or Untitled Letter* that identifies deviations from statutes and regulations that do not meet the threshold of regulatory significance for a Warning Letter. Generally, such letters may request a written response from the clinical investigator.
3. A *Warning Letter* that identifies serious deviations from applicable statutes and regulations. A Warning Letter is issued for violations of regulatory significance. Significant violations are those violations that may lead to enforcement action if not promptly and adequately corrected. Warning Letters are issued to achieve voluntary compliance and include a request for correction and a written response to the agency.[20]
4. A *Notice of Initiation of Disqualification Proceedings and Opportunity to Explain (NIDPOE)*. FDA may initiate a process to disqualify the clinical investigator from further trials of investigational new drugs and/or biologics or investigational devices if the FDA finds the investigator has repeatedly or deliberately failed to comply with applicable regulatory requirements or has deliberately or repeatedly submitted false information to the sponsor or FDA in any required report.

The NIDPOE identifies alleged violations and provides the investigator with an opportunity to explain the matter at an informal conference or in writing to the FDA. If, in response to the NIDPOE, the investigator provides an acceptable explanation to the FDA, and the FDA finds the disqualification is not warranted, FDA executives may explore alternatives such as a detailed corrective action plan, known formally as a *Corrective and Preventive Action Plan*.[21]

If the investigator's explanation is not accepted by the FDA, the agency may issue a Notice of Opportunity for Hearing (NOOH). This hearing provides a clinical team with the opportunity for a hearing on a regulatory action, including a proposed action (such as debarment), before a presiding officer designated by the FDA Commissioner at: https://www.fda.gov/downloads/regulatoryinformation/guidances/ucm126553.pdf.

There is useful fact sheet at: https://www.fda.gov/downloads/regulatoryinformation/guidances/ucm214282.pdf.[22]

With the serious consequences of an FDA inspection outlined above, it is clear—and compelling—that the PI and all members of the clinical trial team are alert to every aspect of their trial. As the FDA executives emphasized, a focus on quality in the operation of a trial site is essential, and a quality environment has key elements: Skilled staff; close adherence to accurate documentation and data entry; accountability in all processes, and rigid adherence to regulations. No site wants to receive a call that an FDA Investigator is on the way; moreover, any site that is audited remains open under statute to re-inspection at any time. By following the guidance given in this chapter and understanding the mechanics of what triggers—and is involved in—an FDA audit, you are well positioned to conduct your trial with the proper regulatory acumen.

### Additional Resources
### Investigational Human Drugs Clinical Investigator Inspection List
(https://www.accessdata.fda.gov/scripts/cder/cliil/index.cfm)

The Clinical Inspection List, maintained by the Center for Drug Evaluation and Research, contains the names, addresses, and other information obtained during FDA inspections of clinical investigators who have performed studies with human investigational drugs. The list contains information on investigators inspected since July 1977 whose files have been closed with a final classification.

### Clinical Investigator List
(https://www.fda.gov/BiologicsBloodVaccines/GuidanceComplianceRegulatoryInformation/ComplianceActivities/ucm165743.htm)

The Clinical Investigator Inspection List, maintained by the Center for Biologics Evaluation and Research, contains names, addresses, and other information gathered from inspections of clinical investigators who have conducted studies with investigational new drugs or investigational devices reviewed by CBER. This list contains information on inspections that were closed after 1989.

### Bioresearch-Monitoring Information System File (BMIS)
(https://www.fda.gov/Drugs/InformationOnDrugs/ucm135162.htm)

BMIS contains information submitted to FDA identifying Clinical Investigators (CIs), Contract Research Organizations (CROs), and IRBs involved in the conduct of Investigational New Drug (IND) studies with human investigational drugs.

### IRBs—Restrictions Imposed Letters and Disqualification Proceedings
(https://www.fda.gov/ScienceResearch/SpecialTopics/RunningClinicalTrials/ComplianceEnforcement/ucm369514.htm)

An IRB—Restrictions Imposed Letter (Restrictions Letter) is a noncompliance letter issued under 21 CFR 56.120(a) that imposes restrictions on the IRB in accordance with 21 CFR 56.103 and 56.120(b). IRBs that refuse or repeatedly fail to comply with any of the applicable regulations and whose noncompliance adversely affects the rights or welfare of the human subjects in a clinical investigation may be subject to an administrative IRB disqualification action. This page indicates the current status of IRBs that have received Restrictions Letters or are the subject of disqualification actions.

**Warning Letters**

(https://www.fda.gov/ICECI/EnforcementActions/WarningLetters/default.htm)

A Warning Letter is an informal advisory to a firm communicating the Agency's position on a matter but does not commit FDA to taking enforcement action. The Agency's policy is that a Warning Letter should be issued for violations, which are of regulatory significance in that failure to adequately and promptly take corrections may be expected to result in enforcement action should the violation(s) continue.

**Clinical Investigator-Disqualification Proceedings**

(https://www.fda.gov/ICECI/EnforcementActions/ucm321308.htm)

FDA's new Clinical Investigator—Disqualification Proceedings database provides a list of clinical investigators who are or have been subject to an administrative clinical investigator disqualification action and indicates the current status of that action.

---

## ENDNOTES

[1] https://www.fda.gov/RegulatoryInformation/Guidances/ucm126420.htm [accessed 28.03.18].

[2] http://www.ich.org/fileadmin/Public_Web_Site/ICH_Products/Guidelines/Efficacy/E6/E6_R2__Step_4_2016_1109.pdf [accessed 28.03.18].

[3] https://www.accessdata.fda.gov/scripts/cdrh/cfdocs/cfcfr/CFRSearch.cfm?fr=56.107 [accessed 28.03.18].

[4] https://www.fda.gov/downloads/RegulatoryInformation/Guidances/ucm127013.pdf [accessed 28.03.18].

[5] https://osp.od.nih.gov/ufaqs/what-is-the-difference-between-a-central-irb-and-a-single-irb/ [accessed 28.03.18].

[6] https://www.accessdata.fda.gov/scripts/cdrh/cfdocs/cfcfr/CFRSearch.cfm?fr=312.56 [accessed 28.03.18].

[7] https://www.fda.gov/RegulatoryInformation/Guidances/ucm127073.pdf [accessed 28.03.18].

[8] https://www.fda.gov/downloads/Drugs/Guidances/UCM464506.pdf [accessed 28.03.18].

[9] www.aahrpp.org [accessed 29.0318].

[10] https://www.fda.gov/downloads/aboutfda/centersoffices/officeofmedicalproductsandtobacco/cder/ucm438250.pdf [accessed 28.03.18].

[11] https://www.fda.gov/downloads/regulatoryinformation/guidances/ucm126553.pdf [accessed 28.03.18].

[12] Ibid.

[13] Ibid.

[14] Ibid.

[15] Ibid.

[16] Ibid.

[17] Ibid.

[18] Ibid.

[19] Ibid.

[20] Ibid.

[21] Ibid.

[22] Ibid.

# EXCEPTIONAL CIRCUMSTANCES IN CLINICAL RESEARCH

# 6

*Purpose of chapter*:

- Explains Expanded Access (Compassionate Use)
- Describes charging for an Investigational New Drug (IND) in a clinical trial
- Provides overview of emergency use of a test article
  - **a.** Introduces the Checklist for Emergency Use of a Test Article in Appendix 31
  - **b.** Introduces the sample letter to the IRB for notification of emergency use in Appendix 32
- Describes research on decedents and PHI in clinical research
- Defines vulnerable populations
- Defines legally authorized representative and witness
- Provides guidance on actions when PI departs from a study or Institution
- Outlines consequences of clinical research non-compliance
- Provides guidance on how to respond to clinical research non-compliance

## 6.1 EXPANDED ACCESS (COMPASSIONATE USE)

*Purpose of section*:

- Explains how Expanded Access (also known as Compassionate Use) works
- Explains the difference between an Expanded Access IND and an Expanded Access protocol
- Explains the three categories of Expanded Access
- Provides FDA contact information for Expanded Access requests

According to the FDA, "Expanded Access" is the use of an investigational drug when the primary purpose is to diagnose, monitor, or treat a patient's disease or condition. This is significant because investigational drugs used during a clinical trial are never to be confused with "diagnosing" or "treating" a subject because the investigational drugs are being tested. The efficacy outcomes of the drugs are inconclusive during research studies.

Please note, Expanded Access has been nicknamed "Compassionate Use" nationally and internationally. The FDA only recognizes the term "Expanded Access" so that is what we will reference here.

**Useful Points on Expanded Access**

- Expanded Access use is not intended to collect safety or efficacy data. The Sponsor of the IND *can* collect this information if the regulations are followed for the Expanded Access use.
- Expanded Access can be initiated when there is no current clinical trial available at the physician's location with the investigational drug of interest and the physician wants to use the particular investigational drug for a patient. Additionally, Expanded Access is relevant for

The Sourcebook for Clinical Research. https://doi.org/10.1016/B978-0-12-816242-2.00006-0

patients who do not meet the inclusion and exclusion criteria of a clinical trial, or they failed screening, or a trial is closed, so they are unable to enroll in a trial.

> **Expanded Access use can only occur under an IND. There either needs to be a new IND submission or a protocol amendment to an existing IND.**

- When a new IND is submitted, the Expanded Access becomes known as an "Expanded Access IND." When a protocol amendment is created to an existing IND, the Expanded Access becomes known as an "Expanded Access Protocol."[1]

The patients who are allowed to be treated under an Expanded Access IND must meet ALL of the following criteria:

- The patients have a serious or immediately life-threatening disease or condition.
  - A "*serious disease or condition*" is defined as: a disease or condition associated with morbidity that has substantial impact on day-to-day functioning. Short-lived and self-limiting morbidity will usually not be sufficient, but the morbidity need not be irreversible, provided it is persistent or recurrent. Whether a disease or condition is serious is a matter of clinical judgment, based on its impact on such factors as survival, day-to-day functioning, or the likelihood that the disease, if left untreated, will progress from a less severe condition to a more serious one.
  - An "*Immediately life-threatening disease or condition*" is defined as: a stage of disease in which there is reasonable likelihood that death will occur within a matter of months or in which premature death is likely without early treatment.
- There is no comparable or satisfactory alternative therapy to diagnose, monitor, or treat the disease or condition.
- The potential patient benefit justifies the potential risks of the treatment use and those potential risks are not unreasonable in the context of the disease or condition to be treated.
- Providing the investigational drug for the requested use will not interfere with the initiation, conduct, or completion of clinical investigations that could support marketing approval of the expanded access use or otherwise compromise the potential development of the expanded access use.[2]

There are three (3) categories of Expanded Access. They are:

1. Expanded Access for individual patients, including for emergency use; found at 21 CFR 312.310
2. Expanded Access for intermediate-size patient populations; found at 21 CFR 312.315
3. Expanded Access for widespread treatment use in larger patient populations, found at 21 CFR 312.320.

Of note, the FDA does not quantify "intermediate-size" and "larger" patient populations.[3]

The "Sponsor" is the one who submits the Expanded Access request to the FDA. That will either be the Industry Sponsor/manufacturer of the drug, or a singular physician who is requesting Expanded Access. If the physician creates the IND submission, he/she will be the Sponsor-Investigator. (The Sponsor-Investigator scenario typically applies when an Industry Sponsor does not want to submit an Expanded Access use for its IND, but allows an individual physician to use the drug and to submit a new IND.)[4]

"If you are a physician and have questions about completing an application or submitting a request for expanded access for an investigational drug or biologic, contact the Division of Drug Information at 301-796-3400 or druginfo@fda.hhs.gov.[5]"

When an Expanded Access protocol is active at an Institution, the <u>Investigator</u> is responsible for the same tasks as a regular IND. They include:

1. Reporting Adverse Events and Serious Adverse Events;
2. Informed consent requirements
   a. including obtaining consent for Expanded Access emergency use
3. Attainment of IRB reviews
   a. For emergency expanded access when there is no time for prospective IRB review, the IRB must be notified of the emergency expanded access use within 5 working days of the emergency use;
4. Maintaining "accurate case histories" through Case Report Forms/EDCs or other documented means;
5. Maintaining drug disposition records;
6. Record retention requirements;
7. ✎ Other responsibilities found in 21 CFR 312 Subpart D "Responsibilities of Sponsors and Investigators" may apply dependent upon the Expanded Access category.[6]

### Expanded Access Emergency Use for an Individual Patient

When a patient's condition is immediately life threatening and there is no time to submit a new IND or protocol amendment to an existing IND for Expanded Access use for an Individual Patient, a physician will have to call the drug manufacturer to ask if they would be willing to have their investigational drug immediately shipped for an individual patient for Expanded Access emergency use. If the manufacturer is willing and can ship immediately, clarify who will take on Sponsorship. A new IND can be sponsored by the manufacturer, OR by a Principal Investigator as a Sponsor-Investigator. If it is a protocol amendment to an existing IND, the sponsor of the existing IND will be the sponsor of the amendment.

Whoever is declared as the Sponsor, will need to call the FDA next for authorization of the single patient emergency use. The contact information as of February 2018 is:

**Weekdays from 8 a.m. to 4:30 p.m.:**
**The Center for Drug Evaluation and Research (CDER) Division of Drug Information,**
**telephone: 1-855-543-3784 or 1-301-796-3400**
**e-mail: druginfo@fda.hhs.gov**

**After 4:30 p.m. weekdays and on weekends:**
**FDA Emergency Call Center, telephone: 866-300-4374**
**e-mail: emergency.operations@fda.hhs.gov**

The sponsor must then submit a written Expanded Access IND or Expanded Access Protocol amendment to the FDA within <u>15</u> working days.[7]

### Institutional Reviews

The physician may have time to submit the Expanded Access Emergency Use for an individual patient to the IRB while he/she is waiting for the drug to be shipped. However, if there is not enough time to secure IRB review before treatment begins, the emergency use must be reported to the IRB by the physician within five (5) working days of the emergency use. Only one emergency use is allowed per IND without prior IRB review. Any subsequent emergency use of the same IND will need prospective IRB review (21 CFR 56.104(c)). (However, see Question 15 in the *Expanded Access to Investigational Drugs for Treatment Use—Questions and Answers* Guidance document for more information.)[8]

The physician will also need to contact his/her Institution's Investigational Drug Services (IDS) Pharmacy to notify the pharmacist that an Expanded Access investigational drug for emergency use for one patient is being shipped. The IDS will need a contact name and number for the manufacturer so that they may discuss drug preparation, storage, and dispensation.

Whether a new IND or protocol amendment is created for Expanded Access Emergency Use for an Individual Patient, a contract or contract amendment from the Sponsor will be forthcoming. Make sure your contracts office receives it. Let the contracts office know if the emergency use is forthcoming and the date by when the use will occur. The contracts office should have a procedure for expediting emergency use cases. If the emergency use already occurred and there was no time for a contract review, let your contracts office know this as well, so that the office does not commence their emergency use procedure.

👍 It is a best practice to have a Research Coordinator or Clinical Trials Office Manager centrally track and orchestrate the various notifications, approvals, and coordination among departments for emergency use. If you choose this practice, exchange "physician" for "Research Coordinator" or "Clinical Trials Office Manager" in the paragraphs of this "Institutional Reviews" section.

## AUTHOR'S CORNER

At one hospital, a physician contacted the Clinical Trials Department to say that he wanted to perform a procedure on a patient in 5 days and use an investigational drug under Expanded Access for this one patient.

The Clinical Trials Department Manager took charge and rallied all necessary hospital departments and the sponsor to orchestrate the steps needed. The sponsor was the manufacturer who already had an IND for Expanded Access for an Intermediate-Size Patient Population and a protocol written. Therefore, it was a matter of getting a contract from them for this hospital location, a consent form for the patient, and getting the Investigational Pharmacy quickly in touch with the sponsor for a quick training in preparation, dispensing, and storing of the drug. Coordination for overnight shipping of the drug to the Investigational Pharmacy was also arranged. The physician already had the protocol in hand from the sponsor. (He called them first and reviewed it before contacting the Clinical Trials Department.)

The sponsor wanted to retain data from the singular patient use. The data elements for capture were delineated in the protocol. The supply and shipment of the drug, the data ownership, and other terms were written in a short contract by the sponsor for immediate review and approval between the Legal Department and the contracts office of the hospital. The IRB immediately reviewed the Expanded Access protocol and consent. Everyone was kept informed through multiple group e-mails (inclusive of the IRB contact, the legal contact, the contracts office contact, the physician, and the Investigational Pharmacist and the sponsor contact). We did it! The patient had the procedure in 5 days with all steps accomplished. The physician had to be available for several phone calls for questions about the patient and procedure throughout this quick turnaround with the use of a beeper.

Of note, shipping of the drug was the first priority to make sure it was received on time.

### Expanded Access for intermediate-size patient populations

*Under this section, FDA may permit an investigational drug to be used for the treatment of a patient population smaller than that typical of a treatment IND or treatment protocol. FDA may ask a sponsor to consolidate expanded access under this section when the agency has received a significant number of requests for individual patient expanded access to an investigational drug for the same use.* An Industry Sponsor or other type of manufacturer will request this type of Expanded Access.[9]

**Expanded Access for widespread treatment use in larger patient populations**

*Under this section, FDA may permit an investigational drug to be used for widespread treatment use* under a "Treatment IND or Treatment Protocol" (21 CFR 312.320).[10]

An Industry Sponsor or other type of manufacturer will also request this type of Expanded Access. There is no mention of "Expanded Access" or "Compassionate Use" in ICH GCP.

## 6.2 CHARGING FOR AN INVESTIGATIONAL NEW DRUG IN A CLINICAL TRIAL

*Purpose of section*:

- Explains the process for charging for an IND according to Federal regulations
- Explains when an external Certified Public Accountant (CPA) is needed
- Explains how to develop a letter requesting FDA approval to charge for an IND
- Explains how to establish billing in order to charge for an IND

Charging for an IND

⚠ Please Note: Before going through the steps from the regulations outlined below, know that it may not result in reimbursement from a health insurance company. Your more certain path would be to secure grant funding.

**Regulation:**

- 21 CFR 312.8(a)-(d)[11]

The sponsor of an IND may request approval from the FDA to charge for the direct costs of an IND.

**Direct Costs:**

Source: 21 CFR 312.8 (d)-(1)(ii)

(d) *Costs recoverable when charging for an investigational drug.* (1) A sponsor may recover only the **direct costs** of making its investigational drug available.

(i)   **Direct costs** are costs incurred by a sponsor that can be specifically and exclusively attributed to providing the drug for the investigational use for which FDA has authorized cost recovery. Direct costs include costs per unit to manufacture the drug (e.g., raw materials, labor, and non-reusable supplies and equipment used to manufacture the quantity of drug needed for the use for which charging is authorized) or costs to acquire the drug from another manufacturing source, and direct costs to ship and handle (e.g., store) the drug.

(ii)  **Indirect costs** include costs incurred primarily to produce the drug for commercial sale (e.g., costs for facilities and equipment used to manufacture the supply of investigational drug, but that are primarily intended to produce large quantities of drug for eventual commercial sale) and research and development, administrative, labor, or other costs that would be incurred even if the clinical trial or treatment use for which charging is authorized did not occur.[12]

**Once FDA authorizes a request to charge, whom may the sponsor charge?**

Although FDA determines whether a sponsor may charge for an investigational drug used in a clinical trial or for expanded access, FDA does not decide *how* that charging is to be carried out. FDA anticipates that the sponsor would ordinarily charge a patient directly or would charge a third-party payer if reimbursement were available. FDA notes that it has no authority to require that the Centers for Medicare and Medicaid Services (CMS) reimburse for investigational drugs for which FDA has authorized charging. Similarly, FDA has no authority to dictate reimbursement policy to any other entity, including private health insurance providers. For questions pertaining to third-party payer reimbursement, the third-party payer should be consulted.[13]

**The Process:**

1. Create an itemized budget listing all of your direct costs for which you would like reimbursement from a health insurance company or patient, and your indirect costs for payment by a Sponsor or your internal Medical Center Department.
2. Secure an independent Certified Public Accountant (CPA) who will review your budget and write a letter certifying its accuracy.
   a. An "independent" CPA means one who is not employed by your organization. He/she has to be an external professional.
3. Receive the letter from the CPA and pay for his/her services.
   a. See two CPA template letters of certification for charging for an IND in Appendix 19.
4. Write a letter to the FDA requesting approval to charge for your IND direct costs.
5. Include in the letter as stated in 21 CFR 312.8(b)(1)(i)-(iii):
   a. (i) Provide evidence that the drug has a potential clinical benefit that, if demonstrated in the clinical investigations, would provide a significant advantage over available products in the diagnosis, treatment, mitigation, or prevention of a disease or condition;
   b. (ii) Demonstrate that the data to be obtained from the clinical trial would be essential to establishing that the drug is effective or safe for the purpose of obtaining initial approval of a drug, or would support a significant change in the labeling of an approved drug (e.g., new indication, inclusion of comparative safety information); and
   c. (iii) Demonstrate that the clinical trial could not be conducted without charging because the cost of the drug is extraordinary to the sponsor. The cost may be extraordinary due to manufacturing complexity, scarcity of a natural resource, the large quantity of drug needed (e.g., due to the size or duration of the trial), or some combination of these or other extraordinary circumstances (e.g., resources available to a sponsor).
   d. The itemized budget that clearly manifests what the direct costs are.
   e. The CPA letter of certification.[14]
6. Mail it to:
   **U.S. Food and Drug Administration**
   **Center for Drug Evaluation and Research**
   10903 New Hampshire Avenue
   Silver Spring, MD 20993
   For questions, call:
   **1-888-INFO-FDA (1-888-463-6332)**
7. The FDA will write a letter to you with their decision. If they approve charging for your IND, you will receive a "Cost Recovery Approval" letter. It will state the IND number, the dollar amount the FDA approves, and the period of time the authorization covers (for example, 1 year).

---

**AUTHOR'S CORNER**

A letter one of the authors received from the FDA stated, "In the event you wish to charge for the IND beyond that date, you should submit a new request." FYI! Be aware of your deadline. Also, we were reminded in the letter that only the direct costs were recoverable.

---

Billing

Billing for the IND is quite a different matter.

When figuring out how to operationalize this regulation, it was discovered that there is no written guidance from CMS or MACs as to a code to put on a claim form.

What is definitely known is that you will need to:

1. Do a coverage analysis (reference NCD 310.1). See Chapter 2, Section 2.8.
2. If you have an "applicable clinical trial," register with ClinicalTrials.gov. Or, obtain the NCT number from the ClinicalTrials.gov site for your trial. The NCT number will be put on the claim from your Billing Office.
3. Place the following information on a claim:
   a. The ICD-10 code Z00.6 for the secondary diagnosis
   b. Modifier Q0 (Investigational) or Q1 (Routine) as appropriate. See Clinical Trial Coding in Chapter 4, Section 4.4.
   c. Condition Code 30 (for a qualifying clinical trial)
   d. Value Code D4 (This signifies that the trial has an NCT number and you are reporting it... if the trial is an "applicable clinical trial".) See ClinicalTrials.gov information in Chapter 2, Section 2.9.
   e. Make sure the NCT number from ClinicalTrials.gov is on the claim.
   f. Include a note about the FDA approval for charging.

What was provided as a best guesstimate from a MAC is:

1. Use a Revenue Code.
   a. As an example, if the experimental agent is being delivered via infusion, use the IV Therapy Revenue Code 026X. Fill in the "X."

You can call the Medicare Administrative Contractor (MAC) for your State for more information regarding your specific trial. Please see the MACs by State List in Appendix 8.

Another way to go about it is to have your Medical Center Department set up an internal departmental code. When a claim is created, use this internal code and send the FDA approval letter and the CPA letter with the claim. Include items a through f above on your claims.

These two options shall have to suffice until CMS produces guidance on the coding for charging for an IND by FDA approval.

From the health insurance company perspective, you will need to get pre-authorization for each subject's use of your IND. Health insurance companies will struggle with not having a CPT code to look up, so expect that you will need to educate the subject's insurance company on the regulation.

ICH GCP does not speak to billing or charging.

## 6.3 EMERGENCY USE OF A TEST ARTICLE

*Purpose of section*:

- Provides an overview of the process by which an investigative product or test article may be administered in a clinical trial on an emergency basis
- Introduces the Checklist for Emergency Use of a Test Article in Appendix 31
- Introduces the "Sample letter to the IRB for notification of emergency use of a test article" in Appendix 32

1. EMERGENCY USE OF A TEST Article as it applies to an INVESTIGATIONAL NEW DRUG (IND)

    Emergency use of a test article spans three distinct parts in the Code of Federal Regulations (CFR). They have to be followed TOGETHER to conduct emergency use properly.

    Here is what the CFR states specifically about emergency use:

    *Emergency use* means the use of a test article on a human subject in a life-threatening situation in which no standard acceptable treatment is available, and in which there is not sufficient time to obtain IRB approval. 21 CFR 56.102 (d)

    21 CFR 56.104: Exemptions from IRB requirement:

    Emergency use of a test article, provided that such emergency use is reported to the IRB within 5 working days. Any subsequent use of the test article at the institution is subject to IRB review. 21 CFR 56.104 (c) (Note: This means that subsequent use of the test article requires IRB review and approval. Emergency use for a patient can only occur one time.)[15]

    The PI needs to determine whether the condition of the patient is "life threatening." The FDA definition for "life-threatening" is found in 21 CFR 312.32 (a), which is "immediate risk of death." The adjective "immediate" is the key.[16]

    Add 21 CFR 50.23: Exception from general requirements:

    (1) You must make a concerted effort to obtain the informed consent of the patient or the patient's Legally Authorized Representative prior to use of the test article.

    Note outside of the CFR: The consent may be a short form or abbreviated type of consent furnished by the Sponsor. Ask the sponsor at the time of your Site Initiation Visit (SIV) if they have such a consent and receive a copy of it to have on hand and send to the IRB at the time of your initial review.

    If you are in an emergency situation and have not gone through this preparatory step, use the standard consent form approved by the IRB for the study.

    (2) If the patient is unable to provide consent, the Investigator AND a physician who is not a part of the investigation (Find an available physician colleague.) with the test article must certify in writing ALL of the following (not some of these, but ALL of these): 21 CFR 50.23 (a)

---

(1) The human subject is confronted by a life-threatening situation necessitating the use of the test article.

(2) Informed consent cannot be obtained from the subject because of an inability to communicate with, or obtain legally effective consent from, the subject.

(3) Time is not sufficient to obtain consent from the subject's legal representative.

(4) There is available no alternative method of approved or generally recognized therapy (i.e., there is no FDA-approved medicine available or the physician has tried everything that is approved for the indication and they have not worked) that provides an equal or greater likelihood of saving the life of the subject.

(b) If immediate use of the test article is, in the investigator's opinion, required to preserve the life of the subject, and time is not sufficient to obtain the independent determination (added: of the physician independent from the study/investigation) required in paragraph (a) of this section in advance of using the test article, the determinations of the clinical investigator shall be made and, within 5 working days after the use of the article, be reviewed and evaluated in writing by a physician who is not participating in the clinical investigation. Paraphrased: The PI will need to document 1–4 above if consent cannot be obtained and certification is received from an independent physician, or the PI will need to document 1–4 above and explain why an independent physician was not obtained to evaluate the situation as required in (b) above. The documentation required from 1 to 4 must be submitted to the IRB within 5 working days after the use of the test article. (Note: It is best to write your report as soon as possible after the event so that the circumstances are recalled in their greatest detail and clarity. It can then be reviewed by the writer/Investigator and the independent physician within the 5 working day requirement prior to IRB submission.)[17]

See the *Checklist for Emergency Use of a Test Article* in Appendix 31 to use as a quick, guiding tool while you are in an emergency situation.

IRB Note: Even though the CFR does not require IRB notification prior to the emergency use of a test article, your Institution's IRB may require or request a phone call or other notification method to inform them that emergency use is imminent. Check your IRB policy.
Your IRB may want the opportunity to check whether the test article was ever used in an emergency previously in order to abide by the CFR for one emergency use only.

For IRB notification after Emergency Use, see the "Sample letter to the IRB for notification of emergency use of a test article" in Appendix 32.
One of the big questions in emergency use is whether the data can be used for research or if it only becomes a part of the clinical data. Here is how you determine data use in an emergency use of a test article scenario:

If the Investigator is ABLE to follow the FDA requirements from the CFR for emergency use, the data may be used for research.
If emergency care is rendered without following the CFR for emergency use of a test article, the data from the care can only be clinical data; it cannot be assumed into the research data.

ICH ICH GCP has this to say regarding emergencies (that relate to emergency use):
3.1.7 Where the protocol indicates that prior consent of the trial subject or the subject's legally acceptable representative is not possible (see 4.8.15), the IRB/IEC should determine that the proposed protocol and/or other document(s) adequately addresses relevant ethical concerns and meets applicable regulatory requirements for such trials (i.e., in emergency situations).
1.6.1 Vulnerable Subjects includes "patients in emergency situations."
4.8.15 In emergency situations, when prior consent of the subject is not possible, the consent of the subject's legally acceptable representative, if present, should be requested. When prior consent of the subject is not possible, and the subject's legally acceptable representative is not available, enrolment of the subject should require measures described in the protocol and/or elsewhere, with documented approval/favorable opinion by the IRB/IEC, to protect the rights, safety and well-being of the subject and to ensure compliance with applicable regulatory requirements. The subject or the subject's legally acceptable representative should be informed about the trial as soon as possible and consent to continue and other consent as appropriate (see 4.8.10) should be requested.[18]

## DEVICES

### Emergency Use as it applies to an INVESTIGATIONAL DEVICE EXEMPTION (IDE)

Emergency situations may arise in which there will be a need to use an investigational device in a manner inconsistent with the approved investigational plan or by a physician who is not part of the clinical study. Emergency use of an unapproved device may occur before an IDE is approved. The sponsor must notify the FDA of the emergency use within 5 days through a submission of an IDE Report describing the details of the case and the patient protection measures that were followed.

**Criteria**:

- Life-threatening or serious disease or condition
- No alternative
- No time to obtain FDA approval

*Source:* www.fda.gov/medicaldevices/deviceregulationandguidance, *updated 3/26/2015.*[19]

### TREATMENT USE OF AN IDE

"Treatment use" of an IDE includes use for a serious or immediately life-threatening disease or condition.

The definition from 21 CFR 812.36 (a) is as follows [20]:

(An) "immediately life-threatening" disease means a stage of a disease in which there is a reasonable likelihood that death will occur within a matter of months or in which premature death is likely without early treatment.

⚠️ Please note, this is NOT an immediate process like the IND emergency use. The Sponsor of the device has to submit a treatment IDE application to the FDA and an Agreement must be signed by each individual PI that will be using the IDE for treatment.

The regulations are found here:

---

21 CFR 812.36 Treatment use of an investigational device:

(a) *General.* A device that is not approved for marketing may be under clinical investigation for a serious or immediately life-threatening disease or condition in patients for whom no comparable or satisfactory alternative device or other therapy is available. During the clinical trial or prior to final action on the marketing application, it may be appropriate to use the device in the treatment of patients not in the trial under the provisions of a treatment IDE. The purpose of this section is to facilitate the availability of promising new devices to desperately ill patients as early in the device development process as possible, before general marketing begins, and to obtain additional data on the device's safety and effectiveness. In the case of a serious disease, a device ordinarily may be made available for treatment use under this section after all clinical trials have been completed. In the case of an immediately life-threatening disease, a device may be made available for treatment use under this section prior to the completion of all clinical trials. For the purpose of this section, an "immediately life-threatening" disease means a stage of a disease in which there is a reasonable likelihood that death will occur within a matter of months or in which premature death is likely without early treatment. For purposes of this section, "treatment use" of a device includes the use of a device for diagnostic purposes.

(b) *Criteria.* FDA shall consider the use of an investigational device under a treatment IDE if:

(1) The device is intended to treat or diagnose a serious or immediately life-threatening disease or condition;

(2) There is no comparable or satisfactory alternative device or other therapy available to treat or diagnose that stage of the disease or condition in the intended patient population;

(3) The device is under investigation in a controlled clinical trial for the same use under an approved IDE, or such clinical trials have been completed; and

(4) The sponsor of the investigation is actively pursuing marketing approval/clearance of the investigational device with due diligence.

(c) *Applications for treatment use.* (1) A treatment IDE application shall include, in the following order:

(i) The name, address, and telephone number of the sponsor of the treatment IDE;

(ii) The intended use of the device, the criteria for patient selection, and a written protocol describing the treatment use;

(iii) An explanation of the rationale for use of the device, including, as appropriate, either a list of the available regimens that ordinarily should be tried before using the investigational device or an explanation of why the use of the investigational device is preferable to the use of available marketed treatments;

(iv) A description of clinical procedures, laboratory tests, or other measures that will be used to evaluate the effects of the device and to minimize risk;

(v) Written procedures for monitoring the treatment use and the name and address of the monitor;

(vi) Instructions for use for the device and all other labeling as required under 812.5(a) and (b);

(vii) Information that is relevant to the safety and effectiveness of the device for the intended treatment use. Information from other IDEs may be incorporated by reference to support the treatment use;

(viii) A statement of the sponsor's commitment to meet all applicable responsibilities under this part and part 56 of this chapter and to ensure compliance of all participating investigators with the informed consent requirements of part 50 of this chapter;

(ix) An example of the agreement to be signed by all investigators participating in the treatment IDE and certification that no investigator will be added to the treatment IDE before the agreement is signed; and

(x) If the device is to be sold, the price to be charged and a statement indicating that the price is based on manufacturing and handling costs only.

(2) A licensed practitioner who receives an investigational device for treatment use under a treatment IDE is an "investigator" under the IDE and is responsible for meeting all applicable investigator responsibilities under this part and parts 50 and 56 of this chapter.

(d) *FDA action on treatment IDE applications*—(1) *Approval of treatment IDE's.* Treatment use may begin 30 days after FDA receives the treatment IDE submission at the address specified in 812.19, unless FDA notifies the sponsor in writing earlier than the 30 days that the treatment use may or may not begin. FDA may approve the treatment use as proposed or approve it with modifications.

(2) *Disapproval or withdrawal of approval of treatment IDEs.* FDA may disapprove or withdraw approval of a treatment IDE if:

(i) The criteria specified in 812.36(b) are not met or the treatment IDE does not contain the information required in 812.36(c);

(ii) FDA determines that any of the grounds for disapproval or withdrawal of approval listed in 812.30(b)(1) through (b)(5) apply;

(iii) The device is intended for a serious disease or condition and there is insufficient evidence of safety and effectiveness to support such use;

(iv) The device is intended for an immediately life-threatening disease or condition and the available scientific evidence, taken as a whole, fails to provide a reasonable basis for concluding that the device:

(A) May be effective for its intended use in its intended population; or

(B) Would not expose the patients to whom the device is to be administered to an unreasonable and significant additional risk of illness or injury;

(v) There is reasonable evidence that the treatment use is impeding enrollment in, or otherwise interfering with the conduct or completion of, a controlled investigation of the same or another investigational device;

(vi) The device has received marketing approval/clearance or a comparable device or therapy becomes available to treat or diagnose the same indication in the same patient population for which the investigational device is being used;

(vii) The sponsor of the controlled clinical trial is not pursuing marketing approval/clearance with due diligence;

(viii) Approval of the IDE for the controlled clinical investigation of the device has been withdrawn; or

(ix) The clinical investigator(s) named in the treatment IDE are not qualified by reason of their scientific training and/or experience to use the investigational device for the intended treatment use.

(3) *Notice of disapproval or withdrawal.* If FDA disapproves or proposes to withdraw approval of a treatment IDE, FDA will follow the procedures set forth in 812.30(c).

(e) *Safeguards.* Treatment use of an investigational device is conditioned upon the sponsor and investigators complying with the safeguards of the IDE process and the regulations governing informed consent (part 50 of this chapter) and institutional review boards (part 56 of this chapter).

(f) *Reporting requirements.* The sponsor of a treatment IDE shall submit progress reports on a semiannual basis to all reviewing IRBs and FDA until the filing of a marketing application.[20]

These reports shall be based on the period of time since initial approval of the treatment IDE and shall include the number of patients treated with the device under the treatment IDE, the names of the investigators participating in the treatment IDE, and a brief description of the sponsor's efforts to pursue marketing approval/clearance of the device. Upon filing of a marketing application, progress reports shall be submitted annually in accordance with 812.150(b)(5). The sponsor of a treatment IDE is responsible for submitting all other reports required under 812.150.[21]

## 6.4 RESEARCH ON DECEDENTS AND PHI IN CLINICAL RESEARCH

*Purpose of section*:

- Defines decedent research
- Describes requirements for accessing PHI
- Defines organ and cadaver donation

Research on Decedents

Decedent research means medical research conducted with the use of deceased persons' protected health information.

Decedent research is not mentioned in ICH GCP, 45 CFR 46, 21 CFR 50, or 21 CFR 56. It is only mentioned in the Privacy Rule at 45 CFR 164.512.[22]

To use or disclose PHI of the deceased for research, covered entities are <u>not</u> required to obtain:

- Authorizations from the personal representative or next of kin;
- A (HIPAA) waiver or an alteration of the Authorization; or,
- A data use agreement.

However, the researcher who is seeking access to decedents' PHI must provide the covered entity with the following:

**(1)** Oral or written representations that the use and disclosure is sought solely for research on the PHI of decedents;

**(2)** Oral or written representations that the PHI for which use or disclosure is sought is necessary for the research purposes; and

**(3)** Documentation, at the request of the covered entity, of the death of the individuals whose PHI is sought by the researchers.[23]

Here is the actual regulation:

PHI of Decedents
45 CFR 164.512
(i)(1)(iii) Research on decedent's information. The covered entity obtains from the researcher:

**(A)** Representation that the use or disclosure sought is solely for research on the protected health information of decedents;

**(B)** Documentation, at the request of the covered entity, of the death of such individuals; and

**(C)** Representation that the protected health information for which use or disclosure is sought is necessary for the research purposes.[24]

Of note, the HIPAA Privacy Rule applies to protections of the individually identifiable health information for 50 years past the deceased person's actual date of death. After the 50 years, the decedent's health information is no longer protected under the Privacy Rule.

The use of organs and tissue for cadaver research is completely separate. For this type of research, you can see if a decedent has an Advance Directive or Living Will, which clearly specifies donation of their body to cadaver research or organ donation. The decedent's next of kin will have hopefully been informed by the decedent prior to death of his/her wishes for donation.

See the "Anatomical Gift Act" (2006) for more information regarding organ and cadaver donation. The Act has been ratified by the following States:

Alabama, Alaska, Arizona, Arkansas, California, Colorado, Connecticut, District of Columbia, Georgia, Hawaii, Idaho, Illinois, Indiana, Iowa, Kansas, Kentucky, Louisiana, Maine, Maryland, Massachusetts, Michigan, Minnesota, Mississippi, Missouri, Montana, Nebraska, Nevada, New Hampshire, New Jersey, New Mexico, North Carolina, North Dakota, Ohio, Oklahoma, Oregon, Rhode Island, South Carolina, South Dakota, Tennessee, Texas, U.S. Virgin Islands, Utah, Vermont, Virginia, Washington, West Virginia, Wisconsin, Wyoming

You can also check your State Law regarding whole body donation.

Under Maryland law, if a person does not stipulate in an Advance Directive or Living Will whether they wish to donate their organs after death, or if they do not wish to donate their organs after death, the right to make this decision falls to the following people in this order:

- The decedent's health care agent, if one is appointed, unless the appointing document explicitly withholds this power
- The decedent's spouse or registered domestic partner
- The decedent's adult children
- The decedent's parents
- The decedent's adult siblings
- The decedent's grandparents
- An adult who exhibited special care and concern for the decedent, or
- Any other person who has the authority to handle the disposition of the decedent's body.[25]

## 6.5 VULNERABLE POPULATIONS

*Purpose of section*:

- Outlines the categories of populations considered vulnerable
- Describes why these populations are considered vulnerable

A clinical research study may have in its inclusion criteria a certain vulnerable population endemic to the purposes of the study, or a subject enrolls in a study who happens to be a member of a vulnerable population. To identify persons included in a "vulnerable population," here are the categories and their definitions:

- Pregnant women
- Human fetuses
  - Definition: prenatal human beings between the embryonic stage and birth/unborn human baby; and

- Definition per HHS (The U.S. Department of Health and Human Services): the product of conception from implantation until delivery 45 CFR 46.202(c)
- Neonates of uncertain viability or non-viable neonates
  - Neonate Definition: A newborn child/an infant less than four weeks old;
  - Uncertain viability: A state in which it is unclear, or it cannot be determined, whether a fetus (or unborn baby) will be born alive;
  - Non-viable neonate: The fetus (or unborn baby) has no chance of being born alive.
- Children
  - Child definition: Persons from birth to the legal age of majority. (State law determines the "legal age of majority." In most US States, this is 18 years of age.)
- Prisoners
  - "Prisoner" is defined by HHS regulations at 45 CFR part 46.303(c) as "any individual involuntarily confined or detained in a penal institution. The term is intended to encompass individuals sentenced to such an institution under a criminal or civil statute, individuals detained in other facilities by virtue of statutes or commitment procedures which provide alternatives to criminal prosecution or incarceration in a penal institution, and individuals detained pending arraignment, trial, or sentencing.[26]"
- Cognitively impaired persons
  - E.g., birth defects, such as Down's Syndrome
- Students
- Employees
- Educationally disadvantaged persons
  - "Educationally disadvantaged" is defined as:
    - Lack of or limited proficiency in a person's language of origin
    - The inability to read or /and write
- Persons with Impaired Decision Making Capacity
  - E.g., Persons experiencing trauma, such as a patient in the Emergency Room after a car accident or heart attack;
  - E.g., Psychiatric patients who have not been compliant with their medications, and are consequently unstable, e.g., schizophrenics who are off their medicine and experiencing hallucinations; and
  - E.g., Intoxicated individuals.

**Why are these persons or conditions considered "vulnerable"?**

For pregnant women, human fetus, and neonates, it is unknown what the effects of investigational products will have on each. The risks of research need to be carefully considered, because the research may be a benefit to the pregnant woman, but may harm the fetus or neonate, or the research may benefit the fetus or neonate, but may harm the pregnant woman. Families need to consider the risks and treatment alternatives carefully. And, human fetuses and neonates cannot speak for themselves.

- Children

Children are considered too cognitively and emotionally immature to make serious decisions for their healthcare, including the inability to determine long-term consequences.

- Prisoners

Federal regulations note: "…prisoners may be under constraints because of their incarceration which could affect their ability to make a truly voluntary and uncoerced decision whether or not to participate as subjects in research,…" (45 CFR 46.302).[27]

Cognitively Impaired Persons
Protections must be in place for persons who are unable to make healthcare decisions for themselves.

- Students
  Students, such as college students, are placed in a vulnerable position when they are asked by a Teacher or Faculty Member to participate in research. Students may feel pressure that they need to participate in order to receive a good grade or receive a teacher recommendation in the future.
  Medical students who are asked to participate in research by a supervisor or Faculty Member may feel uncomfortable in declining participation, which might appear unsupportive of the research of their supervisor. Or, academic credits may be offered for participation in research, placing medical students in an uncomfortable position to decline. Indeed, protocol design, consent forms and the consenting process need to be carefully reviewed by an IRB for lack of coercion, and freedom of choice by the students.
- Employees
  Employees can be placed in a vulnerable position when their employers ask them to participate in research. Employees may feel they need to comply in order to receive a good performance review, forestall a negative review, or feel pressure that participation is connected to career advancement. In addition, employees at medical institutions may feel uncomfortable revealing their lab test results or a medical condition to their employer through a research study. And, employees may feel vulnerable regarding the confidentiality of their medical records.
- Educationally Disadvantaged Persons
  If a person is unable to read or write, he/she is considered vulnerable, because of the dependence on others to understand information and make informed decisions.
- Persons with Impaired Decision Making Capacity (IDMC)
  A person with IDMC is unable to make an informed decision in full awareness at the time needed due to a medical condition or an altered state of mind. Protections are needed in recognition of the temporal condition or state of mind.
  **Regulations for Vulnerable Populations:**

---

**45 CFR 46 Subpart B. Additional Protections for Pregnant Women, Human Fetuses, and Neonates Involved in Research, 45 CFR 46.201-.207**

---

**45 CFR 46 Subpart C. Additional Protections Pertaining to Biomedical and Behavioral Research Involving Prisoners as Subjects, 45 CFR 46.301-.306**

---

**45 CFR 46 Subpart D. Additional Protections for Children Involved as Subjects in Research, 45 CFR 46.401-.409**

---

**What Medical Institutions and Study Teams can do to manage research with vulnerable populations:**

1. Keep consent forms at the 7th grade reading level.

2. Develop and maintain comprehensive safety-monitoring plans with a Data Safety Monitoring Board (DSMB) for trials requiring a DSMB. See Chapter 5, Section 5.2.
3. Be willing to revise monitoring plans as a result of data reviewed by a DSMB during an ongoing study with vulnerable populations.
4. Train and test your IRB members periodically (such as biannually) in various regulatory competencies including safeguards for vulnerable populations. Make sure your IRB members are knowledgeable and that you have an adequate training plan for new IRB members.
5. Develop a contact database for the IRB that includes industry experts or professionals who can serve as consultants for IRB meetings. These contacts will provide consultation for studies and representation for vulnerable populations, such as schizophrenics, non-viable neonates, children, cognitively impaired persons, prisoners, and so on.
6. Utilize Legally Authorized Representatives (see Section 6.6), Witnesses (see Section 6.6), and Research Subject Advocates (see Chapter 2, Section 2.5 in "Consent Extras").
7. Provide Assents as well as Parental Permission Forms (see Chapter 2, Section 2.5).
8. Ensure your IRB understands the regulatory criteria for Waivers of Consent (see Chapter 2, Section 2.5.1).
9. Ensure your IRB understands and governs appropriately that an FDA-approved drug has to become an IND, and needs a study protocol, when the drug is tested in a new subject population for which the FDA has not previously given approval, such as children.
10. IRB members can observe the consenting process. The IRB should exercise this option periodically and make certain, in the case of vulnerable populations, that there is no pressure nor persuasion exacted on potential research subjects.
11. Where prisoners are concerned, the IRB must follow HHS regulation 45 CFR 46.304(b), which states: *At least one member of the Board shall be a prisoner, or a prisoner representative with appropriate background and experience to serve in that capacity, except that where a particular research project is reviewed by more than one Board, only one Board need satisfy this requirement.*[28]
12. Ensure that study teams are sufficiently trained regarding vulnerable populations and know what regulations apply. Include in the training that those subjects with IDMC may regain their reasoning capacity at some point during the study, in which case they can be led through the consenting process themselves at that time, in addition to the initial consent with the LAR signature.

## AUTHOR'S CORNER

Scenario 1:

During one trial, a subject became a "prisoner" who was not a prisoner when he initially enrolled. Fortunately, the subject disclosed this information. The study team had to adjust for this new vulnerable population member in their trial and the IRB had to find a prisoner representative. Remember that HHS has a broad definition for "prisoner"; the term does not include only those who are incarcerated.

Scenario 2:

Be aware that if your protocol design includes research with prisoners who are transported to a medical facility for a study visit or visits, prisoners may see a trip outside of the prison as an opportunity for escape. At one hospital, a few prisoners got past the prison guards accompanying them and were crawling through the HVAC system in the ceiling trying to escape.

It is highly recommended that if incarcerated prisoners are being transported to a medical facility, that medical facility security guards are present in addition to the prison guards, and that only your male study team members meet with the (male and female) prisoners for visits.

Scenario 3:

For a study involving pregnant women and fetuses, the protocol read throughout that a "Brain MRI" was needed. However, the writers meant that a brain MRI of the fetus was needed. Therefore, this translates to an "Abdominal MRI" of the mother. There are different CPT codes and different charges for various body parts that are imaged. Be aware of the need for practical translation when reading a protocol for a study with fetuses.

---

**Sections in this book speak further on topics relevant to vulnerable populations.**
For more information on Assent, see Chapter 2, Section 2.5.
For more information on Legally Authorized Representatives, see Section 6.6.
For more information on Witnesses, see Section 6.6.

---

## 6.6 LEGALLY AUTHORIZED REPRESENTATIVE AND WITNESS

*Purpose of section*:

- Defines a Legally Authorized Representative (LAR)
- Provides explanation on what individuals need an LAR
- Explains who can be an LAR
- Defines "Witness"
- Explains when a Witness must be present

**Legally Authorized Representatives**

Legally Authorized Representative defined:

A legally authorized representative is "an individual or judicial or other body authorized under applicable law to consent on behalf of a prospective subject to the subject's participation in the procedure(s) involved in the research." (21 CFR 50.3(l), 45 CFR 46.102(c)).[29]

---

**45 CFR 46.102(i) the New Common Rule**

*Legally authorized representative* **means an individual or judicial or other body authorized under applicable law to consent on behalf of a prospective subject to the subject's participation in the procedure(s) involved in the research. If there is no applicable law addressing this issue,** *legally authorized representative* **means an individual recognized by institutional policy as acceptable for providing consent in the non-research context on behalf of the prospective subject to the subject's participation in the procedure(s) involved in the research.**

---

The ICH GCP changes the title and provides this similar definition:

1.37 Legally Acceptable Representative

ᛰ<sup>ICH</sup> An individual or juridical or other body authorized under applicable law to consent, on behalf of a prospective subject, to the subject's participation in the clinical trial.

**Who needs an LAR?**

**1.** A patient with Impaired Decision Making Capacity (IDMC)

   **a.** This means that an individual loses the ability to make health care decisions on his or her own.

     **i.** Examples are (This is not all-inclusive.):

       **1.** A patient is sedated or on a high dose of pain medication from an automobile accident;

       **2.** A patient has bipolar disorder and is off medication. When they are taking medication, they may be able to make their own decisions;

       **3.** A patient has an addiction. When they are using the substance, they are impaired. When they are "clean" or not using, they may be able to make their own decisions;

       **4.** A patient is highly emotionally distraught from an accident;

**2.** Intellectually disabled individuals

   **a.** For example, a patient with Down's syndrome;

**3.** A patient with dementia or Alzheimer's;

**4.** A patient with a debilitating psychiatric disorder;

**5.** A patient with a debilitating neurologic disorder; and/or,

**6.** An educationally disadvantaged person.

**Determining decision-making capacity:**

Determine the decision-making capacity of the person you are interested in consenting. In some cases, it will be straightforward, such as a person presenting with Down's Syndrome, or a patient who is unconscious.

For those patients for whom decision-making capacity is in question, have an assessment tool handy.

NIH states, "Instead of trying to quantify the cognitive and other abilities that might relate to decision-making capacity, some methods now involve questions about consent-related aspects of the particular study being considered." NIH uses the term "consent-capacity" in this regard.[30]

Your site can create a Question-and-Answer form that tests a patient's understanding of what is reviewed with them in a consent form during consenting or you can use the one in this book. (See the Consent Question and Answer Form in Appendix 20.) The patient can write his or her own answers, or the Q&A form can be presented orally while a study team member writes the responses of the patient on the form.

If the patient is not able to answer the Q&A form satisfactorily, finding or designating an LAR is the next step.

Note that there are varying names for an LAR as defined by each state. For example:

- "Healthcare" or "health care" proxy
- Health care agent (Maryland)
- Surrogate

See if the individual has an Advance Directive in which a surrogate/healthcare proxy/Legally Authorized Representative is named. A surrogate can also be known as a Durable Power of Attorney for Health Care.

If an Advance Directive does not exist or the surrogate is not available, see your state law for who can be a healthcare proxy. Note that the states define who can be an overall healthcare proxy/LAR. It is not for research purposes only; it applies to research studies and clinical care.

You can get information for most states via each state's website. The url convention is (State Name).gov. For example, Delaware.gov or Nebraska.gov or Montana.gov. Place "authorized representative" in the search field. There are other ways to obtain state LAR information; this is one possibility and a place to start.

You can also look up your state statutes. For example:

Arizona Revised Statutes 36-3231
Florida Statutes 765.401
Minnesota Statutes 253B.03 Subd. 6

✎ There is an extremely well-written handbook from the State of Maryland about the role of a health care proxy. It is recommended reading. Even if this is not your state, it contains the information you will need to understand the role of a health care proxy (LAR) and the questions you will need to ask. (It goes beyond research.) It is called "Making Medical Decisions for Someone Else: A Maryland Handbook". The url where you can find the link to the Handbook is: http://www.marylandattorneygeneral.gov/Pages/HealthPolicy/proxyguide.aspx

You can also request this handbook via mail by calling 410-576-7000 or by e-mailing proxies@oag.state.md.us[31]

Examples of who can be an LAR are:

Florida

A person can be appointed as an LAR <u>in the following order</u>:

1. Judicially appointed guardian of the patient;
2. Patient's spouse;
3. Adult child of the patient
   a. If there is more than one adult child, "a majority of the adult children who are reasonably available for consultation";
4. A parent of the patient;
5. Adult sibling of the patient;
   a. If there is more than one adult sibling, "a majority of the adult siblings who are reasonably available for consultation";
6. Adult relative of the patient who has maintained regular contact with the patient;
7. A close friend of the patient;
8. A licensed clinical social worker or a social worker who has graduated from a court-approved guardianship program who is selected by a bioethics committee.

Minnesota

"(b) If the patient is subject to guardianship which includes the provision of medical care, the written, informed consent of the guardian for the treatment is sufficient.

(c) If the head of the treatment facility determines that the patient is not competent to consent to the treatment and the patient has not been adjudicated incompetent, written, informed consent for the surgery or medical treatment shall be obtained from the nearest proper relative. For this purpose, the following persons are proper relatives, in the order listed: the patient's spouse, parent, adult child, or adult sibling. If the nearest proper relatives cannot be located, refuse to consent to the procedure, or are unable to consent, the head of the treatment facility or an interested person may petition the committing court for approval for the treatment or may petition a court of competent jurisdiction for the appointment of a guardian. The determination that the patient is not competent, and the reasons for the determination, shall be documented in the patient's clinical record."

Maryland
An LAR can be one of the following in this order:

1. Health care agent
2. Court-appointed guardian
3. Patient's spouse
4. Adult child of patient
   a. If there is more than one adult child, these children can decide together.
5. A parent of the patient
6. Adult sister or adult brother
7. Friend or more distant relative of patient
   a. The friend or distant relative must sign a statement referencing his/her regular contact with the patient and knowledge of the patient's personal beliefs and health care wishes.

**Practical application:**

"When LARs are involved, their role should be documented and, after the elements of consent have been reviewed, their consent should be recorded in the informed consent document in the same manner as if the subject were giving consent directly. In addition to receiving information about the study, it is important for LARs to be informed about the role of an LAR and provided information about the health status of the research subject.[32]"

Mentioned above, "Making Medical Decisions for Someone Else: A Maryland Handbook" is a great resource for informing an LAR about their role.[33]

**How LARs are to make decisions on behalf of the patient/subject:**

It is advised that LARs make decisions for an Impaired Decision Making Capacity (IDMC) patient based upon something called "substituted judgment." This means that empathy is employed by the LAR making the decision that the patient would have made if he or she were able to make decisions.

The next best way LARs are to make decisions is to act in the "best interest" of the patient. LARs are to review the facts of the research, such as the risks and benefits, the subject's medical condition and prognosis, and make a decision that will benefit the patient the most. NIH provides this comment,

"LARs who make research decisions on the basis of *substituted judgment* should be guided by their knowledge of the beliefs, views, and preferences of the subject. Basing decisions on a substituted judgment standard is considered preferable from an ethical standpoint because it is consistent with the principles of respect for persons and autonomy, which are central to informed consent. In the absence of knowledge of subject values, the *best interest* standard is typically used in making decisions on behalf of the subject. While there are some data from studies suggesting that LARs who make clinical care decisions are not always able to predict patient treatment preferences in the research setting, the substituted judgment approach is still favored over the best interest standard. In situations where LARs make consent decisions on behalf of prospective subjects, the autonomy of the subjects is further respected by seeking their assent for participation and by honoring their objection to participation or, subsequently, a desire to withdraw.[34]"

Consenting is an ongoing process, so keep these points in mind from NIH:

"Consent capacity can be affected by disorders with progressive or fluctuating courses. In cases where a subject's cognitive condition is expected to deteriorate or fluctuate, it may make sense to re-evaluate consent capacity (and, as appropriate, strategies for consent enhancement) at several intervals during the study, especially in long-term studies that may involve multiple phases. In addition, such changes in clinical status may affect, for example, the risk/benefit considerations, appropriate alternatives to study participation, and need for additional safeguards or monitoring."

"When consent capacity could diminish during the course of a study, it may be most appropriate to transition to LAR consent and decision-making. In these cases, involving at the start of the study an individual who could serve as an LAR later on may be most prudent. For individuals with conditions that bring about fluctuating levels of consent capacity, it is important to consider the timing of the assessment and consent; it may make sense to time the initial consent carefully to avoid periods when prospective subjects may be experiencing heightened impairments, e.g., an individual with schizophrenia who is refusing medication or acute drug intoxication. In all cases, respecting a subject's right to withdrawal from a research study is a continuation of the initial consent process, and consideration should be given to ensuring that diminished capacity does not limit this right. The right to discontinue participation in HHS-funded or FDA-regulated research at any time without penalty or loss of benefits to which the subject is otherwise entitled is protected in the HHS and FDA regulations. See 45 CFR 46.116(a)(8) and 21 CFR 50.25(a)(8), respectively.[35]"

---

**45 CFR 46.116(b)(8) the New Common Rule: The language is exactly the same as the Common rule 45 CFR 46.116(a)(8).**

A statement that participation is voluntary, refusal to participate will involve no penalty or loss of benefits to which the subject is otherwise entitled, and the subject may discontinue participation at any time without penalty or loss of benefits to which the subject is otherwise entitled.

---

**The regulations mentioning the use of an LAR are as follows:**
**21 CFR 50.20:**
…no investigator may involve a human being as a subject in research covered by these regulations unless the investigator has obtained the legally effective informed consent of the subject or the subject's legally authorized representative.[36]
**45 CFR 46.117 Documentation of informed consent & 21 CFR 50.27**
(b)…the consent form may be either of the following:

**(1)** A written consent document that embodies the elements of informed consent required by §46.116. This form may be read to the subject or the subject's legally authorized representative, but in any event, the investigator shall give either the subject or the representative adequate opportunity to read it before it is signed; or

**(2)** A short form written consent document stating that the elements of informed consent required by §46.116 have been presented orally to the subject or the subject's legally authorized representative. When this method is used, there shall be a witness to the oral presentation. Also, the IRB shall approve a written summary of what is to be said to the subject or the representative. Only the short form itself is to be signed by the subject or the representative. However, the witness shall sign both the short form and a copy of the summary, and the person actually obtaining consent shall sign a copy of the summary. A copy of the summary shall be given to the subject or the representative, in addition to a copy of the short form.[37]

**45 CFR 46.117(b)(1)-(2) the New Common Rule:**

...the *informed* consent form may be either of the following:

**(1)** A written *informed* consent *form that meets the requirements of*

**§__.116.** The investigator shall give either the subject or the *subject's legally authorized* representative adequate opportunity to read *the informed consent form* before it is signed; *alternatively*, this form may be read to the subject or the subject's legally authorized representative.

**(2)** A short form written *informed* consent *form* stating that the elements of informed consent required by **§__.116** have been presented orally to the subject or the subject's legally authorized representative, *and that the key information required by §ll.116(a)(5)(i) was presented first to the subject, before other information, if any, was provided.* The IRB shall approve a written summary of what is to be said to the subject or the *legally authorized* representative. When this method is used, there shall be a witness to the oral presentation. Only the short form itself is to be signed by the subject or the *subject's legally authorized* representative. However, the witness shall sign both the short form and a copy of the summary, and the person actually obtaining consent shall sign a copy of the summary. A copy of the summary shall be given to the subject *or the subject's legally authorized* representative, in addition to a copy of the short form.

**(The italicized font represents the added language in the New Common Rule. See Appendix 28.)**

### 21 CFR 56.111:

(4) Informed consent will be sought from each prospective subject or the subject's legally authorized representative, in accordance with and to the extent required by part 50.[38]

 ICH **ICH GCP "Informed Consent of Trial Subjects" speaks to the Legally Acceptable Representative, Section 4.8**

4.8.2 ... The subject or the subject's legally acceptable representative should be informed in a timely manner if new information becomes available that may be relevant to the subject's willingness to continue participation in the trial. The communication of this information should be documented.

4.8.4 None of the oral and written information concerning the trial, including the written informed consent form, should contain any language that causes the subject or the subject's legally acceptable representative to waive or to appear to waive any legal rights, or that releases or appears to release the investigator, the institution, the sponsor, or their agents from liability for negligence.

4.8.6 The language used in the oral and written information about the trial, including the written informed consent form, should be as non-technical as practical and should be understandable to the subject or the subject's legally acceptable representative and the impartial witness, where applicable.

4.8.7 Before informed consent may be obtained, the investigator, or a person designated by the investigator, should provide the subject or the subject's legally acceptable representative ample time and opportunity to inquire about details of the trial and to decide whether or not to participate in the trial. All questions about the trial should be answered to the satisfaction of the subject or the subject's legally acceptable representative.

4.8.8 Prior to a subject's participation in the trial, the written informed consent form should be signed and personally dated by the subject or by the subject's legally acceptable representative, and by the person who conducted the informed consent discussion.

4.8.9 If a subject is unable to read or if a legally acceptable representative is unable to read, an impartial witness should be present during the entire informed consent discussion. After the written informed consent form and any other written information to be provided to subjects, is read and explained to the subject or the subject's legally acceptable representative, and after the subject or the subject's legally acceptable representative has orally consented to the subject's participation in the trial and, if capable of doing so, has signed and personally dated the informed consent form, the witness should sign and personally date the consent form. By signing the consent form, the witness attests that the information in the consent form and any other written information was accurately explained to, and apparently understood by, the subject or the subject's legally acceptable representative, and that informed consent was freely given by the subject or the subject's legally acceptable representative.

4.8.10(n) That the monitor(s), the auditor(s), the IRB/IEC, and the regulatory authority(ies) will be granted direct access to the subject's original medical records for verification of clinical trial procedures and/or data, without violating the confidentiality of the subject, to the extent permitted by the applicable laws and regulations and that, by signing a written informed consent form, the subject or the subject's legally acceptable representative is authorizing such access.

4.8.10 (p) ...the subject or the subject's legally acceptable representative will be informed in a timely manner if information becomes available that may be relevant to the subject's willingness to continue participation in the trial.

Additionally, ICH GCP speaks to the use of an LAR for non-therapeutic trials. (Examples of non-therapeutic research include Laboratory studies, behavioral studies, observational studies, prevention studies, screening studies, medical chart reviews, and supportive care studies (e.g., stress management techniques)). Non-therapeutic research purposes to obtain information that may benefit the health of patients in the future. See "non-therapeutic research" in Chapter 1, Section 1.2: *Defining the Types of Research Studies.*

4.8.14 Non-therapeutic trials may be conducted in subjects with consent of a legally acceptable representative provided the following conditions are fulfilled:

   (a)   The objectives of the trial cannot be met by means of a trial in subjects who can give informed consent personally.
   (b)   The foreseeable risks to the subjects are low.
   (c)   The negative impact on the subject's well-being is minimized and low.
   (d)   The trial is not prohibited by law.
   (e)   The approval/favorable opinion of the IRB/IEC is expressly sought on the inclusion of such subjects, and the written approval/ favorable opinion covers this aspect.

Such trials, unless an exception is justified, should be conducted in patients having a disease or condition for which the investigational product is intended. Subjects in these trials should be particularly closely monitored and should be withdrawn if they appear to be unduly distressed.

4.8.11 Prior to participation in the trial, the subject or the subject's legally acceptable representative should receive a copy of the signed and dated written informed consent form and any other written information provided to the subjects. During a subject's participation in the trial, the subject or the subject's legally acceptable representative should receive a copy of the signed and dated consent form updates and a copy of any amendments to the written information provided to subjects.

4.8.12 When a clinical trial (therapeutic or non-therapeutic) includes subjects who can only be enrolled in the trial with the consent of the subject's legally acceptable representative (e.g., minors, or patients with severe dementia), the subject should be informed about the trial to the extent compatible with the subject's understanding and, if capable, the subject should sign and personally date the written informed consent.

4.8.15 In emergency situations, when prior consent of the subject is not possible, the consent of the subject's legally acceptable representative, if present, should be requested. When prior consent of the subject is not possible, and the subject's legally acceptable representative is not available, enrolment of the subject should require measures described in the protocol and/or elsewhere, with documented approval/favorable opinion by the IRB/IEC, to protect the rights, safety and well-being of the subject and to ensure compliance with applicable regulatory requirements. The subject or the subject's legally acceptable representative should be informed about the trial as soon as possible and consent to continue and other consent as appropriate (see 4.8.10) should be requested.[39]

**WITNESS**

🏃ICH A witness is defined as

**ICH GCP E6 R2: 1.26**

Impartial Witness

A person, who is independent of the trial, who cannot be unfairly influenced by people involved with the trial, who attends the informed consent process if the subject or the subject's legally acceptable representative cannot read, and who reads the informed consent form and any other written information supplied to the subject

A witness is required in the following circumstances:

- When consenting an illiterate (a person unable to read or write) English-speaking subject (per FDA);
- When the short (consent) form is used (per FDA and HHS); and,
- If a subject is unable to read or if a legally acceptable representative is unable to read (per ICH GCP).[40]

Here are the references:

**Illiterate English-Speaking Subjects**

A person who speaks and understands English, but does not read and write, can be enrolled in a study by "making their mark" on the consent document, when consistent with applicable state law.

A person who can understand and comprehend spoken English, but is physically unable to talk or write, can be entered into a study if they are competent and able to indicate approval or disapproval by other means. If (1) the person retains the ability to understand the concepts of the study and evaluate the risk and benefit of being in the study when it is explained verbally (still competent) and (2) is able to indicate approval or disapproval to study entry, they may be entered into the study.

---

📝 The consent form should document the method used for communication with the prospective subject and the specific means by which the prospective subject communicated agreement to participate in the study. An impartial third party should witness the entire consent process and sign the consent document. A video tape recording of the consent interview is recommended.[41]

---

(Also, see "Short Form" consent in Chapter 2, Section 2.5.3.)

The Code of Federal Regulations references:

21 CFR 50.27 (b)(2) and 45 CFR 46.117 (b)(2)

(2) A *short form* written consent document stating that the elements of informed consent required by 50.25(46.116) have been presented orally to the subject or the subject's legally authorized representative. When this method is used, there shall be a witness to the oral presentation. Also, the IRB shall approve a written summary of what is to be said to the subject or the representative. Only the short

form itself is to be signed by the subject or the representative. However, the witness shall sign both the short form and a copy of the summary, and the person actually obtaining the consent shall sign a copy of the summary. A copy of the summary shall be given to the subject or the representative in addition to a copy of the short form.

---

**45 CFR 46.117(b)(2) the New Common Rule:**
  A short form written *informed* consent *form* stating that the elements of informed consent required by §__.116 have been presented orally to the subject or the subject's legally authorized representative, *and that the key information required by §ll.116(a)(5)(i) was presented first to the subject, before other information, if any, was provided.* The IRB shall approve a written summary of what is to be said to the subject or the *legally authorized* representative. When this method is used, there shall be a witness to the oral presentation. Only the short form itself is to be signed by the subject or the *subject's legally authorized* representative. However, the witness shall sign both the short form and a copy of the summary, and the person actually obtaining consent shall sign a copy of the summary. A copy of the summary shall be given to the subject *or the subject's legally authorized* representative, in addition to a copy of the short form.
  **(The italicized font represents the added language in the New Common Rule. See Appendix 28.)**

---

In the context of the short form:

"A witness is required to attest to the adequacy of the consent process and to the subject's voluntary consent. Therefore, the witness must be present during the entire consent interview, not just for signing the documents.[42]"

ᛁCH **ICH GCP E6 R2 references:**

4.8.6 The language used in the oral and written information about the trial, including the written informed consent form, should be as non-technical as practical and should be understandable to the subject or the subject's legally acceptable representative and the impartial witness, where applicable.

4.8.9 If a subject is unable to read or if a legally acceptable representative is unable to read, an impartial witness should be present during the entire informed consent discussion. After the written informed consent form and any other written information to be provided to subjects, is read and explained to the subject or the subject's legally acceptable representative, and after the subject or the subject's legally acceptable representative has orally consented to the subject's participation in the trial and, if capable of doing so, has signed and personally dated the informed consent form, the witness should sign and personally date the consent form. By signing the consent form, the witness attests that the information in the consent form and any other written information was accurately explained to, and apparently understood by, the subject or the subject's legally acceptable representative, and that informed consent was freely given by the subject or the subject's legally acceptable representative.[43]

Logistics

1. A witness, being a person who is independent of the trial, cannot be a study team member. A witness can be a friend, family member, or caregiver that is accompanying the patient. A witness can also be a hospital nurse or technician or other hospital staff member that is <u>not</u> involved with the trial in any way.

2. 👍 A study team member will need to advise the witness as to what they are expected to do in accordance with the CFR and ICH GCP.

3. 👍 Since the witness is to "… witness the entire consent process and sign the consent document", the witness signature line should be the very LAST one on the consent form so that he or she can witness the consent process and the signing of all other necessary parties.
4. Create two lines in the witness signature area of the consent form to document:
    a. the method used to communicate with the subject
    b. the specific means by which the subject communicated agreement to participate in the study

## 6.7  WHAT TO DO WHEN A PI DEPARTS FROM A STUDY OR INSTITUTION

*Purpose of section*:

- Suggests a Plan of Action when a PI leaves the Institution, but the study remains with the Institution
- Suggests a Plan of Action when the PI steps down from a study or the PI leaves the Institution and the study closes
- Suggests a Plan of Action when a PI leaves the Institution and transfers the study to the new work location
- Outlines grant requirements for a "Change of Grantee Organization" when a study is transferred to a new location
- Provides tips on Institutional Project Management when a PI leaves or steps down

There are no federal regulations that speak to this occurrence.
ICH GCP has the following to say:
ICH GCP E6 R2
🎯ICH 4.12 Premature Termination or Suspension of a Trial
If the trial is prematurely **terminated or suspended for any reason**, the investigator/institution should promptly **inform the trial subjects**, should assure appropriate therapy and follow-up for the subjects, and, where required by the applicable regulatory requirement(s), should inform the regulatory authority(ies). In addition:
4.12.1 If the **investigator terminates or suspends** a trial without prior agreement of the sponsor, the investigator should inform the institution where applicable, and the investigator/institution should promptly inform the sponsor and the IRB/IEC, and should provide the sponsor and the IRB/IEC a detailed written explanation of the termination or suspension.
4.12.2 If the **sponsor terminates or suspends** a trial (see 5.21), the investigator should promptly inform the institution where applicable and the investigator/institution should promptly inform the IRB/IEC and provide the IRB/IEC a detailed written explanation of the termination or suspension.
4.12.3 If the **IRB/IEC terminates or suspends** its approval/favorable opinion of a trial (see 3.1.2 and 3.3.9), the investigator should inform the institution where applicable and the investigator/institution should promptly notify the sponsor and provide the sponsor with a detailed written explanation of the termination or suspension.[44]
We will explore a few scenarios below and the steps you can take. For all scenarios, check the following first:

1. Your Institutional Policy regarding PI departure;

2. Your IRB Policy regarding PI departure; and,
3. The contract or award signed with a Sponsor. Read the "Termination" clauses and the "Data Ownership" clauses.

If your Institution or IRB does not have a current policy or procedure, or if there is a policy or procedure, but it lacks sufficient detail, the following is recommended:

SCENARIO ONE

The PI steps down from a study but the study continues at the Institution, or the PI leaves the Institution while the study remains at the Institution

1. **Start planning and notification at least TWO MONTHS in advance of the planned step down or departure**.
2. The PI needs to contact the IRB to let them know of his intention to depart from the study.
   a. Typically, the PI or a study team member will need to submit notification of the PI departure, along with an explanation, to the IRB through the IRB's electronic submission software program.
3. The PI should ask colleagues if any of them would like to become the Principal Investigator for the trial.
   a. If the study has a Co-Investigator or Sub-Investigator, they cannot automatically take on the role of the Principal Investigator, but would be first choices to become the PI.
4. Your Institution may have a process whereby a PI nominee needs to be vetted to make sure he or she has the qualifications and training to be a Principal Investigator. This could be through a Medical Department Chair, or a committee or the IRB. Check your Institution's policy.
   a. If the study has a Co-Investigator, he or she would have been vetted at the time of joining the study. Transitioning the role of the Principal Investigator to a Co-Investigator will be the easiest and smoothest transition.
5. The PI will need to speak with the Sponsor to inform the Sponsor of his/her decision to step down and to provide a name of a suggested new PI if a colleague is willing to take over the study, or if a Co-I is willing to become the singular PI, or if a Sub-I is willing to step up.
   a. The Sponsor may request the PI write a letter of resignation from the study and the reasons for the departure (in keeping with ICH GCP).
   b. If the Sponsor accepts another PI, the Sponsor will write an Amendment to the Study naming the new PI along with the effective date.

   i. Some Sponsors want a new contract ratified rather than an Amendment, but most create an Amendment.
   ii. Typically, contracts have a "no reassignment" or "no substitution" clause stating that the PI or Institution may not reassign the study to another PI without the Sponsor's or CRO's approval.
   iii. When the study is funded by a grant, there is an option for the grantee (meaning the Institution that received the award) to issue a subaward for the remainder of the study to another person who will become the PI if the awarding agency approves of the PI nominee.
   c. If the study is an IND study, FDA Form 1572 will need to be updated with the new PI's name and sent to the Sponsor.
   i. The FDA requires the knowledge of who the PI is for IND studies. (The Sponsor takes care of this step.)

6. Have your Compliance Department perform an internal audit of study data, CRFs/eCRFs, IDS drug inventory or device inventory if applicable, Regulatory Binder, IRB review documentation, etc. at least 2 months prior to the PI stepping down or leaving. Resolve all questions, data entry errors, and needed corrections before transitioning to the new PI.
   a. This allows the current PI to leave with a good reputation and to resolve any issues with his/her knowledge of the history of the study, and it protects the new PI by starting with a documented study status.
7. Have the new PI fill out a Conflict of Interest form and report it pursuant to Federal regulation, Institutional, and Sponsor policy.
8. If the study continues with a new PI, the Responsible Party will need to update ClinicalTrials. gov if the study is an "applicable clinical trial" and has, therefore, been registered on this site.
9. If the trial continues, the *Delegation of Authority* (see Chapter 4, Section 4.5.1) will need to be updated with the new PI's name and responsibilities.
10. The informed consent form will have to be amended to name the new PI, and study subjects will need to be notified by the study team. The revised consent form will need to be used from the effective date of the new consent onward and the previous consent form retired.
   a. **IRB** Follow your IRB's procedure for re-consenting all active subjects or providing them a one-page amendment to sign.
11. The study team will need to notify all stakeholders within the Institution of the change in PI and update all forms and advertising materials naming the PI. (Anything subject facing will have to be submitted to the IRB for approval.)
12. Your Contracts Office/Legal Department will need to clarify which PI has the right to publish the results of the trial. This point should be addressed in the revised contract or amendment naming the new PI.

## SCENARIO TWO
**The PI steps down from a study or leaves the Institution and the study closes.**

1. Start planning and notification at least **TWO MONTHS** in advance of the planned step down or departure.
2. The PI needs to contact the IRB to let them know of his intention to depart from the study.
   a. Typically, the PI or a study team member will need to submit notification of the PI departure to the IRB through the IRB's electronic submission software program.
3. The PI will need to speak with the Sponsor to inform them of her decision to step down.
   a. The Sponsor may request the PI write a letter of resignation from the study.
4. Have your Compliance Department perform an internal audit of study data, CRFs/eCRFs, IDS drug inventory or device inventory if applicable, Regulatory Binder, IRB review documentation, etc. at least 2 months prior to the PI stepping down or leaving. Resolve all questions, data entry errors, and needed corrections.
   a. If there is an Industry Monitor for the study, the Compliance review will be in addition to the Industry Monitor's review, and **prior** to the Monitor's review and close out of your site.
5. The Sponsor will write a formal closure letter.
6. When the study closes, the Responsible Party will need to update ClinicalTrials.gov if the study is an "applicable clinical trial" and has, therefore, been registered on this site.

7. If the Sponsor chooses to close the study, ALL Institutional systems will need to reflect the change. Make sure notifications go to the following (This list is not exhaustive.):
   a. Grants Office or Contracts Office (If the study was funded by a grant, then the Grants office needs notification. If the study was funded by an Industry contract, then the Contracts office will need notification.)
   b. Finance Office
      i. The financial account for the study should be closed after final invoicing and receipt of funds, and final reconciliation.
   c. The office responsible for Study ID retirement
      i. This office/party makes sure the Study ID is withdrawn from all hospital systems.
   d. IRB
      i. Send the formal Sponsor letter of closure.
   e. The Research Pharmacy, if applicable
   f. Any other office or party with a need-to-know according to your Institution's infrastructure.
8. A plan will need to be developed by the departing PI, the Sponsor, and IRB (meaning the Institutional Office of Human Research Protections that supports the IRB) regarding the safe exit of subjects from the study.
9. Study subjects will have to be notified. It is typically the study team that sends the notification and is available for questions.

SCENARIO THREE
The PI is leaving the Institution and is transferring the study to the new Medical Center where he/she is going.

**FUNDING CONSIDERATIONS**
**GRANTS**

For the transfer of an NIH grant to a new Institution, there are application instructions that must be followed. The transfer is seen as a "Funding Opportunity," which must be applied for rather than it being a guaranteed right to the funds at the new Institution. The Title for it is "Change of Grantee Organization (Type 7 Parent)." Additionally, the Grant Form PHS 398, known as the "Grant Application Kit," must be filled out. Instructions and forms for downloading can be found here: https://grants.nih.gov/grants/funding/phs398/phs398.html.[45]

The forms may need to route through the current Institution for review and approval prior to being sent to the new Institution. Check your IRB and Grants office policies.

**Here is NIH's stated position:**

*Although requests for change of grantee organization may be submitted through this FOA, there is no guarantee that an award will be transferred to the new organization. All applicants are encouraged to discuss potential requests with the awarding IC before submission.* (Source: DHHS Overview Information through grants.nih.gov)

"FOA" means Funding Opportunity Announcement.

"IC" means the NIH Institute or Center (For example, NIAID, the National Institute for Allergy and Infectious Diseases).

The best time to transfer a grant is on its anniversary date, when yearly reconciliation is performed.

**The overview and application for the Change of Grantee Organization Funding Opportunity can be found here:** https://grants.nih.gov/grants/guide/pa-files/PA-18-590.html Contact your Grants Administration Office for their procedure and assistance.

### INDUSTRY

For transitioning Industry Sponsor funding, talk with the CRO if the CRO has been assigned contracting and financial responsibilities. Otherwise, talk to the Sponsor. If the new site has the potential to enroll subjects at a better or equal rate to your current Institution, you will want to speak to this point (because you have already done your Feasibility Analysis for the new site).

Ask the CRO/Sponsor if they are willing to contract and finance the PI at the new Institution and close out the contract and budget at the current Institution.

Get in touch with your Institution's Industry Clinical Trials Office to take you through their process. The best time for you to transfer will be:

- prior to enrollment, or
- after your research subjects have completed all follow-up visits and you have not enrolled anyone new, or
- when your follow-up visits consist of phone call follow-ups only, or
- when you are at the data analysis stage.

Otherwise, your research subjects will have to be willing to travel to the new Medical Center.

### INSTITUTIONAL REVIEW BOARD CONSIDERATIONS

If your study is being reviewed and followed by a Single IRB outside of your Institution or by a Central IRB, it will be easy to ask for a change in study location by a simple Amendment (after Sponsor/funding approval of the transfer).

If your study is being reviewed and followed by your local IRB, the PI needs to contact the local IRB to let them know of his upcoming departure when the transfer is official.

Typically, the PI or a study team member will need to submit notification of the PI departure, along with an explanation, to the IRB through the IRB's electronic submission software program.

Additionally, the PI will need to contact the IRB at the Institution where she will be going to submit the study for IRB review and approval. This will have to be accomplished prior to the transfer, ideally, (to avoid delays) or prior to any study research activity at the new location.

See the *Guidance for IRBs, Clinical Investigators, and Sponsors:*
*Considerations When Transferring Clinical Investigation Oversight to Another IRB*
https://www.fda.gov/downloads/RegulatoryInformation/Guidances/UCM307779.pdf.[46]

### DATABASE CONSIDERATIONS

If your research data are housed on a server through a Sponsor's software application, the research data ownership will be described in your contract/Clinical Trial Agreement.

Typically, the source data in the form of electronic medical records, lab reports, and the like are the sole property of the medical center. The research data documented within Sponsor Case Report Forms are the sole property of the Sponsor. See your contract for the exact language.

If the research database is in the Cloud or web-based, wherever the PI transfers, the data will be accessible. There will be no particular "transfer" requirements as the data ownership is already specified in the contract and there are no physical files to move. The Data section of the study contract will not need to be amended as there will be no change to where and how the research data will be housed and secured.

If the research database is local to an Institution, a Data Transfer Agreement (DTA) will need to be written and signed between your current Institution and the new Institution. See the DTA definition in the Glossary.

A DTA will be needed for identifiable information, Limited Data Sets, and De-identified information as "data" are still being transferred regardless of its form.

The study consent form will need to be amended to inform subjects that their PHI and study data will be moved—inclusive of how, where, and the security measures to be employed.

**Source Data (This is a Best Practice. Your Institutional Policy may differ.)**

The cleanest way to deal with source data is to perform a study close out visit in the current location, which will include examining source documents against CRFs/eCRFs. Complete and finalize the close out, including resolution of all queries. Make sure all source data are captured, and captured correctly on the Case Report Forms. The close out should be performed by an internal Compliance Department Associate or a seasoned Research Coordinator, as well as a Monitor from the Sponsor's company or CRO (if an Industry study). The PI should oversee the close out or the PI should delegate the oversight to a highly trusted study team member, such as a Co-I or Sub-I. Have this step signed off by the PI and Sponsor Monitor, if applicable, before transfer. Do not take any source data with you to the new location. It is the property of the current Institution.

## HUMAN BIOLOGICAL SAMPLES CONSIDERATIONS

Human biological samples include all types of human tissue, body fluids, organ biopsies, urine, stools, and cells.

To transfer human biological samples from one Institution to another, a Materials Transfer Agreement (MTA) is required. See your Legal or MTA office within your Institution for the creation and ratification of an MTA. (See the Glossary for the definition of an MTA.)

A Data Transfer Agreement will need to accompany the MTA if data are transferred along with the biological samples.

## EQUIPMENT TRANSFER CONSIDERATIONS

### Industry

If an Industry Sponsor loaned you equipment for your study, the Sponsor can retrieve the equipment from your current location and arrange to have it sent to your new location.

We have experienced only one Industry Sponsor that was willing to donate equipment to an Institution after study completion. As this is rare, it is not likely, but you can always ask if the Sponsor would like to donate the equipment to the current location if your new Institution has the equipment needed.

### Grants/Awards

Check with the Institution to which you are transferring. They may have financial support available for the transfer of equipment with the onboarding of new Faculty members.

If not, write the name of the equipment you purchased with your grant funds, the model, any tag/identifier put on it by your Institution, and where it is located. Contact your Property Management Department or your Department Chair (pursuant to your Institutional Policy) to request the process for transferring equipment.

## MANUSCRIPT WRITING AND PUBLISHING CONSIDERATIONS

The PI should determine:

- whether anyone from the current Institution should be named as an author or be acknowledged on future manuscripts

- whether anyone from the current Institution should be contacted after database lock and data analysis to assist in the writing of manuscripts

These decisions should be made prior to departure and communicated to the individuals affected and to the current Institution's Department Chair for documentation.

## 6.8 CONSEQUENCES OF CLINICAL RESEARCH NON-COMPLIANCE AND HOW TO RESPOND TO NON-COMPLIANCE

*Purpose of section*:

- **Provides overview of common non-compliance issues found in FDA audits**
- **Suggests responses to non-compliance for Institutions**
- **Information on FDA clinical investigator disqualification proceedings**

What is research non-compliance?

Research non-compliance is the failure or refusal to comply with a federal law, federal regulation, state law, IRB policy, Institutional policy, or study protocol regarding clinical research conduct and/or human subjects protections.

In Fiscal Year 2017, the FDA conducted 700 medical institution audits. Examples of common non-compliance found were:

- Failure to follow the investigational plan/agreement or regulations, or both;
- Protocol deviations;
- Inadequate recordkeeping;
- Inadequate subject protection, such as informed consent issues or failure to report Adverse Events (AEs);
- Inadequate accountability for the investigational product;
- Inadequate communication with the IRB; and
- The investigational product was represented as safe or effective.[47]

Neither the FDA nor the Code of Federal Regulations informs or advises Institutions on what the specific internal institutional processes for managing non-compliance should be beyond what is written in the regulations. The FDA does expect that each Institution will have "written procedures" for handling non-compliance. Therefore, it is the responsibility of the Institution, through its IRB (Human Research Protections Office) or Compliance Department, to create policies and procedures for the steps the Institution will take if a PI is non-compliant in the research under his/her supervision.

However, some Institutions lack policies and procedures where the regulations are silent.

For example, at a hospital where one of the author's worked, there was a compliance review procedure, but no procedure for what action to take if a PI were found deficient! What should have been a two-day process for rolling out next steps and communicating with all parties necessary, became a two-month scramble with a flurry of e-mails ensuing. Suffice it to say, if your Institution needs ideas for the creation of written procedures for non-compliance, or needs to improve upon the ones it does have, here are some ideas.

1. Severity Scale

(1) First, create a scale to define each level of non-compliance severity.
   a. For example:
      i. Minor—First infraction that is not serious or an infraction that does not increase risk to subjects
         1. Example: protocol deviation (defined as a variation from processes or procedures defined in a protocol)
            a. Seeing a subject outside of a time window
         2. Example: Data were retained for a few months shorter than the period required by Federal regulation
      ii. Serious—Human Subjects are not protected as they should be and are exposed to risk.
         1. Example: Enrolling one subject in two (2) IND trials simultaneously
         2. Example: Enrolling a subject who did not meet the inclusion or exclusion criteria
         3. Example: Neglecting to get the consent of a subject
         4. Example: Protocol violation (defined as a significant departure from processes or procedures that were required by the protocol)
            a. For example, providing a medication to a subject that is not allowed (This medication may not increase risk to the subject, but may interfere with the intervention to the point that the subject will have to be withdrawn from the study.)
         5. Example: A Breach of confidentiality
      iii. Continuing—There is a repetitive pattern and the infraction is serious.
         1. Example: The PI and study team repeatedly miss the yearly IRB continuing review deadline, creating a suspension in their research each time. They do not stop research activities during the suspension.
         2. Comments: This could either be very poor project management/operations or a blatant disregard for IRB policy and human subjects protections.
      iv. Intentional—The PI is aware and intentionally performed, approved of, or refused to intervene to stop, fraud.
         1. Example: falsifying data
         2. Example: Using a specimen from one patient who met the enrollment criteria for multiple subjects' screening

2. Department Ownership

   Second, determine which Hospital Department will impose the consequences for non-compliance and report to the IRB. Will it be the Compliance Department or the Human Research Protections Office supporting the IRB? It can be either; the responsibility must have an "owner." Matters for consideration: Which Department has the staff and time available, and the Operations expertise to follow through on disciplinary action? Non-compliance should be quite infrequent at your Institution, but when it occurs, the designated staff will need to be able to take action immediately and confront persons with power in your Institution.

3. Plan of Action

   Third, determine a plan for disciplinary action for each level of non-compliance.
   **For example, for minor non-compliance:**

The Department taking ownership will gather evidence, decide on the Plan of Action, retain documentation, and confirm satisfactory completion of the Plan of Action.

**If the infraction was protocol related:**

The designated Department will require the study team to meet with the relevant Sponsor/CRO contact to review significant points in the protocol again and as an action step, require the creation of laminated cards for the team to keep and serve as reminders of those points. This non-electronic solution is suggested so that study team members have instant access to necessary information as the team provides research care for subjects in clinics, surgical suites, and the lab. (It is very difficult to remember all the necessary details of a specific protocol when a study team conducts multiple studies. Reminders help compliance!)

**If the infraction was GCP or conduct related:**

The Department taking ownership will require the study team members to take a course in ICH GCP and provide the certificate to acknowledge completion and a passing score.

**For serious or continuing non-compliance:**

The Department taking ownership will promptly notify the PI if he/she was not informed at the time of the discovery of non-compliance and will gather all evidence and documentation from the PI and the internal audit records, and/or other mechanism that revealed the non-compliance, and will promptly report the non-compliance to the IRB for review and adjudication of the infraction(s).

The IRB will prioritize any non-compliance reviews. After review, the IRB may require one or more of the following consequences or/and establish their own consequences:

**(a)** Internal monitoring of the research study;
**(b)** Witnessing the informed consent process for subjects;
**(c)** More frequent continuing reviews;
**(d)** Warning Letter (notifying the individual/s that the infraction can never happen again) without further consequence;
**(e)** Notification to current subjects in the study;
**(f)** Notification to current and completed subjects of the study;
**(g)** Training/Retraining of the PI and Study Team;
**(h)** Suspension of any future initial study reviews until the current infraction(s) is(are) addressed;
**(i)** Suspension of the study until resolution;
**(j)** Placing restrictions on publication;
**(k)** Allow follow-up visits with active subjects, but suspend new subject enrollments;
**(l)** Revising the Consent Form and reconsenting subjects;
**(m)** Replacing the PI of the study;
**(n)** Terminating approval of the study;
**(o)** Stricter or revised DSMB review plan;
**(p)** Improved confidentiality controls;
**(q)** Submission of periodic status reports from the PI to the IRB or Compliance Department;
**(r)** Request for Letter of Explanation and Plan of Action from the PI; and,
**(s)** IRB meeting with the PI in attendance to present his/her Plan of Action inclusive of deadlines.

The Code of Federal Regulations has clear instruction regarding:

**i.** suspension of approval
**ii.** termination of approval
**iii.** reporting

**iv.** serious non-compliance

**v.** continuing non-compliance

**Here are the references:**

**21 CFR 56.108 IRB functions and operations**

(b) Follow written procedures for **ensuring prompt reporting to the IRB, appropriate institutional officials, and the Food and Drug Administration of:** (1) Any unanticipated problems involving risks to human subjects or others; **(2) any instance of serious or continuing noncompliance with these regulations or the requirements or determinations of the IRB; or (3) any suspension or termination of IRB approval.**[48]

---

**21 CFR 56.113 Suspension or termination of IRB approval of research.**

**An IRB shall have authority to suspend or terminate approval of research** that is not being conducted in accordance with the IRB's requirements or that has been associated with unexpected serious harm to subjects. Any suspension or termination of approval shall include a statement of the reasons for the IRB's action and shall be **reported promptly to the investigator, appropriate institutional officials, and the Food and Drug Administration.**[49]

---

## ϽϹ<sup>ICH</sup> ICH GCP E6 R2

### 5.20 Noncompliance

5.20.1 Noncompliance with the protocol, SOPs, GCP, and/or applicable regulatory requirement(s) by an investigator/institution, or by member(s) of the sponsor's staff should lead to prompt action by the sponsor to secure compliance.

**ADDENDUM**

If noncompliance that significantly affects or has the potential to significantly affect human subject protection or reliability of trial results is discovered, the sponsor should perform a root cause analysis and implement appropriate corrective and preventive actions.

5.20.2 If the monitoring and/or auditing identifies serious and/or persistent noncompliance on the part of an investigator/institution, the sponsor should terminate the investigator's/institution's participation in the trial. When an investigator's/institution's participation is terminated because of noncompliance, the sponsor should notify promptly the regulatory authority(ies).[50]

**For Intentional non-compliance:**

The legal definition of fraud is: "A false representation of a matter of fact—whether by words or by conduct, by false or misleading allegations, or by concealment of what should have been disclosed. Farlex Legal Dictionary

Laws against fraud vary from state to state and can be criminal or civil in nature. Criminal fraud requires criminal intent on the part of the perpetrator, and is punishable by fines or imprisonment. http://criminal.findlaw.com/criminal-charges/fraud.html

Because of the very serious nature of fraud/intentional non-compliance, consultation with your Institute's Legal Department is recommended.

**FDA Audits and Resulting Investigator Restriction or Disqualification:**

In certain situations, in which FDA alleges a clinical investigator has violated applicable regulations, FDA may initiate a clinical investigator disqualification proceeding. https://www.fda.gov/ICECI/EnforcementActions/ucm321308.htm.[51]

**Here are the FDA terms used in the context of clinical investigator disqualification proceedings:**

**NIDPOE**—A Notice of Initiation of Disqualification Proceedings and Opportunity to Explain (NIDPOE) letter informs the recipient clinical investigator that FDA is initiating an administrative proceeding to determine whether the clinical investigator should be disqualified from receiving investigational products pursuant to the Food and Drug Administration's regulations.

**NOOH**—The Notice of Opportunity for Hearing (NOOH) provides an individual with the opportunity for a hearing on a regulatory action, including a proposed action (such as disqualification), before a presiding officer designated by the Commissioner.

**Not Disqualified Clinical Investigator**—FDA may discontinue a disqualification proceeding when an investigator offers an explanation in response to the NIDPOE that is accepted by the applicable Center. If an explanation is offered by an investigator but not accepted by the applicable Center, the investigator is given an opportunity for an informal regulatory hearing to determine whether the investigator should remain eligible to receive FDA-regulated test articles. After review of the administrative record of a regulatory disqualification proceeding, the Commissioner of Food and Drugs may determine that the investigator should continue to be eligible to receive FDA-regulated test articles and to conduct any clinical investigation that supports an application for a research or marketing permit for products regulated by FDA.

**Disqualified Clinical Investigator**—FDA may disqualify a clinical investigator if the clinical investigator has repeatedly or deliberately failed to comply with applicable regulatory requirements or the clinical investigator has repeatedly or deliberately submitted false information to the sponsor or, if applicable, to FDA, in any required report. A disqualified clinical investigator is not eligible to receive investigational drugs, biologics, or devices, and is not eligible to conduct any clinical investigation that supports an application for a research or marketing permit for products regulated by FDA (including drugs, biologics, devices, new animal drugs, foods, including dietary supplements, that bear a nutrient content claim or a health claim, infant formulas, food and color additives, and tobacco products). In the past, the phrase "totally restricted" was also used to refer to clinical investigators who had been disqualified. Where an investigator has been reinstated, it is so noted.

**Totally Restricted Clinical Investigator**—In the past, the phrase "totally restricted" was also used to refer to clinical investigators who had been disqualified. It is important to underscore the difference between "totally restricted" clinical investigators and "restricted" clinical investigators. "Totally restricted" investigators are ineligible to receive investigational products (absent reinstatement).

**Restricted Clinical Investigator**—FDA may, in some instances, allow a clinical investigator to enter into a restricted agreement when the agency believes that lesser sanctions than disqualification would be adequate to protect the public health. The decision to offer a restricted agreement is within the discretion of FDA. A restricted clinical investigator is still eligible to receive investigational products, provided the investigator conducts regulated studies in accordance with the restrictions specified in their agreement with FDA and all applicable regulatory requirements.

https://www.fda.gov/ICECI/EnforcementActions/ucm321308.htm.[52]

Code of Federal Regulation reference: 21 CFR 312.70 (IND) and 21 CFR 812.119 (IDE) "Disqualification of a Clinical Investigator".[53]

## ENDNOTES

[1] 21 CFR 312 Subpart I, which is 21 CFR 312.300-320, https://www.accessdata.fda.gov/scripts/cdrh/cfdocs/cfCFR/CFRSearch.cfm?fr=312.300 [accessed 28.03.18].

[2] https://www.fda.gov/NewsEvents/PublicHealthFocus/ExpandedAccessCompassionateUse/default.htm [accessed 28.03.18].

[3] Ibid.

[4] 21 CFR 312.305(b), https://www.accessdata.fda.gov/scripts/cdrh/cfdocs/cfcfr/CFRSearch.cfm?CFRPart=312&showFR=1&subpartNode=21:5.0.1.1.3.9 [accessed 28.03.18].

[5] https://www.fda.gov/NewsEvents/PublicHealthFocus/ExpandedAccessCompassionateUse/default.htm [accessed 28.03.18].

[6] Ibid.

[7] https://www.fda.gov/regulatoryinformation/guidances/ucm126491.htm [accessed 28.03.18].

[8] https://www.fda.gov/aboutfda/centersoffices/officeofmedicalproductsandtobacco/cder/contactcder/default.htm [accessed 28.03.18].

[9] *Expanded Access to Investigational Drugs for Treatment Use—Questions and Answers,* https://www.fda.gov/downloads/drugs/guidancecomplianceregulatoryinformation/guidances/ucm351261.pdf [accessed 28.03.18].

[10] 21 CFR 312.315 https://www.gpo.gov/fdsys/granule/CFR-2013-title21-vol5/CFR-2013-title21-vol5-sec312-315 [accessed 28.03.18].

[11] 21 CFR 312.320, https://www.accessdata.fda.gov/scripts/cdrh/cfdocs/cfcfr/CFRSearch.cfm?fr=312.320 [accessed 28.03.18].

[12] Ibid.

[13] Ibid.

[14] *Charging for Investigational Drugs Under an IND—Questions and Answers Guidance for Industry June 2016* https://www.fda.gov/downloads/Drugs/GuidanceComplianceRegulatoryInformation/Guidances/UCM351264.pd [accessed 28.03.18].

[15] 21 CFR 312.8(b)(1)(i)-(iii), https://www.gpo.gov/fdsys/granule/CFR-2014-title16-vol1/CFR-2014-title16-vol1-part312 [accessed 28.03.18].

[16] 21 CFR 56.104 (c) https://www.accessdata.fda.gov/scripts/cdrh/cfdocs/cfcfr/CFRSearch.cfm?fr=56.104 [accessed 28.03.18].

[17] 21 CFR 312.32 (a), https://www.accessdata.fda.gov/scripts/cdrh/cfdocs/cfcfr/CFRSearch.cfm?fr=312.32">https://www.accessdata.fda.gov/scripts/cdrh/cfdocs/cfcfr/CFRSearch.cfm?fr=312.32 [accessed 28.03.18].

[18] 21 CFR 50.23 (a), https://www.accessdata.fda.gov/scripts/cdrh/cfdocs/cfcfr/CFRSearch.cfm?fr=50.23.

[19] www.fda.gov/medicaldevices/deviceregulationandguidance [accessed 28.03.18].

[20] 21 CFR 812.36 (a), https://www.accessdata.fda.gov/scripts/cdrh/cfdocs/cfcfr/CFRSearch.cfm?fr=812.36 [accessed 28.03.18].

[21] https://www.accessdata.fda.gov/scripts/cdrh/cfdocs/cfcfr/CFRSearch.cfm?fr=812.150 [accessed 28.03.18].

[22] Privacy Rule at 45 CFR 164.512., https://www.gpo.gov/fdsys/granule/CFR-2004-title45-vol1/CFR-2004-title45-vol1-sec164-512 [accessed 28.03.18].

[23] https://privacyruleandresearch.nih.gov/pr_08.asp [accessed 28.03.18].

[24] https://www.hhs.gov/hipaa/for-professionals/privacy/guidance/disclosures-public-health-activities/index.html [accessed 28.03.18].

[25] https://law.justia.com/codes/maryland/2013/article-gho/ [accessed 28.03.18].

[26] https://www.hhs.gov/ohrp/regulations-and-policy/guidance/prisoner-research-ohrp-guidance-2003/index.html [accessed 28.03.18].

[27] https://www.hhs.gov/ohrp/regulations-and-policy/guidance/prisoner-research-ohrp-guidance-2003/index.html [accessed 28.03.18].

[28] Ibid.

[29] https://www.hhs.gov/ohrp/regulations-and-policy/regulations/45-cfr-46/index.html [accessed 38.02.18].

[30] https://grants.nih.gov/grants/policy/questionablecapacity.htm#_ftn11 [accessed 28.03.18].

[31] http://www.marylandattorneygeneral.gov/Pages/HealthPolicy/default.aspx [accessed 28.03.18].

[32] Ibid.

[33] https://grants.nih.gov/grants/policy/questionablecapacity.htm#_ftn11 [accessed 28.03.18].

[34] Ibid.

[35] Ibid.

[36] 21 CFR 50.20.

[37] https://www.fda.gov/RegulatoryInformation/Guidances/ucm126431.htm [accessed 28.03.18].

[38] https://www.hhs.gov/ohrp/regulations-and-policy/regulations/45-cfr-46/index.html5 [accessed 28.03.18]

[39] 21 CFR 56.111, https://www.accessdata.fda.gov/scripts/cdrh/cfdocs/cfcfr/CFRSearch.cfm?fr=56.111 [accessed 28.03.18].

[40] http://ichgcp.net/48-informed-consent-of-trial-subjects [accessed 28.03.18].

[41] ICH GCP E6 R2: 1.26, https://www.fda.gov/downloads/Drugs/Guidances/UCM464506.pdf [accessed 28.03.18].

[42] https://www.fda.gov/RegulatoryInformation/Guidances/ucm126431.htm [accessed 28.03.18].

[43] ICH    GP    E6,    https://www.fda.gov/downloads/Drugs/GuidanceComplianceRegulatoryInformation/Guidances/UCM464506.pdf [accessed 28.03.18].

[44] ICH GCP E6 R2 4.12 Premature Termination or Suspension of a Trial, http://www.ema.europa.eu/docs/en_GB/document_library/Scientific_guideline/2009/09/WC500002874.pdf [accessed 28.03.18].

[45] Additionally, the Grant Form PHS 398, known as the "Grant Application Kit" must be filled out. Instructions and forms for downloading can be found here: https://grants.nih.gov/grants/funding/phs398/phs398.html [accessed 28.03.18].

[46] *Guidance for IRBs, Clinical Investigators, and Sponsors: Considerations When Transferring Clinical Investigation Oversight to Another IRB* https://www.fda.gov/downloads/RegulatoryInformation/Guidances/UCM307779.pdf [accessed 28.03.18].

[47] https://www.fda.gov/downloads/aboutfda/centersoffices/officeofmedicalproductsandtobacco/cder/ucm438250.pdf    [accessed 28.0-3.18].

[48] 21 CFR 56.108, https://www.accessdata.fda.gov/scripts/cdrh/cfdocs/cfcfr/CFRSearch.cfm?fr=56.108 [accessed 28.03.18].

[49] 21    CFR    56.113,    https://www.accessdata.fda.gov/scripts/cdrh/cfdocs/cfcfr/CFRSearch.cfm?CFRPart=56    [accessed 28.03.18].

[50] ICH GCP E6 R2—5.20 Noncompliance, https://www.ich.org/fileadmin/Public_Web_Site/ICH_Products/Guidelines/Efficacy/E6/E6_R2__Addendum_Step2.pdf [accessed 29.03.18].

[51] https://www.fda.gov/ICECI/EnforcementActions/ucm321308.htm [accessed 28.03.18].

[52] Ibid.

[53] https://www.accessdata.fda.gov/scripts/cdrh/cfdocs/cfCFR/CFRSearch.cfm?fr=312.70    and    https://www.accessdata.fda.gov/scripts/cdrh/cfdocs/cfcfr/CFRSearch.cfm?fr=812.119

# EDUCATION AND CERTIFICATION IN CLINICAL RESEARCH

*Purpose of chapter:*

- Describes Bachelor and Master's Degree programs in Clinical Research
- Outlines certification training programs in Clinical Research
- Provides overview of regulations for participation in Clinical Research
- Reviews policy on Good Clinical Practice Training for NIH Awardees Involved in NIH-funded Clinical Trials
- Suggests training for Key Personnel in clinical research

**Overview**

Clinical trials and clinical research are prevalent worldwide; ClinicalTrials.gov currently lists 248,088 studies with locations in all 50 States and in 201 countries. Clinical research positions provide individuals with valuable experience in medical institutions, laboratories, and pharmaceutical companies. As well, clinical research provides individuals contact with patients and, personal and professional rewards in the discovery of new medical treatments.

## 7.1 BACHELORS AND MASTERS DEGREE PROGRAMS IN CLINICAL RESEARCH

*Purpose of chapter:*

- Provides an overview of current Bachelors and Master's Degree Programs in Clinical Research

Following is a list of some of the prominent colleges and universities that offer a 4-year degree in various aspects of Clinical Research:

1. University of North Carolina, Wilmington, N.C.; College of Health and Human Services; Bachelor of Science (B.S.) in Clinical Research. The program website notes:
   "This undergraduate program will prepare health science professionals to participate in the science and business of developing health care products and protocols, from discovery to market and human utilization. This 4-year undergraduate program includes a didactic curriculum and a mentored experience or internship in clinical research during the senior year. The university studies, collaterals, and electives (64 h) and core curriculum (60 h) are designed to provide essential knowledge and skills to promote competency for professional practice."
   Website: http://catalogue.uncw.edu/preview_program.php?catoid=3&poid=201&returnto=128
   Contact: UNCW CHHS, McNeill Hall 3080, 601 South College Road, Wilmington, NC 28403-5685; Phone: 910.962.3317; Email: chhs@uncw.edu

The Sourcebook for Clinical Research. https://doi.org/10.1016/B978-0-12-816242-2.00007-2

2. Boston University Metropolitan College, Boston University School of Medicine; Bachelor of Science in Biomedical Laboratory & Clinical Sciences. The program website notes: "Offered by Metropolitan College in collaboration with Boston University School of Medicine, the Bachelor of Science in Biomedical Laboratory & Clinical Sciences (BLCS) prepares students for jobs and careers in the fields of biotechnology and clinical research. Boston is one of the world's preeminent biomedical centers; the rapid pace of innovation in these industries and the high demand for trained professionals ensures continual growth and means a broad range of exciting opportunities at the forefront of life sciences research."
Contact: Mail: Undergraduate Student Services, 755 Commonwealth Avenue, Room 102, Boston, MA 02215; Phone: 617.353.2980; Email: metuss@bu.edu
Website: http://www.bu.edu/met/programs/undergraduate/biomedical-laboratory-clinical-sciences/

3. Campbell University, Buies Creek, N.C.; College of Pharmacy & Health Sciences; B.S. in Clinical Research. The program website notes: "This novel program, developed through the efforts of Campbell University's College of Pharmacy & Health Sciences (CPHS), provides students with the didactic and experiential training necessary for the development of careers as clinical monitors or coordinators to work in contract research organizations (CROs), pharmaceutical companies, or academia. The objective of the major is to prepare students for distinguished careers in clinical research. Graduates of this program are expected to play a wide variety of roles in the clinical research and drug development process."
Website: https://cphs.campbell.edu/academic-programs/clinical-research/bs-in-clinical-research/
Contact: College of Pharmacy and Health Science, P.O. Box 1090, Buies Creek, NC 27506; Phone: 800.760.9734 or 910.893.1690

4. Washington University in St. Louis, St. Louis, MO; College of Arts and Sciences; B.S. in Clinical Research Management. The program website notes: "The Bachelor of Science in Clinical Research Management is designed for students in the early stages of a career in clinical research, as well as more experienced individuals such as investigators, coordinators, or sponsor representatives who want to expand their knowledge and skills in the field. The program lays a foundation in principles and applications from the basic sciences, and then covers in greater depth the processes necessary in the management of studies that develop drugs, devices, and treatment protocols for patient care. This customized undergraduate program focuses on the scientific methods of clinical research, good clinical practice, research ethics, and the regulatory guidelines that protect human subjects—all integral components of clinical trial management in academic research or pharmaceutical industry settings."
Contact: Office of Admissions and Student Services, Washington University in St. Louis University College Campus, 11 N. Jackson Road, Suite 1000, St. Louis, MO 63105; Phone: 314.935.6700; Email: ucollege@wustl.edu
Website: https://ucollege.wustl.edu/programs/undergraduate/bachelors-clinical-research-management

5. Kent State University, Kent, OH; College of Public Health; Bachelors of Science in Public Health (B.S.P.H.) in Clinical Trials Research. The program website notes: "Bachelor of Science in Public Health students with a concentration in Clinical Trials Research prepare to obtain a position as a Clinical Research Associate or Clinical Trials Manager. This is an ideal degree for students interested in epidemiology and health research. With experience, there is room for advancement and the clinical research field is growing."

Contact: Mailing address: College of Public Health, Office of Provost, P.O. Box 5190, Kent, OH 44242-0001; Phone: 330.672.6500; Email: publichealth@kent.edu

Website: https://www.kent.edu/publichealth/bachelor-science-public-health-bsph-clinical-trials-research

6. National University, La Jolla, CA; School of Health and Human Services; B.S. in Healthcare Administration. The program website notes:

"The Bachelor of Science, Major in Healthcare Administration (BSHA), is an undergraduate professional degree designed to prepare students for entry-level administrative/management positions in healthcare organizations. Ideal candidates for the healthcare administration degree program are those students looking for career entry in administration and supervisory roles in the healthcare system. Graduates will enhance their opportunities for professional growth and job placement through carefully planned internships and a capstone experience. The BSHA program emphasizes the conceptual and analytical skills required to manage in contemporary healthcare organizations. The program features opportunities in project management, teamwork and leadership. The BSHA program is an associate member institution of the Association of University Programs in Health Administration (AUPHA)."

Website: https://www.nu.edu/OurPrograms/SchoolOfHealthAndHumanServices/CommunityHealth/Programs/Bachelor-Science-Healthcare-Administration.html

Contact Information: Program Lead, Dr. Peggy Ranke, Phone: 858.309.3451; Email: PRanke@nu.edu

7. Massachusetts College of Pharmacy and Health Sciences, Boston, MA; B.S. in Pharmaceutical Sciences. The program website notes:

"This program provides students with a broad-based education in the basic and biological and pharmaceutical sciences with a focus on core areas of industrial pharmacy including drug discovery, research and development, and manufacturing. During this full time 4-year undergraduate program, you'll have the opportunity to work alongside professional experts in modern laboratories equipped with advanced technology for hands-on education and research."

Contact: To request information, go to: https://www.mcphs.edu/admission-and-aid/request-information

Website: https://www.mcphs.edu/academics/school-of-pharmacy/pharmaceutical-sciences/pharmaceutical-sciences-bs

8. George Washington University, Washington, D.C.; School of Medicine and Health Sciences; B.S.in Health Sciences (B.S.H.S.) with a major in Clinical Research Administration. The program website notes:

"Clinical Research Administration is a vast and expanding field that involves the processes in which products (drugs, devices, biologics) and treatment protocols are developed for improving patient care. The online BSHS in Clinical Research Administration prepares health sciences professionals to participate in the industry of developing new therapeutics.

Further information can be found here: https://smhs.gwu.edu/clinical-research-administration/

Contact: Becky Karlin, M.Ed. Assistant Director of Admissions and Enrollment Services, Phone: 202.994.6844; Email: beckykarlin@gwu.edu

**Online Bachelor Programs**

An online bachelor's degree program in clinical research can prepare you for a career in the biopharmaceutical industry or in medical research. Programs will teach you about regulatory compliance, clinical research methods, data collection, and ethics in research and protocol development. They generally take about 4 years to complete. A comprehensive list can be found here: http://www.onlineeducation.net/programs/clinical-research/online.

**Schools Offering a Master's of Science in Clinical Research**

Following is a list of universities offering an advanced degree in various aspects of Clinical Research:

1. St. Cloud University, St. Cloud, MN; School of Health and Human Services; Masters of Science (M.S.) in Applied Clinical Research. The program website notes:

   "As an Applied Clinical Research student you will receive the necessary knowledge and skills to design, conduct and evaluate human clinical trials of medical devices. You will learn how medical device products affect the human body, how new products are developed and brought to market and how to design and conduct ethical and scientific medical research. Upon completion of this program, you will have the knowledge and competencies industry executives identify as essential to the successful clinical research leader including the science of medical research, medical product regulations, research ethics, study management and operations and risk management as well as effective communication and leadership."

   Contact: School of Health and Human Services, 720 4th Avenue South, St. Cloud, MN 56301-4498; Phone: 320.308.0121

   For more information, please go here: https://stcloudg.askadmissions.net/emtinterestpage.aspx?ip=graduate

   Website: https://www.stcloudstate.edu/graduate/applied-clinical-research/default.aspx

2. Campbell University, Buies, NC; College of Pharmacy & Health Sciences; offers an M.S. in Clinical Research. The program website notes:

   "The MS in Clinical Research curriculum provides students with an in-depth understanding of producing and interpreting medical evidence in a variety of practice settings. Graduates are prepared for leadership positions in pharmaceutical and biotechnology industries, government agencies, medical institutions, academic institutions and hospitals. Within these fields, graduates are qualified to work as clinical research associates, project managers, data managers, clinical monitors, biostatisticians and many other positions. Faculty members in the Department of Clinical Research are recognized experts, published scientists, committed mentors and proven professionals."

   Contact: P.O. Box 1090, Buies Creek, NC 27506; Phone: 800.760.9734 or 910.893.1690

   Website: https://cphs.campbell.edu/academic-programs/clinical-research/ms-in-clinical-research/?academic-programs/ms-clinical-research/

3. San Jose State University, San Jose, CA; College of International and Extended Studies; M.S. in Medical Product Development Management (MPDM). The program website notes:

   "The Masters of Science degree in Medical Product Development Management (MPDM) is a Special Sessions graduate program offered by SJSU's College of Science, in collaboration with the College of International and Extended Studies and the Lucas Graduate School of Business. The MPDM MS program combines customized clinical, regulatory and technical classes with MBA-level business and management courses. The industry-relevant curriculum was designed in collaboration with experts from biomedical companies in the greater San Francisco Bay area. The MPDM Program Mission: applying leadership, management and decision-making skills in a regulated environment; understanding and conversing with others in key disciplines involved in medical product development; understanding ethical, business, financial, global, and strategic implications in medical product development."

Contact: Director Tonja Green; Phone: 408.924.4853; Email: tonja.green@sjsu.edu

Website: http://www.medproddev.sjsu.edu/

4. University of Vermont, Burlington, Vermont—Masters of Science in Clinical and Translational Science. The program website notes:

   "This program is designed to effectively and efficiently transform clinicians and other young academics drawn from the large array of disciplines contributing to health into successful independent clinical and translational science investigators. It's designed for individuals who have an interest in becoming research coordinators, patient advocates, research administrators, study nurses and other science professionals."

   Website: http://catalogue.uvm.edu/graduate/clinicaltranslational/clinicalandtranslationalsciencems/

5. Thomas Jefferson University, Philadelphia, PA; College of Biomedical Sciences; Masters of Science in Clinical Research. The website notes:

   "The Master of Science in Clinical Research was created by clinical researchers to train scientists with a variety of backgrounds. This program is well suited for career changers with a background in life, physical or clinical sciences that would like to break into the field of clinical research. It is also appropriate for individuals already in the industry and looking for additional graduate-level training. The field of clinical research is expanding and well-trained professionals are needed to coordinate, manage, and administer clinical research and trials. This Master of Science degree will provide students with the foundation that they need to be an effective clinical research scientist. Students completing the MS in Clinical Research will: Understand the experimental design, statistical analysis and interpretation, and regulatory and ethical issues pertaining to human clinical research and trials; be able to read, understand, and critique published reports of clinical trials; acquire management skills that will enable them to develop a human clinical research project or trial from the idea phase to implementation to completion; and, be prepared for employment in the academic industrial or hospital clinical research setting."

   Contact: Office of Admissions; Phone: 215.503.4400; E-mail: jgsbs-info@jefferson.edu

   Website: http://www.jefferson.edu/university/biomedical-sciences/degrees-programs/master-programs/clinical-research-MS/MS-Clinical-research-overview.html

6. University of Virginia, Charlottesville, VA; Department of Health Sciences; Masters of Science in Clinical Research. The program website notes:

   "This is an interdisciplinary graduate degree designed to meet the changing needs of the current health care field, particularly the increasing need for trained professionals with well-developed quantitative and analytic skills. The MS-CR program provides training to health and medical professionals who desire and need quantitative and analytic skills in patient-oriented and translational research, as well as more traditional clinical investigation."

   Contact: University of Virginia School of Medicine, Health Sciences, P.O. Box 800717, Charlottesville, VA 22908; Phone: 434.924.8430

   Website: https://med.virginia.edu/phs/education-programs-in-public-health-sciences/masters-in-clinical-research-university-of-virginia/

7. Duke University, Durham, NC; School of Medicine; Masters of Health Sciences in Clinical Research (MHSCR). The program website notes:

   "The Duke University School of Medicine's Clinical Research Training Program (CRTP) provides physicians, investigators and other healthcare professionals with the rigorous academic training in the quantitative and methodological principles of clinical research required to excel in

today's dynamic clinical research environment. The Program's degree option leads to a Master of Health Sciences in Clinical Research awarded by the Duke School of Medicine."
Contact: Office of Admissions, DUMC 3710, Durham, NC 27710; Phone: 919.684.2985; E-mail: medadm@mc.duke.edu
Website: https://medschool.duke.edu/education/degree-programs-and- admissions/clinical-research-training-program

8. Rush University, Chicago, IL; Graduate College; Masters of Science in Clinical Research. The program website notes:
"The Master of Science in Clinical Research is a 2-year program that aims to provide the tools and guidance necessary to undertake clinical research. Clinical research courses include the following: Clinical Trials I & II, Biostatistics I & 2, Bioinformatics 1 & 2, Introduction to Drug & Device Development: the U.S. Regulatory Process, Epidemiology, Tools for Research, Craftsmanship, Ethics and the IRB."
Contact: Marisol Vega; Phone: 312.942.3589; Email: gc_admissions@rush.edu
Website: https://www.rushu.rush.edu/graduate-college/academic-programs/master-science-clinical-research

9. University of Pittsburgh, Pittsburgh, PA; Institute of for Clinical Research Education; Masters of Science in Clinical Research. The program website notes:
"The Institute for Clinical Research Education (ICRE) is the home for the University of Pittsburgh's premier clinical and translational research training programs as well as the home for the Research Education and Career Development Core of the Clinical and Translational Science Institute (CTSI). The ICRE's primary objectives are to develop, nurture, and support a cadre of clinical and translational scientists by building on the University of Pittsburgh's existing clinical research training programs to establish a comprehensive program with activities ranging from early research exposure for high school students to programs for faculty."
Contact: Institute for Clinical Research Education, 200 Meyran Avenue, Suite 300, Pittsburgh, PA 15213; Phone: 412.586.9632; E-mail: icre@pitt.edu
Website: https://www.icre.pitt.edu/

## 7.2 CERTIFICATION ORGANIZATIONS

*Purpose of chapter*:

- **Provides overview of organizations providing Certifications in Clinical Research**
Certificates in clinical research coordination are focused on teaching research skills and knowledge of industry practices. Unlike associates or bachelor's degree programs, they do not usually include classes that are not specifically related to clinical research, such as theoretical science and mathematics or general education classes. You will learn about industry standards for clinical research, such as Good Clinical Practice (GCP), and the legal and ethical issues surrounding medical research. Other topics in a certification program may include documentation, institutional review board submissions, drug compliance, Principal Investigator responsibilities, regulatory knowledge, Food and Drug Administration audits and informed consent.

**Certification Organizations**

1. The Society of Clinical Research Associates (SOCRA)
   SOCRA offers the "Certified Clinical Research Professional" certification (CCRP). To become certified, you must be a member of the association and provide evidence of experience as a Clinical Research Professional. The amount of experience you are required to have is dependent upon the level of education you have completed. The CCRP is available for clinical research coordinators, principal investigators, researchers, and others working in clinical research. Website: http://www.socra.org/

2. The Association for Clinical Research Professionals (ACRP)
   ACRP offers a clinical research coordinator certification. To qualify for the ACRP certification, you must provide documentation that you have performed the "Essential Duties" of a Clinical Research Coordinator. The number of hours performing CRC Essential Duties you are required to have is dependent upon the level of education you have completed. ACRP also has a substitution for work experience. ACRP also offers other certifications, such as Clinical Research Associate (CRA), Certified Principal Investigator (CPI), and Association of Clinical Research Professionals—Certified Professional (ACRP-CP). Each certification requires that you meet eligibility qualifications and pass an examination. Website: https://www.acrpnet.org/

3. Model Agreements and Guidelines International (MAGI)
   MAGI offers Clinical Research Contract Professional (CRCP) certification. The certification exam takes 1 hour. There are 20 short-answer questions. Questions often relate to common topics of negotiation between sponsors and sites. You should be familiar with negotiations and contracts in general, legal concepts and terms in Clinical Trial Agreements (CTAs), the business implications of CTA provisions, sponsor and site perspectives on common negotiation issues, and how to create and negotiate study budgets. Website: www.magiworld.org

---

## 7.3 TRAINING REQUIREMENTS FOR PERSONNEL CONDUCTING CLINICAL TRIALS

*Purpose of section*:

- Outlines training requirements for conducting clinical trials
- The Code of Federal Regulations and ICH GCP do not define who should be trained beyond the PI and "each individual involved in conducting a trial." This section addresses those individuals who should be trained, among all the people who interact with subjects during trials, with the help of the regulations, Good Clinical Practice, and the Guidances that exist.
- WHAT should be taught is not defined in ICH GCP nor in the Code of Federal Regulations, except for a few specific notations. This section tackles <u>what</u> should be taught.

Let's look at the Federal regulations first:

45 CFR 46—no mention of training or education for study team members
21 CFR 50—no mention of training or education for study team members
21 CFR 56—no mention of training or education for study team members

In 21 CFR 312.53(a) "*Selecting investigators.* A sponsor shall select only investigators qualified by training and experience as appropriate experts to investigate the drug."

21 CFR 312.53( c)(2) *Curriculum vitae.* A curriculum vitae or other statement of qualifications of the investigator showing the education, training, and experience that qualifies the investigator as an expert in the clinical investigation of the drug for the use under investigation.

**21 CFR 312.120 Foreign clinical studies not conducted under an IND**

21 CFR 312.120 (B)(11) A description of how investigators were trained to comply with GCP (as described in paragraph (a)(1)(i) of this section) and to conduct the study in accordance with the study protocol, and a statement on whether written commitments by investigators to comply with GCP and the protocol were obtained.

21 CFR 812.43 (a) *Selecting investigators.* A sponsor shall select investigators qualified by training and experience to investigate the device.

ĴC ICH **Now, let's look at ICH GCP E6 R2:**

ICH GCP is equally not forthcoming in the details needed.

2.8 Each individual involved in conducting a trial should be qualified by education, training, and experience to perform his or her respective task(s).

**4.1 Investigator's Qualifications and Agreements**

*4.1.1* The investigator(s) should be qualified by education, training, and experience to assume responsibility for the proper conduct of the trial, should meet all the qualifications specified by the applicable regulatory requirement(s), and should provide evidence of such qualifications through up-to-date curriculum vitae and/or other relevant documentation requested by the sponsor, the IRB/IEC, and/or the regulatory authority(ies).

5. SPONSOR 5.0 Quality Management

*5.0.4 Risk Control*

The sponsor should decide which risks to reduce and/or which risks to accept. The approach used to reduce risk to an acceptable level should be proportionate to the significance of the risk. Risk reduction activities may be incorporated in protocol design and implementation, monitoring plans, agreements between parties defining roles and responsibilities, systematic safeguards to ensure adherence to standard operating procedures, and training in processes and procedures.

5.5.3 When using electronic trial data handling and/or remote electronic trial data systems, the sponsor should: (b) Maintain SOPs for using these systems.

**ADDENDUM**

The SOPs should cover system setup, installation, and use. The SOPs should describe system validation and functionality testing, data collection and handling, system maintenance, system security measures, change control, data backup, recovery, contingency planning, and decommissioning. The responsibilities of the sponsor, investigator, and other parties with respect to the use of these computerized systems should be clear, and the users should be provided with training in their use.

**5.6 Investigator Selection**

5.6.1 The sponsor is responsible for selecting the investigator(s)/institution(s). Each investigator should be qualified by training and experience and should have adequate resources (see 4.1, 4.2) to properly conduct the trial for which the investigator is selected.

**Training for NIH-Funded Clinical Trials**

For NIH research, the following Policy Statement is articulated:

This policy establishes the expectation that all NIH-funded investigators and staff who are involved in the conduct, oversight, or management of clinical trials should be trained in Good Clinical Practice (GCP), consistent with principles of the International Conference on Harmonisation (ICH) E6 (R2).

This policy went into effect on January 1, 2017: https://grants.nih.gov/grants/guide/notice-files/NOT-OD-16-148.html

**We now have the answer to our question as to what curriculum needs to be trained, which is ICH GCP, but only definitively for NIH-funded trials.**

Note that the course or degree or other means of training a person is not mentioned. Following is the relevant NIH guidance on this point:

**Does NIH specify which educational programs should be used to fulfill the protection of human subjects education requirement?**

No. The NIH does not endorse any specific educational programs. We believe that institutions are in the best position to determine what programs are appropriate for fulfilling the education requirement. Institutions may require a particular program or may choose to develop a program to meet the requirement.

As a public service, the NIH Office of Extramural Research offers a free tutorial on "Protecting Human Research Participants" that institutions may elect to use to meet the human subjects protections education requirement. It can be found here: https://humansubjects.nih.gov/requirement-education.

Your medical center may utilize CITI training or another program.

Here are some FAQs from the NIH website regarding the "Policy on Good Clinical Practice Training for NIH Awardees Involved in NIH-funded Clinical Trials."

We have included the most relevant in order to address our next question of <u>WHO must be trained</u>:

**Who needs to receive required education on the protection of human subjects?**

Individuals who will be involved in the design or conduct of NIH-funded human subjects research must fulfill the education requirement. These individuals are considered to be "Key Personnel" on NIH awards and contracts that include research involving human subjects. This includes the Principal Investigator(s), all individuals responsible for the design or conduct of the study, and those individuals identified as key personnel of consortium participants or alternate performance sites.

**Do individuals identified as Key Personnel who are not involved in the design and conduct of the human subjects portion of an award need to comply with the education requirement?**

No. Investigators who are identified as Key Personnel, but are not involved in the design and conduct of human subjects research do not need to comply with this requirement. For example, those involved solely in the analysis of de-identified data.

**Do third-party (subcontract) Key Personnel or consultants need to comply with the education requirement?**

Yes. Third-party Key Personnel and consultants must comply with the education requirement if they are involved in the design and conduct of research involving human subjects.

The full list of FAQs is here: https://humansubjects.nih.gov/requirement-education

Let's look a little more closely at who must be trained by reiterating the key language:

1. Individuals who will be involved in the design or conduct of NIH-funded human subjects research must fulfill the education requirement. These individuals are considered to be "Key Personnel"…
2. This includes the Principal Investigator(s), all individuals responsible for the design or conduct of the study, and those individuals identified as key personnel of consortium participants or alternate performance sites
3. Third-party Key Personnel and consultants must comply with the education requirement if they are involved in the design and conduct of research involving human subjects.

"Key personnel" are defined by NIH as: "The program director/principal investigator (PD/PI) and other individuals who contribute to the scientific development or execution of a project in a substantive, measurable way, whether or not they request salaries or compensation."

https://grants.nih.gov/grants/policy/senior_key_personnel_faqs.htm#1660

Applying all of this to your medical center, it means that:

1. The study team must be trained in the <u>protocol</u> and <u>good clinical practice</u> and in <u>regulations.</u>
   a. Anyone on your Delegation of Authority or Delegation of Responsibility Log will become a part of the study team, and we can logically deduce are considered "Key Personnel" by contributing "substantive, measurable" tasks to the study.
   b. These Key Personnel must have training in the protocol, the regulations, and ICH GCP. Indeed, on the NIH Delegation of Authority Log in Appendix 15, the PI signature statement on the form reads the following, "I certify that the above individuals are appropriately trained, have read the Protocol and pertinent sections of 21 CFR 50 and 56 and ICH GCPs, and are authorized to perform the above study-related tasks/procedures."

      i. See the Delegation of Authority in the Forms section. Chapter 4, Section 4.5.1.
      ii. For Investigator-Initiated studies, and subawards with Universities, for which a Delegation of Authority Form (DOA) is not provided (as they are in Industry studies), it is highly recommended that you use a DOA in order to document your Key Personnel for your study and ensure each person on the log is properly trained. There are two templates for Delegation of Authority Forms in Appendix 15.
   c. If your Institution has a Federal Wide Assurance, your Institution is legally bound to comply with the Common Rule, which is 45 CFR 46 Subpart A. Therefore, training in 45 CFR 46 Subpart A is prudent. See Chapter 1, Section 1.3.
   d. If there are any vulnerable populations in your research study, the study team should be well versed in 45 CFR 46 Subparts B, C, or D as applicable.

# THE NEWEST CHANGES IN CLINICAL RESEARCH

# 8

*Purpose of chapter*:

This chapter provides updates on the new rulings and changes affecting clinical research, including:

- FDA Final Rule on Acceptance of Data From Clinical Investigations for Medical Devices—*Effective date 2-21-19*
- Common Rule changes—*Effective date 1-21-19*
- FDA guidance on Payment and Reimbursement to Research Subjects—*Effective date: 1-25-18*
- sIRB (Single IRB)—*Effective date: 1-25-18*
- Certificate of Confidentiality—*Effective date 10-01-17*
- ICH GCP E6 R2—*Effective date 6-14-17*
- Electronic Common Technical Document (eCTD)—*Effective dates: 5-05-17 and 5-05-18*
- Clinicaltrials.gov registration and reporting—*Effective date: 1-18-17*

## 8.1 HUMAN SUBJECTS PROTECTION: ACCEPTANCE OF DATA FROM CLINICAL INVESTIGATIONS FOR MEDICAL DEVICES

The FDA issued this Final Rule on 2/21/18. It will become effective on 2/21/2019.

Here is FDA's Summary:

"The Food and Drug Administration (FDA or we) is amending its regulations on acceptance of data from clinical investigations for medical devices. We are requiring that data submitted from clinical investigations conducted outside the United States intended to support an investigational device exemption (IDE) application, a premarket notification (510(k)) submission, a request for De Novo classification, a premarket approval (PMA) application, a product development protocol (PDP) application, or a humanitarian device exemption (HDE) application be from investigations conducted in accordance with good clinical practice (GCP), which includes obtaining and documenting the review and approval of the clinical investigation by an independent ethics committee (IEC) and obtaining and documenting freely given informed consent of subjects, which includes individuals whose specimens are used in investigations of medical devices. The final rule updates the criteria for FDA acceptance of data from clinical investigations conducted outside the United States to help ensure the quality and integrity of data obtained from these investigations and the protection of human subjects. As part of this final rule, we are also amending the IDE, 510(k), and HDE regulations to address the requirements for FDA acceptance of data from clinical investigations conducted inside the United States. The final rule provides consistency in FDA requirements for acceptance of data from clinical investigations, whatever the application or submission type."

The Sourcebook for Clinical Research. https://doi.org/10.1016/B978-0-12-816242-2.00008-4

Here is the url for the Federal Register announcement: https://www.federalregister.gov/documents/2018/02/21/2018-03244/human-subject-protection-acceptance-of-data-from-clinical-investigations-for-medical-devices?utm_campaign=FDA%20releases%20final%20rule%20on%20Acceptance%20of%20Data%20from%20Clinical%20Investigations%20for%20Medical%20Devices&utm_medium=email&utm_source=Eloqua&elqTrackId=A790E62E93937FE7627879A3C630AA39&elq=9e8a9f19bd4f400c81ef2d0d678cd829&elqaid=2484&elqat=1&elqCampaignId=1788.[1]

FAQs for Medical Devices can be found here: https://www.fda.gov/downloads/MedicalDevices/DeviceRegulationandGuidance/GuidanceDocuments/UCM597273.pdf?utm_campaign=FDA%20releases%20final%20rule%20on%20Acceptance%20of%20Data%20from%20Clinical%20Investigations%20for%20Medical%20Devices&utm_medium=email&utm_source=Eloqua&elqTrackId=F4F5E63809CD6EC32B7CD25DAE698BDF&elq=9e8a9f19bd4f400c81ef2d0d678cd829&elqaid=2484&elqat=1&elqCampaignId=1788.[2]

## 8.2 THE NEW COMMON RULE

The "Common Rule" is the nickname for 45 CFR 46 Subpart A. The regulation covers the protection of human subjects in clinical research. The federal government entity with the responsibility for this rule, the U.S. Department of Health and Human Services, has revised the Common Rule and people are referring to the revised Subpart A as the "New Common Rule." The changes will become effective on January 21, 2019 unless another delay occurs.

**The New Common Rule applies to:**

45 CFR 46.101 (a): this policy applies to all research involving human subjects conducted, supported, or otherwise subject to regulation by any Federal department or agency…It also includes research conducted, supported, or otherwise subject to regulation by the Federal Government outside the United States.

**New Definitions**

**Following are definitions of new terms introduced in the New Common Rule. These new terms are not spelled out in a "Definitions" section of the regulation. They had to be found throughout the writing and are only explained very briefly. Here is what is available:**

**broad consent**—i.e., seeking prospective consent to unspecified future research (found in the Federal Register summary)

**secondary research**—collected for either research studies other than the proposed research or non-research purposes (found in 45 CFR 46.116(d))

"…**limited IRB review** to ensure that there are adequate privacy safeguards for identifiable private information and identifiable biospecimens." (found in the Federal Register summary).

An *identifiable biospecimen* is a biospecimen for which the identity of the subject is or may readily be ascertained by the investigator or associated with the biospecimen (found in 45 CFR 46.102).[3]

**Revised Definitions**

**Following are revised definitions in the New Common Rule (found in 45 CFR 46.102):**

1. The definitions of "human subject" and "intervention" have been expanded to include biospecimens.
   *Human subject* means a living individual about whom an investigator (whether professional or student) conducting research:

**(i)** Obtains information or biospecimens through intervention or interaction with the individual, and uses, studies, or analyzes the information or biospecimens; or

**(ii)** Obtains, uses, studies, analyzes, or generates identifiable private information or identifiable biospecimens.

2. *Intervention* includes both physical procedures by which information or biospecimens are gathered (*e.g.*, venipuncture) and manipulations of the subject or the subject's environment that are performed for research purposes.

   *Public health authority* means an agency or authority of the United States, a state, a territory, a political subdivision of a state or territory, an Indian tribe, or a foreign government, or a person or entity acting under a grant of authority from or contract with such public agency, including the employees or agents of such public agency or its contractors or persons or entities to whom it has granted authority, that is responsible for public health matters as part of its official mandate.[4]

### Misinformation on the Common Rule

Beware of outdated or incomplete information posted on the Internet, i.e., links to the proposed New Common Rule rather than the final New Common Rule as the rule went through the HHS and U.S. Office of Management and Budget review and comment process. Ensure your institution has the most current Common Rule, that is, the Rule that goes into effect on January 21, 2019 unless another delay occurs. (The Authors have seen some Internet sites that blend the proposed terms with the final terms.)

### Which Common Rule should you follow?

### Currently active studies

All active studies will maintain the IRB determinations made prior to January 21, 2019 as currently written, unless another delay occurs.

### New studies

Any research (IRB) reviewed on or after 1-21-19, shall follow the New Common Rule regulations unless another delay occurs.

### Continuing reviews

Continuing reviews on or after January 21, 2019 will follow the New Common rule. Note that this means your currently active studies that were IRB approved prior to 1-21-19 that have been following the previous Common Rule regulations, must comply with the New Common Rule when the Continuing Review occurs on or after January 21, 2019 unless another delay occurs.

### Following are the notable changes in the New Common Rule:

1. The definitions of "human subject" and "intervention" have been expanded to include biospecimens.
2. Federal Agency responsibilities have been broadened to include periodic examination of new terms, assessment of analytic technologies, and expedited review categories.
3. A Reliance Agreement is required between a site IRB and the IRB of record.
4. A new type of intervention has been coined: *benign behavioral intervention*.
5. There are new categories for exempt research—*secondary research* and *broad consent*.
6. There is an addition to Expedited Reviews.
7. IRB Continuing Review is NOT required any longer for:
   a. expedited studies
   b. the new limited IRB review studies
   c. Studies in the status of:

      **i.** Data analysis

     **ii.** Data collection or access from clinical care only

**8.** There is mandatory broad consent for secondary research use of biospecimens.

**9.** A Single IRB (sIRB) is mandatory for multisite studies. (See sIRB in this chapter, Section 8.4.)

**10.** Informed consent must begin with a concise and focused presentation of key information.

**11.** There is one addition to the Basic Elements of Informed Consent.

**12.** There are three additions to the Additional Elements of Informed Consent.

**13.** Broad Consent is explained.

**14.** There are new IRB waiver of consent provisions for identifiable private information or identifiable biospecimens.

**15.** *"Screening, recruiting, or determining eligibility"* without informed consent has been added.

**16.** Clinical trial consent forms must be posted to a federal website.

**17.** A new type of review has been coined: *Limited IRB review* (found under the Reliance Agreement, Exempt Research, Continuing Review and Broad Consent).

    Here are the regulatory references that support the list of notable changes in the New Common Rule:

**1.** The definitions have been provided above.

**2.** In 45 CFR 46.102.e.7.i, Federal Agencies will reexamine the meaning of "identifiable private information," and "identifiable biospecimen," within one (1) year (of the New Common Rule going into effect) and regularly thereafter (at least every four (4) years).

In 45 CFR 46.102.e.7.ii, Federal Agencies will assess whether there are analytic technologies or techniques that should be considered by investigators to generate "identifiable private information," or an "identifiable biospecimen" within one (1) year (of the New Common Rule going into effect) and regularly thereafter (at least every four (4) years).

In 45 CFR 46.110, the HHS Secretary will evaluate a list of categories of research that may be reviewed by the IRB through an expedited review procedure at least every eight (8) years and amend it as appropriate.[5]

**3.** A Reliance Agreement is Required Between a Site IRB and the IRB of Record

**Reliance Agreement between IRBs (found in .103.e):** (e) For non-exempt research involving human subjects covered by this policy (or exempt research for which limited IRB review takes place pursuant to §ll.104(d)(2)(iii), (d)(3)(i)(C), or (d)(7) or (8)) that takes place at an institution in which IRB oversight is conducted by an IRB that is not operated by the institution, the institution and the organization operating the IRB shall document the institution's reliance on the IRB for oversight of the research and the responsibilities that each entity will undertake to ensure compliance with the requirements of this policy (e.g., in a written agreement between the institution and the IRB, by implementation of an institution-wide policy directive providing the allocation of responsibilities between the institution and an IRB that is not affiliated with the institution, or as set forth in a research protocol).[6]

**4.** A new type of intervention has been defined: *benign behavioral interventions*.

**New: "benign behavioral interventions"** (found in .104(d)(3)(ii)): (ii) For the purpose of this provision, **benign behavioral interventions** are brief in duration, harmless, painless, not physically invasive, not likely to have a significant adverse lasting impact on the subjects, and the investigator has no reason to think the subjects will find the interventions offensive or embarrassing. Provided all such criteria are met, examples of such benign behavioral interventions would include having the subjects play an online game, having them solve puzzles under various noise conditions, or having them decide how to allocate a nominal amount of received cash between themselves and someone else.

5. There are new categories for exempt research—*secondary research* and *broad consent*

   **Under Exempt Research .104(d)(7): Secondary research & broad consent**

   (7) Storage or maintenance for secondary research for which broad consent is required: Storage or maintenance of identifiable private information or identifiable biospecimens for potential secondary research use if an IRB conducts a limited IRB review and makes the determinations required by §ll.111(a)(8).

   (8) Secondary research for which broad consent is required: Research involving the use of identifiable private information or identifiable biospecimens for secondary research use, if the following criteria are met: (i) Broad consent for the storage, maintenance, and secondary research use of the identifiable private information or identifiable biospecimens was obtained in accordance with §ll.116(a)(1) through (4), (a)(6), and (d).[7]

6. There is an addition to Expedited Reviews.

   **Expedited review now includes (found in .109):** (A) Data analysis, including analysis of identifiable private information or identifiable biospecimens.

7. IRB Continuing Review is NOT required any longer for the following:

   **IRB Continuing review is not required (found in .109.f):** (f)(1) Unless an IRB determines otherwise, continuing review of research is not required in the following circumstances:

   (i) Research eligible for expedited review in accordance with §ll.110;

   (ii) Research reviewed by the IRB in accordance with the limited IRB review described in §ll.104(d)(2)(iii), (d)(3)(i)(C), or (d)(7) or (8);

   (iii) Research that has progressed to the point that it involves only one or both of the following, which are part of the IRB-approved study:

   (A) Data analysis, including analysis of identifiable private information or identifiable biospecimens, or

   (B) Accessing follow-up clinical data from procedures that subjects would undergo as part of clinical care.

8. There is mandatory broad consent for secondary research use of biospecimens.

   **Broad Consent Under .111(a)(8):** (8) For purposes of conducting the limited IRB review required by §ll.104(d)(7)), the IRB need not make the determinations at paragraphs (a)(1) through (7) of this section, and shall make the following determinations:

   (i) Broad consent for storage, maintenance, and secondary research use of identifiable private information or identifiable biospecimens is obtained in accordance with the requirements of §ll.116(a)(1)–(4), (a)(6), and (d);

   (ii) Broad consent is appropriately documented or waiver of documentation is appropriate, in accordance with §ll.117; and

   (iii) If there is a change made for research purposes in the way the identifiable private information or identifiable biospecimens are stored or maintained, there are adequate provisions to protect the privacy of subjects and to maintain the confidentiality of data.

9. A Single IRB (sIRB) is mandatory for multisite studies.

   **Single IRB (found in .114.b.1):** (b)(1) Any institution located in the United States that is engaged in cooperative research must rely upon approval by a single IRB for that portion of the research that is conducted in the United States. The reviewing IRB will be identified by the Federal department or agency supporting or conducting the research or proposed by the lead institution subject to the acceptance of the Federal department or agency supporting the research.

**10.** Informed consent must begin with a concise and focused presentation of key information.
   **Start of consent (found in .116(a)(5)(i)):**
   **(i)** Informed consent must begin with a **concise and focused presentation of the key information** that is most likely to assist a prospective subject or legally authorized representative in understanding the **reasons why one might or might not want to participate** in the research. This part of the informed consent must be organized and presented in a way that **facilitates comprehension**.
   **(ii)** Informed **consent as a whole** must present information in **sufficient detail** relating to the research, and must be **organized** and presented in a way that does not merely provide lists of isolated facts, but rather **facilitates** the prospective subject's or legally authorized representative's **understanding of the reasons why one might or might not want to participate**

**11.** There is one addition to the Basic Elements of Informed Consent.
   **One Addition to Basic Elements of Informed Consent (found in .116(b)):** (9) **One of the following statements** about any research that involves the collection of identifiable private information or identifiable biospecimens:
   **(i)** A statement that identifiers might be removed from the identifiable private information or identifiable biospecimens and that, after such removal, the information or biospecimens could be used for future research studies or distributed to another investigator for future research studies without additional informed consent from the subject or the legally authorized representative, if this might be a possibility; or
   **(ii)** A statement that the subject's information or biospecimens collected as part of the research, even if identifiers are removed, will not be used or distributed for future research studies.

**12.** There are three additions to the Additional Elements of Informed Consent.
   **Three Additions to Additional Elements of Informed Consent (found in .116.c):**
   (7) A statement that the subject's biospecimens (even if identifiers are removed) may be used for commercial profit and whether the subject will or will not share in this commercial profit;
   (8) A statement regarding whether clinically relevant research results, including individual research results, will be disclosed to subjects, and if so, under what conditions; and
   (9) For research involving biospecimens, whether the research will (if known) or might include whole genome sequencing (i.e., sequencing of a human germline or somatic specimen with the intent to generate the genome or exome sequence of that specimen).

**13.** Broad Consent is explained.
   **Broad Consent (found in .116 (d)):** (d) *Elements of broad consent for the storage, maintenance, and secondary research use of identifiable private information or identifiable biospecimens.* Broad consent for the storage, maintenance, and secondary research use of identifiable private information or identifiable biospecimens (collected for either research studies other than the proposed research or non-research purposes) is permitted as an alternative to the informed consent requirements in paragraphs (b) and (c) of this section. If the subject or the legally authorized representative is asked to provide broad consent, the following shall be provided to each subject or the subject's legally authorized representative:

**(1)** The information required in paragraphs (b)(2), (b)(3), (b)(5), and (b)(8) and, when appropriate, (c)(7) and (9) of this section;

**(2)** A general description of the types of research that may be conducted with the identifiable private information or identifiable biospecimens. This description must include sufficient information such that a reasonable person would expect that the broad consent would permit the types of research conducted;

**(3)** A description of the identifiable private information or identifiable biospecimens that might be used in research, whether sharing of identifiable private information or identifiable biospecimens might occur, and the types of institutions or researchers that might conduct research with the identifiable private information or identifiable biospecimens;

**(4)** A description of the period of time that the identifiable private information or identifiable biospecimens may be stored and maintained (which period of time could be indefinite), and a description of the period of time that the identifiable private information or identifiable biospecimens may be used for research purposes (which period of time could be indefinite);

**(5)** Unless the subject or legally authorized representative will be provided details about specific research studies, a statement that they will not be informed of the details of any specific research studies that might be conducted using the subject's identifiable private information or identifiable biospecimens, including the purposes of the research, and that they might have chosen not to consent to some of those specific research studies;

**(6)** Unless it is known that clinically relevant research results, including individual research results, will be disclosed to the subject in all circumstances, a statement that such results may not be disclosed to the subject; and

**(7)** An explanation of whom to contact for answers to questions about the subject's rights and about storage and use of the subject's identifiable private information or identifiable biospecimens, and whom to contact in the event of a research-related harm.

14. There are new IRB waiver of consent provisions for identifiable private information or identifiable biospecimens.
    **New IRB waiver of consent provisions for identifiable private information or identifiable biospecimens (found in .116.e and .116.f):** .116 (e) *Waiver or alteration of consent in research involving public benefit and service programs conducted by or subject to the approval of state or local officials AND* (f) *General waiver or alteration of consent*:
    If an individual was asked to provide broad consent for the storage, maintenance, and secondary research use of identifiable private information or identifiable biospecimens in accordance with the requirements at paragraph (d) of this section, and refused to consent, an IRB cannot waive consent for the storage, maintenance, or secondary research use of the identifiable private information or identifiable biospecimens.
    **Requirements for waiver and alteration added (found in .116.f.3.iii):** (3) *Requirements for waiver and alteration.* In order for an IRB to waive or alter consent as described in this subsection, the IRB must find and document that:
    (iii) If the research involves using identifiable private information or identifiable biospecimens, the research could not practicably be carried out without using such information or biospecimens in an identifiable format;

15. *Screening, recruiting, or determining eligibility* without informed consent has been added (found in .116.g): **(g) *Screening, recruiting, or determining eligibility.*** An IRB may approve

a research proposal in which an investigator will obtain information or biospecimens for the purpose of screening, recruiting, or determining the eligibility of prospective subjects without the informed consent of the prospective subject or the subject's legally authorized representative, if either of the following conditions is met:

**(1)** The investigator will obtain information through oral or written communication with the prospective subject or legally authorized representative, or

**(2)** The investigator will obtain identifiable private information or identifiable biospecimens by accessing records or stored identifiable biospecimens.

**(Of note, the HIPAA Privacy Rule requirement for Representations at 45 CFR 164.512(i)(ii) still stands with the adoption of the New Common Rule. See Chapter 3, Section 3.1.)**

**16.** Clinical trial consent forms must be posted to a federal website.

   **Posting of Consent form (found in .116.h):** (h) *Posting of clinical trial consent form.*

**(1)** For each clinical trial conducted or supported by a Federal department or agency, one IRB-approved informed consent form used to enroll subjects must be posted by the awardee or the Federal department or agency component conducting the trial on a publicly available Federal Web site that will be established as a repository for such informed consent forms.

**(2)** If the Federal department or agency supporting or conducting the clinical trial determines that certain information should not be made publicly available on a Federal Web site (e.g., confidential commercial information), such Federal department or agency may permit or require redactions to the information posted.

**(3)** The informed consent form must be posted on the Federal Web site after the clinical trial is closed to recruitment, and no later than 60 days after the last study visit by any subject, as required by the protocol.

**17.** "Limited IRB review" has been defined above.[8]

---

> **Please reference the *45 CFR 46 Common Rule Changes Comparison Document*, which compares the new and old regulatory language side-by-side, in Appendix 28.**

---

Current eCFR for the full 45 CFR 46 regulation: https://www.ecfr.gov/cgi-bin/text-idx?SID=1619c64383ac85189ffcb78213115cbc&mc=true&node=pt45.1.46&rgn=div5#se45.1.46_1111.

January 21, 2019 effective eCFR for the New Common Rule: https://www.gpo.gov/fdsys/pkg/FR-2017-01-19/pdf/2017-01058.pdf. (Note: It has the original effective date of January 19, 2018 written within it, and the date of the original Federal Register notice of January 19, 2017.)

On June 18, 2018, HHS released a final rule, which delayed the effective date of the New Common Rule until January 21, 2019.

**The Federal Register states:**

As a result of this delay, regulated entities will be required, with an exception, to continue to comply with the requirements of the pre-2018 version of the Federal Policy for the Protection of Human Subjects (the "pre-2018 Requirements") until January 21, 2019. The one exception to this general rule is that institutions will be permitted (but not required) to implement, for certain research, three burden-reducing provisions of the 2018 Requirements during the delay period (July 19, 2018, through January 20, 2019). Those three provisions are: The revised definition of "research," which deems certain activities not to be research covered by the Common Rule; the elimination of the requirement for annual continuing review with respect to certain categories of research; and the elimination of the requirement that institutional review boards (IRBs) review grant applications or other funding proposals related to the research. Institutions taking advantage of the three-burden reducing provisions must comply with all other pre-2018 Requirements during the delay period.

https://www.gpo.gov/fdsys/pkg/FR-2018-06-19/pdf/2018-13187.pdf.

## 8.3 PAYMENT AND REIMBURSEMENT TO RESEARCH SUBJECTS

The FDA published an Information Sheet with new guidance on this topic on 1/25/2018. The link is here: https://www.fda.gov/RegulatoryInformation/Guidances/ucm126429.htm.

Salient points are as follows:

"FDA does not consider reimbursement for travel expenses to and from the clinical trial site and associated costs such as airfare, parking, and lodging to raise issues regarding undue influence. Other than reimbursement for reasonable travel and lodging expenses, IRBs should be sensitive to whether other aspects of proposed payment for participation could present an undue influence, thus interfering with the potential subjects' ability to give voluntary informed consent."

"The amount and schedule of all payments should be presented to the IRB at the time of initial review. The IRB should review both the amount of payment and the proposed method and timing of disbursement to assure that neither are coercive or present undue influence [21 CFR 50.20]."

"Any credit for payment should accrue as the study progresses and not be contingent upon the subject completing the entire study."

"…payment of a small proportion as an incentive for completion of the study is acceptable to FDA, providing that such incentive is not coercive."

"All information concerning payment, including the amount and schedule of payment(s), should be set forth in the informed consent document."[9]

## 8.4 THE SINGLE INSTITUTIONAL REVIEW BOARD (sIRB)

**NIH has created a policy for the use of a single IRB for NIH-funded trials. The policy states that** all sites participating in multisite studies involving non-exempt human subjects research funded by the National Institutes of Health (NIH) will use a single Institutional Review Board (sIRB) to conduct the ethical review required by the U.S. Department of Health and Human Services regulations for the Protection of Human Subjects at 45 CFR Part 46.[10]

**Effective Date: January 25, 2018**

The policy will apply to all competing grant applications for due dates on or after January 25, 2018. For Research and Development (R&D) contracts, the policy will apply to all solicitations issued on or after this effective date.

**Scope and Applicability**

The policy applies to the domestic sites of NIH-funded multi-site studies where each site will conduct the same protocol involving non-exempt human subjects research, whether supported through grants, cooperative agreements, contracts, or the NIH Intramural Research Program. It does not apply to career development, research training, or fellowship awards.

The policy applies to domestic awardees and participating domestic sites. Foreign sites participating in NIH-funded, multi-site studies will not be expected to follow this policy.

<u>Purpose</u>

The purpose of this policy is to **streamline** the IRB review process and **reduce inefficiencies** so that research can proceed as **expeditiously** as possible without compromising ethical principles and protections for human research participants.

For local IRBs, the purpose is to create a shift in workload away from conducting redundant reviews in order to allow (local) IRBs to concentrate more time and attention on the review of single-site protocols, thereby enhancing research oversight.

<u>How it will work</u>

Grant applicants will be expected to include a plan for the use of an sIRB that will be selected to serve as the IRB of record for all study sites in the applications/proposals they submit to the NIH.

The NIH funding Institute or Center (IC) must approve the sIRB. The NIH's acceptance of the submitted plan will be incorporated as a term and condition in the Notice of Award or in the Contract Award.

The sIRB may serve as a Privacy Board, as applicable, to fulfill the requirements of the HIPAA Privacy Rule for use or disclosure of protected health information for research purposes. The sIRB will collaborate with the awardee to establish a mechanism for communication between the sIRB and the participating sites.

The applicant may request direct cost funding for the additional costs associated with the establishment and review of the multi-site study by the sIRB, with appropriate justification; all such costs must be reasonable and consistent with cost principles, as described in the NIH Grants Policy Statement and the Federal Acquisition Regulation (FAR) 31.302 (Direct Costs) and FAR 31.203 (Indirect Costs).

Final NIH Policy on the Use of a Single Institutional Review Board for Multi-Site Research **(and the source of this section's information):** Notice Number: NOT-OD-16-094 https://grants.nih.gov/grants/guide/notice-files/NOT-OD-16-094.html.[11]

The compliance date for §ll.114(b) (cooperative research) for a single IRB is January 20, 2020.

Which IRB should serve as the Single IRB?

An NIH award recipient has several possible options for complying with the NIH single IRB policy including having the **IRB at one of the participating sites** agree to serve as the single IRB, using an **independent IRB**, including the **IRB of a non-participating site**, or **using the IRB as required in the Funding Opportunity Announcement (FOA) or Request for Proposal (RFP)** (for example, certain cancer clinical trials funded by the National Cancer Institute (NCI) are required to use the NCI Central IRB (CIRB)). As required in the federal Protection of Human Subjects regulations (45 CFR 46 Part E), the IRB must be registered with the Office for Human Research Protections (OHRP) and must have the appropriate membership, including the professional competence necessary to review the proposed research."[12] https://grants.nih.gov/grants/policy/faq_single_IRB_policy_research.htm#5167.

Guidance and Frequently Asked Questions to assist in the implementation of the policy will be available at: https://osp.od.nih.gov/clinical-research/irb-review/.[13]

Direct all inquiries to:

NIH Office of Science Policy

Telephone: 301-496-9838

Email: SingleIRBPolicy@mail.nih.gov

## 8.5  NEW CHANGES TO CERTIFICATES OF CONFIDENTIALITY

A Certificate of Confidentiality ensures the following research subject rights:

- Protects the privacy of subjects enrolled in research studies from anyone not connected to the research except when the subject consents or:
  - As required by Federal, State or local laws
    - i.e., State laws that require the reporting of communicable diseases to State and local health departments
  - The disclosure is "for the purposes of other scientific research that is in compliance with applicable Federal regulations governing the protection of human subjects in research".
- Prohibits the disclosure of subjects':
  - Names
  - Study documents
  - Biospecimens
  - identifiable, sensitive information
    https://grants.nih.gov/grants/guide/notice-files/NOT-OD-17-109.html[14]

NIH states that "… the term 'identifiable, sensitive information' means information about an individual that is gathered or used during the course of biomedical, behavioral, clinical, or other research, where the following may occur:

- An individual is identified; or
- For which there is at least a very small risk, that some combination of the information, a request for the information, and other available data sources could be used to deduce the identity of an individual." A revised policy regarding Certificates of Confidentiality **came into effect on October 1, 2017** for all research that began on or after December 13, 2016 or has been ongoing as of December 13, 2016. It was issued by the U.S. National Institutes of Health (NIH) for research, which is NIH-funded. However, a PI or Institution that is conducting a study, which is not NIH funded, may still apply for a Certificate of Confidentiality under this revision. Prior to this revision, all Principal Investigators were required to <u>apply</u> for a Certificate of Confidentiality for NIH-supported studies in order to protect subjects engaged in, what was considered to be <u>sensitive research</u>, such as HIV studies.

Now, the application requirement has been expanded to include all research studies defined by 45 CFR 46 except for de-identified studies. Here is the language from the revision:

- "Human subjects research as defined in the Federal Policy for the Protection of Human Subjects (45 CFR 46), including exempt research except for human subjects research that is determined to be exempt from all or some of the requirements of 45 CFR 46 if the information obtained is recorded in such a manner that human subjects cannot be identified or the identity of the human subjects cannot readily be ascertained, directly or through identifiers linked to the subjects;
- Research involving the collection or use of biospecimens that are identifiable to an individual or for which there is at least a very small risk that some combination of the biospecimen, a request for the biospecimen, and other available data sources could be used to deduce the identity of an individual;

- Research that involves the generation of individual level, human genomic data from biospecimens, or the use of such data, regardless of whether the data is recorded in such a manner that human subjects can be identified or the identity of the human subjects can readily be ascertained as defined in the Federal Policy for the Protection of Human Subjects (45 CFR 46); or
- Any other research that involves information about an individual for which there is at least a very small risk, as determined by current scientific practices or statistical methods, that some combination of the information, a request for the information, and other available data sources could be used to deduce the identity of an individual, as defined in subsection 301(d) of the Public Health Service Act."[15] https://grants.nih.gov/grants/guide/notice-files/NOT-OD-17-109.html
- In addition to greater study design inclusion, Certificates of Confidentiality will now be <u>automatically provided</u> within grant awards for any NIH-funded studies that meet the requirements in the four bullets directly above.

**Here's how to determine if this applies to your NIH research:**
"To determine if this Policy applies to research conducted or supported by NIH, investigators will need to ask, and answer the following question:

- Is the activity biomedical, behavioral, clinical, or other research?

If the answer to this question is no, then the activity is not issued a Certificate. If the answer is yes, then investigators will need to answer the following questions:

- Does the research involve Human Subjects as defined by 45 CFR Part 46?
- Are you collecting or using biospecimens that are identifiable to an individual as part of the research?
- If collecting or using biospecimens as part of the research, is there a small risk that some combination of the biospecimen, a request for the biospecimen, and other available data sources could be used to deduce the identity of an individual?
- Does the research involve the generation of individual level, human genomic data?

If the answer to any one of these questions is yes, then this Policy will apply to the research."[16]
**Certificate of Confidentiality Recipient Responsibilities:**
"... in accordance with subsection 301(d) of the Public Health Service Act, the recipient of the Certificate shall not:

- Disclose or provide, in any Federal, State, or local civil, criminal, administrative, legislative, or other proceeding, the name of such individual or any such information, document, or biospecimen that contains identifiable, sensitive information about the individual and that was created or compiled for purposes of the research, unless such disclosure or use is made with the consent of the individual to whom the information, document, or biospecimen pertains; or
- Disclose or provide to any other person not connected with the research the name of such an individual or any information, document, or biospecimen that contains identifiable, sensitive information about such an individual and that was created or compiled for purposes of the research."

**To learn how to obtain a Certificate of Confidentiality for HHS non-NIH funded research, Non-HHS funded research, and non-Federal funded research, you will find useful information at:** https://humansubjects.nih.gov/coc/index.[17]

Scroll down to see the boxes for each funding choice. Click on the box that pertains to your research. **You can send questions to:**

Office of Extramural Research
Email: NIH-CoC-Coordinator@mail.nih.gov

Source: https://grants.nih.gov/grants/guide/notice-files/NOT-OD-17-109.html.[18]

## 8.6 NEW ICH GCP E6 R2 (REVISION 2) GUIDELINES

New guidelines for ICH GCP E6 R2 were published on December 15, 2016 and took effect on June 14, 2017. The formal name of the revised document is the **Integrated Addendum to ICH E6(R1), guideline for Good Clinical Practice E6 (R2).**

Changes to the International Council on Harmonisation (ICH) GCP are marked by the word, "Addendum" throughout the ICH GCP document. They are collected together here for easy reference (Figs. 8.1–8.15).

| 20 | **ADDENDUM** |
|---|---|
| 21 | Since the development of the ICH GCP Guideline, the scale, complexity, and cost of clinical |
| 22 | trials have increased. Evolutions in technology and risk management processes offer new |
| 23 | opportunities to increase efficiency and focus on relevant activities. This guideline has been |
| 24 | amended to encourage implementation of improved and more efficient approaches to clinical |
| 25 | trial design, conduct, oversight, recording and reporting while continuing to ensure human |
| 26 | subject protection and data integrity. Standards regarding electronic records and essential |
| 27 | documents intended to increase clinical trial quality and efficiency have also been updated. |
| 28 | This ICH GCP Guideline integrated Addendum provides a unified standard for the European |
| 29 | Union (EU), Japan, the United States, Canada and Switzerland to facilitate the mutual |
| 30 | acceptance of clinical data by the regulatory authorities in these jurisdictions. |

**FIG. 8.1**

Introduction.

| 81 | **ADDENDUM** |
|---|---|
| 82 | **1.11.1 Certified Copy** |
| 83 | A paper or electronic copy of the original record that has been verified (e.g., by a dated |
| 84 | signature) or has been generated through a validated process to produce an exact copy having |
| 85 | all of the same attributes and information as the original. |

**FIG. 8.2**

Case report form.

| 206 | ADDENDUM |
| 207 | **1.38.1 Monitoring Plan** |
| 208 | A description of the methods, responsibilities and requirements for monitoring the trial. |
| 209 | **1.39 Monitoring Report** |
| 210 | A written report from the monitor to the sponsor after each site visit and/or other trial-related |
| 211 | communication according to the sponsor's SOPs. |
| 212 | ADDENDUM |
| 213 | Outcomes of any centralized monitoring should also be reported. |

**FIG. 8.3**

Monitoring plan and report.

| 297 | ADDENDUM |
| 298 | **1.60.1 Validation of computerized systems** |
| 299 | A process of establishing and documenting that the specified requirements of a computerized |
| 300 | system can be consistently fulfilled. Validation should ensure accuracy, reliability and |
| 301 | consistent intended performance, from design until decommissioning of the system or |
| 302 | transition to a new system. |

**FIG. 8.4**

Validation of computerized systems.

| 340 | ADDENDUM |
| 341 | This principle applies to all records (paper or electronic) referenced in this guideline. |

**FIG. 8.5**

Principles of ICH GCP.

| 486 | ADDENDUM |
| 487 | *4.2.5* The investigator is responsible for supervising any individual or party to whom the |
| 488 | investigator delegates study tasks conducted at the trial site. |
| 489 | *4.2.6* If the investigator/institution retains the services of any party to perform study tasks |
| 490 | they should ensure this party is qualified to perform those study tasks and should |
| 491 | implement procedures to ensure the integrity of the study tasks performed and any |
| 492 | data generated. |

**FIG. 8.6**

Investigator.

| 703 | **4.9 Records and Reports** |
| 704 | ADDENDUM |
| 705 | 4.9.0 The investigator should maintain adequate and accurate source documents and trial |
| 706 | records that include all pertinent observations on each of the site's trial subjects. |
| 707 | Source data should be attributable, legible, contemporaneous, original, accurate, and |
| 708 | complete. Changes to source data should be traceable, should not obscure the original |
| 709 | entry and should be explained if necessary (e.g., *via* and audit trail). |

**FIG. 8.7**

Records and reports.

| 783 | **5.** | **SPONSOR** |
|---|---|---|
| 784 | **ADDENDUM** | |

785 **5.0    Quality Management**

786 The sponsor should implement a system to manage quality throughout the design, conduct,
787 recording, evaluation, reporting and archiving of clinical trials.

788 Sponsors should focus on trial activities essential to ensuring human subject protection and
789 the reliability of trial results. Quality management includes the efficient design of clinical trial
790 protocols, data collection tools and procedures, and the collection of information that is
791 essential to decision making.

792 The methods used to assure and control the quality of the trial should be proportionate to the
793 risks inherent in the trial and the importance of the information collected. The sponsor should
794 ensure that all aspects of the trial are operationally feasible and should avoid unnecessary
795 complexity, procedures and data collection. Protocols, case report forms, and other operational
796 documents should be clear, concise and consistent.

797 The quality management system should use a risk-based approach as described below.

798 *5.0.1    Critical Process and Data Identification*
799          During protocol development, the sponsor should identify those processes and data
800          that are critical to assure human subject protection and the reliability of study results.

801 *5.0.2    Risk Identification*
802          Risks to critical study processes and data should be identified. Risks should be
803          considered at both the system level (e.g., facilities, standard operating procedures,
804          computerized systems, personnel, vendors) and clinical trial level (e.g.,
805          investigational product, trial design, data collection and recording).

(Line 806 is blank in ICH GCP E6 R2.)

807 *5.0.3    Risk Evaluation*
808          The identified risks should be evaluated by considering:
809          (a)  The likelihood of errors occurring, given existing risk controls.
810          (b)  The impact of such errors on human subject protection and data integrity.
811          (c)  The extent to which such errors would be detectable.

812 *5.0.4    Risk Control*
813          The sponsor should identify those risks that should be reduced (through mitigating
814          actions) and/or can be accepted. Risk mitigation activities may be incorporated in
815          protocol design and implementation, monitoring plans, agreements between parties
816          defining roles and responsibilities, systematic safeguards to ensure adherence to
817          standard operating procedures, and training in processes and procedures.

818          Predefined quality tolerance limits should be established, taking into consideration
819          the medical and statistical characteristics of the variables as well as the statistical
820          design of the trial, to identify systematic issues that can impact subject safety or data
821          integrity. Detection of deviations from the predefined quality tolerance limits should
822          trigger an evaluation to determine if action is needed.

823 *5.0.5    Risk Communication*
824          The quality management activities should be documented and communicated to
825          stakeholders to facilitate risk review and continual improvement during clinical trial
826          execution.

827 *5.0.6    Risk Review*
828          The sponsor should periodically review risk control measures to ascertain whether
829          the implemented quality management activities remain effective and relevant, taking
830          into account emerging knowledge and experience.

831 *5.0.7    Risk Reporting*
832          The sponsor should describe the quality management approach implemented in the
833          trial and summarize important deviations from the predefined quality tolerance limits
834          in the clinical study report (ICH E3, Section 9.6 Data Quality Assurance).

**FIG. 8.8**

Sponsor.

850 5.2.1 A sponsor may transfer any or all of the sponsor's trial-related duties and functions to a
851 CRO, but the ultimate responsibility for the quality and integrity of the trial data
852 always resides with the sponsor. The CRO should implement quality assurance and
853 quality control.
854 **ADDENDUM**

855 The sponsor should ensure oversight of any trial-related duties and functions carried
856 out on its behalf.

857 5.2.2 Any trial-related duty and function that is transferred to and assumed by a CRO should
858 be specified in writing.
859 **ADDENDUM**

860 The sponsor should document approval of any subcontracting of trial-related duties
861 and functions by a CRO.

**FIG. 8.9**

Contract Research Organization.

888 5.5.3 When using electronic trial data handling and/or remote electronic trial data systems,
889 the sponsor should:
890 (a) Ensure and document that the electronic data processing system(s) conforms to the
891 sponsor's established requirements for completeness, accuracy, reliability, and
892 consistent intended performance (i.e., validation).
893 (b) Maintains SOPs for using these systems.

894 **ADDENDUM**

895 The SOPs should cover system setup, installation and use. The SOPs should
896 describe system validation and functionality testing, data collection and handling,
897 system maintenance, system security measures, change control, data backup,
898 recovery, contingency planning and decommissioning. The responsibilities of the
899 sponsor, investigator and other parties with respect to the use of these
900 computerized systems should be clear, and the users should be provided with
901 training in the use of the systems.

912 **ADDENDUM**

913 (h) Ensure the integrity of the data including any data that describe the context,
914 content and structure of the data. This is particularly important when making
915 changes to the computerized systems, such as software upgrades or migration of
916 data.

**FIG. 8.10**

Trial management.

1115   *5.18.3 Extent and Nature of Monitoring*

1116     The sponsor should ensure that the trials are adequately monitored. The sponsor
1117     should determine the appropriate extent and nature of monitoring. The determination
1118     of the extent and nature of monitoring should be based on considerations such as the
1119     objective, purpose, design, complexity, blinding, size, and endpoints of the trial. In
1120     general there is a need for on-site monitoring, before, during, and after the trial;
1121     however in exceptional circumstances the sponsor may determine that central
1122     monitoring in conjunction with procedures such as investigators' training and
1123     meetings, and extensive written guidance can assure appropriate conduct of the trial in
1124     accordance with GCP. Statistically controlled sampling may be an acceptable method
1125     for selecting the data to be verified.

1126   **ADDENDUM**

1127     The sponsor should develop a systematic, prioritized, risk-based approach to
1128     monitoring clinical trials. The flexibility in the extent and nature of monitoring
1129     described in this section is intended to permit varied approaches that improve the
1130     effectiveness and efficiency of monitoring. A combination of on-site and centralized
1131     monitoring activities may be appropriate. The sponsor should document the rationale
1132     for the chosen monitoring strategy (e.g., in the monitoring plan).

1133     *On*-site monitoring is performed at the sites at which the clinical trial is being
1134     conducted.

1135     Centralized monitoring is a remote evaluation of ongoing and/or cumulative data
1136     collected from trial sites, in a timely manner. Centralized monitoring processes provide
1137     additional monitoring capabilities that can complement and reduce the extent and/or
1138     frequency of on-site monitoring by such methods as:
1139     (a)   Routine review of submitted data.

1140     (b)   Identification of missing data, inconsistent data, data outliers or unexpected lack
1141         of variability and protocol deviations that may be indicative of systematic or
1142         significant errors in data collection and reporting at a site or across sites, or may
1143         be indicative of potential data manipulation or data integrity problems.

1144     (c)   Using statistical analyses to identify data trends such as the range and
1145         consistency of data within and across sites.

1146     (d)   Analyzing site characteristics and performance metrics.

1147     (e)   Selection of sites and/or processes for targeted on-site monitoring.

**FIG. 8.11**

Monitoring.

1232   **ADDENDUM**

1233     (e)   Monitoring results should be provided to the sponsor (including appropriate
1234         management and staff responsible for trial and site oversight) in a timely manner
1235         for review and follow up as indicated. Results of monitoring activities should be
1236         documented in sufficient detail to allow verification of compliance with the
1237         monitoring plan.

**FIG. 8.12**

Monitoring report.

1238
1239 | **ADDENDUM**

1240 | 5.18.7 *Monitoring Plan*

1241 | The sponsor should develop a monitoring plan that is tailored to the specific human
1242 | subject protection and data integrity risks of the trial. The plan should describe the
1243 | monitoring strategy, the monitoring responsibilities of all the parties involved, the
1244 | various monitoring methods to be used and the rationale for their use. The plan
1245 | should also emphasize the monitoring of critical data and processes. Particular
1246 | attention should be given to those aspects that are not routine clinical practice and
1247 | that require additional training. The monitoring plan should reference the applicable
1248 | policies and procedures.

**FIG. 8.13**

Monitoring plan.

1278 | **5.20** **Noncompliance**

1279 | 5.20.1 Noncompliance with the protocol, SOPs, GCP, and/or applicable regulatory
1280 | requirement(s) by an investigator/institution, or by member(s) of the sponsor's staff
1281 | should lead to prompt action by the sponsor to secure compliance.

1282 | **ADDENDUM**

1283 | When significant noncompliance is discovered, the sponsor should perform a root
1284 | cause analysis and implement appropriate corrective and preventive actions. If required
1285 | by applicable law or regulation the sponsor should inform the regulatory authority(ies)
1286 | when the noncompliance is a serious breach of the trial protocol or GCP.

**FIG. 8.14**

Non-compliance.

1694 | **ADDENDUM**

1695 | The sponsor and investigator/institution should maintain a record of the location(s) of their respective essential documents. The storage system
1696 | (irrespective of the media used) should provide for document identification, search and retrieval.
1697 |
1698 | Depending on the activities being carried out, individual trials may require additional documents not specifically mentioned in the essential
1699 | document list. The sponsor and/or investigator/institution should include these as part of the trial master file.

1700 | The sponsor should ensure that the investigator has control of and continuous access to the CRF data reported to the sponsor. The sponsor should
1701 | not have exclusive control of those data.
1702 |
1703 | When a copy is used to replace an original document, the copy should fulfill the requirements for certified copies.
1704 |
1705 | The investigator/institution should have control of all essential documents and records generated by the investigator/institution before, during and
1706 | after the trial.

**FIG. 8.15**

Essential documents.

The link to the information above is here: http://www.ich.org/fileadmin/Public_Web_Site/ICH_Products/Guidelines/Efficacy/E6/E6_R2__Step_4_2016_1109.pdf.[19]

## 8.7 ELECTRONIC COMMON TECHNICAL DOCUMENT (eCTD)

The eCTD is FDA's Center for Drug Evaluation and Research (CDER) and FDA's Center for Biologics Evaluation and Research (CBER) standard format for electronic regulatory submissions. Beginning May 5, 2017, the following submission types: NDA, ANDA, BLA, and Master Files must be submitted in eCTD format. Beginning May 5, 2018, Commercial IND and Commercial Exploratory IND submissions must be submitted in eCTD format. Submissions that do not adhere to the requirements stated in the eCTD Guidance (found at: https://www.fda.gov/downloads/Drugs/GuidanceComplianceRegulatoryInformation/Guidances/UCM333969.pdf) will be subject to rejection. For more information, see: http://www.fda.gov/ectd.[20]

## 8.8 NEW CHANGES IN CLINCIALTRIALS.GOV REGISTRATION AND REPORTING

The National Institutes of Health (NIH) within the U.S. Department of Health and Human Services issued a revised regulation for the submission of registration and summary results information to www.clinicaltrials.gov effective January 18, 2017. However, April 18, 2017 was the date by which compliance with the revised regulation was required. Within the revision, a clinical trial is required to be registered only if it is an "Applicable Clinical Trial" (ACT). See the *Checklist for Evaluating Whether a Clinical Trial or Study is an Applicable Clinical Trial (ACT) Under 42 CFR 11.22(b) for Clinical Trials Initiated on or After January 18, 2017* in Appendix 11.

The revisions to registration and results information, including adverse events, as well as deadlines for submitting updates, are succinctly presented below.

REGISTRATION

As of January 18, 2017, the following data elements are REQUIRED as stated in 42 CFR 11.28(a)(2) when the responsible party **registers** an ACT with www.clinicaltrials.gov (Fig. 8.16).

| # | Data Element | 42 CFR 11.28 (a)(2) Provision |
|---|--------------|-------------------------------|
| 1 | Brief Title | (i)(A) |
| 2 | Official Title | (i)(B) |
| 3 | Brief Summary | (i)(C) |
| 4 | Primary Purpose | (i)(D) |
| 5 | Study Design | (i)(E) |
| 6 | Study Phase | (i)(F) |
| 7 | Study Type | (i)(G) |

**FIG. 8.16**

Clinicaltrials.gov registration.

*(Continued)*

| 8 | Pediatric Postmarket Surveillance of a Device Product | (i)(H) |
|---|---|---|
| 9 | Primary Disease or Condition Being Studied in the Trial, or the Focus of the Study | (i)(I) |
| 10 | Intervention Name(s) | (i)(J) |
| 11 | Other Intervention Name(s) | (i)(K) |
| 12 | Intervention Description | (i)(L) |
| 13 | Intervention Type | (i)(M) |
| 14 | Studies a U.S. FDA-regulated Device Product | (i)(N) |
| 15 | Studies a U.S. FDA-regulated Drug Product | (i)(O) |
| 16 | Device Product Not Approved or Cleared by U.S. FDA | (i)(P) |
| 17 | Post Prior to U.S. FDA Approval or Clearance | (i)(Q) |
| 18 | Product Manufactured in and Exported from the U.S. | (i)(R) |
| 19 | Study Start Date | (i)(S) |
| 20 | Primary Completion Date | (i)(T) |
| 21 | Study Completion Date | (i)(U) |
| 22 | Enrollment | (i)(V) |
| 23 | Primary Outcome Measure Information (Name, Description, Time of Assessment) | (i)(W) |
| 24 | Secondary Outcome Measure Information (Name, Description, Time of Assessment) | (i)(X) |
| 25 | Eligibility Criteria | (ii)(A) |
| 26 | Sex/Gender | (ii)(B) |
| 27 | Age Limits | (ii)(C) |
| 28 | Accepts Healthy Volunteers | (ii)(D) |
| 29 | Overall Recruitment Status | (ii)(E) |
| 30 | Why Study Stopped | (ii)(F) |
| 31 | Individual Site Status | (ii)(G) |
| 32 | Availability of Expanded Access | (ii)(H) |
| 33 | Name of the Sponsor | (iii)(A) |
| 34 | Responsible Party, by Official Title | (iii)(B) |
| 35 | Facility Information (Facility Name, Facility Location, and Facility Contact or Central Contact) | (iii)(C) |
| 36 | Unique Protocol Identification Number | (iv)(A) |
| 37 | Secondary ID (including ID Type) | (iv)(B) |
| 38 | U.S. Food and Drug Administration IND or IDE number (Center, Number, Serial Number) | (iv)(C) |
| 39 | Human Subjects Protection Review Board Status | (iv)(D) |
| 40 | Record Verification Date | (iv)(E) |
| 41 | Responsible Party Contact Information | (iv)(F) |

**FIG. 8.16, CONT'D**

Of the required registration data elements in this table, the new registration data elements that are required as of 1/18/17 are:

- Official Title
- Why the Study Stopped
- Study Start Date

- Study Completion Date
- If the study is a U.S. FDA-regulated Drug Product
- If the study is a U.S. FDA-regulated Device Product
- If the Device Product has not been Approved or Cleared by the U.S. FDA
- Primary Purpose
- Interventional Study Model
- Number of Arms
- Masking
- Allocation
- Enrollment
- Intervention Description
- Accepts Healthy Volunteers
- Facility Name
- Zip code of U.S. Facility
- Responsible Party Contact Information

Definitions for all of the registration data elements (old and new) can be found here: https://prsinfo. clinicaltrials.gov/definitions.html.[21]

RESULTS INFORMATION

As of January 18, 2017, the following data elements are REQUIRED as stated in 42 CFR 11.48(a) when the responsible party submits **results information** for an applicable clinical trial (ACT) with www.clinicaltrials.gov (Fig. 8.17).

| # | Data Element | 42 CFR 11.48(a) Provision |
|---|---|---|
| 1 | Participant Flow Arm Information | (1)(i) |
| 2 | Pre-assignment Information, if any | (1)(ii) |
| 3 | Participant Data (number of human subjects that started and completed the clinical trial, by arm) | (1)(iii) |
| 4 | Baseline Characteristics Arm/Group Information | (2)(i) |
| 5 | Baseline Analysis Population Information | (2)(ii) |
| 6 | Overall Number of Baseline Participants | (2)(ii)(A) |
| 7 | Overall Number of Units Analyzed | (2)(ii)(B) |
| 8 | Analysis Population Description | (2)(ii)(C) |
| 9 | Baseline Measure Information | (2)(iii) |
| 10 | Name and Description of the Measure, including any categories that are used to submit Baseline Measure Data | (2)(iii)(A) |
| 11 | Measure Type and Measure of Dispersion | (2)(iii)(B) |
| 12 | Unit of Measure | (2)(iii)(C) |

**FIG. 8.17**

Clinicaltrials.gov results.

*(Continued)*

| 13 | Baseline Measure Data | (2)(iv) |
|---|---|---|
| 14 | Number of Baseline Participants (and Units) | (2)(v) |
| 15 | Outcome Measure Arm/Group Information | (3)(i) |
| 16 | Analysis Population Information | (3)(ii) |
| 17 | Number of Participants Analyzed | (3)(ii)(A) |
| 18 | Number of Units Analyzed | (3)(ii)(B) |
| 19 | Analysis Population Description | (3)(ii)(C) |
| 20 | Outcome Measure Information | (3)(iii) |
| 21 | Name of the Specific Outcome Measure | (3)(iii)(A) |
| 22 | Description of the Metric Used | (3)(iii)(B) |
| 23 | Time Point(s) at which the Measurement was Assessed | (3)(iii)(C) |
| 24 | Outcome Measure Type | (3)(iii)(D) |
| 25 | Measure Type and Measure of Dispersion or Precision | (3)(iii)(E) |
| 26 | Unit of Measure | (3)(iii)(F) |
| 27 | Outcome Measure Data | (3)(iv) |
| 28 | Statistical Analyses | (3)(v) |
| 29 | Statistical Analysis Overview (including identification of arms compared, type of statistical test conducted, and, for a non-inferiority or equivalence test, a description that includes the power calculation and non-inferiority or equivalence margin) | (3)(v)(B)(1) |
| 30 | One of the following as applicable: | (3)(v)(B)(2) |
| 31 | Statistical Test of Hypothesis (*p*-value and procedure used) | (3)(v)(B)(2)(i) |
| 32 | Method of Estimation (estimation parameter, estimated value, and confidence interval (if calculated)) | (3)(v)(B)(2)(ii) |
| 33 | Information to describe the methods for collecting adverse events | (4)(i) |
| 34 | Time Frame | (4)(i)(A) |
| 35 | Adverse Event Reporting Description | (4)(i)(B) |
| 36 | Collection Approach | (4)(i)(C) |
| 37 | Information for completing three tables summarizing anticipated and unanticipated adverse events collected | (4)(ii) |
| 38 | Table of all serious adverse events grouped by organ system, with the number and frequency of each event by arm or comparison group | (4)(ii)(A) |
| 39 | Table of all adverse events, other than serious adverse events, that exceed a frequency of 5 percent within any arm of the clinical trial, grouped by organ system, with the number and frequency of each event by arm or comparison group. | (4)(ii)(B) |

**FIG. 8.17, CONT'D**

| 40 | Table of all-cause mortality, with the number and frequency of deaths due to any cause by arm or comparison group | (4)(ii)(C) |
|---|---|---|
| 41 | Information for each table specified in paragraph (4)(ii) | (4)(iii) |
| 42 | Adverse Event Arm/Group Information | (4)(iii)(A) |
| 43 | Total Number Affected, by Arm or Comparison Group | (4)(iii)(B) |
| 44 | Total Number at Risk, by Arm or Comparison Group | (4)(iii)(C) |
| 45 | Adverse Event Information for the two tables described in paragraphs (4)(ii)(A) and (B) | (4)(iii)(D) |
| 46 | Descriptive term for the adverse event | (4)(iii)(D)(1) |
| 47 | Organ system associated with the adverse event | (4)(iii)(D)(2) |
| 48 | Adverse Event Data for the two tables described in paragraphs (4)(ii)(A) and (B) | (4)(iii)(E) |
| 49 | Number of human subjects affected by such adverse event | (4)(iii)(E)(1) |
| 50 | Number of human subjects at risk for such adverse event | (4)(iii)(E)(2) |
| 51 | Protocol and Statistical Analysis Plan | (5) |
| 52 | Results Point of Contact | (6)(i) |
| 53 | Name or official title of the point of contact | (6)(i)(A) |
| 54 | Name of the affiliated organization | (6)(i)(B) |
| 55 | Telephone number and email address of the point of contact | (6)(i)(C) |
| 56 | Certain Agreements | (6)(ii) |

**FIG. 8.17, CONT'D**

The "Changes from Current Practice Described in the Final Rule: Final Rule for Clinical Trials Registration and Results Information Submission (42 CFR Part 11)" can be found here: https://prsinfo.clinicaltrials.gov/FinalRuleChanges-16Sept2016.pdf.[22]

**The full final rule can be found at NIH-2011-0003 at www.regulations.gov.**

Table 3. Data Elements for More Rapid Updating for Clinical Trials Initiated On or After January 18, 2017 (42 CFR 11.64(a)(1)(ii))

For clinical trials initiated on or after January 18, 2017, section 11.64(a)(1)(ii) of the Final Rule specifies update requirements. In general, clinical trial information submitted to ClinicalTrials.gov must be updated not less than once every 12 months. The Final Rule further requires that some data elements be updated more rapidly, as summarized in Table 3. In addition, the Final Rule requires that if a protocol is amended in such a manner that changes are communicated to human subjects in the clinical trial, updates to any relevant clinical trial information must be submitted not later than 30 calendar days after the protocol amendment is approved by a human subjects protection review board. See section IV.D.3 of the preamble and 42 CFR 11.64 for a more complete elaboration and specification of these requirements (Fig. 8.18).

| Data Element | Deadline for Updating (i.e., Not Later Than the Specified Date) |
|---|---|
| Study Start Date | 30 calendar days after the first subject is enrolled (if the first human subject was not enrolled at the time of registration). |
| Intervention Name(s) | 30 calendar days after a nonproprietary name is established. |
| Availability of Expanded Access | 30 calendar days after expanded access becomes available (if available after registration); and 30 calendar days after an NCT number is assigned to a newly created expanded access record. [1] |
| Expanded Access Status | 30 calendar days after a change in the availability of expanded access. |
| Expanded Access Type | 30 calendar days after a change in the type(s) of available expanded access. |
| Overall Recruitment Status | 30 calendar days after a change in overall recruitment status. [2] |
| Individual Site Status | 30 calendar days after a change in status of any individual site. |
| Human Subjects Protection Review Board Status | 30 calendar days after a change in status. |
| Primary Completion Date | 30 calendar days after the clinical trial reaches its actual primary completion date. |
| Enrollment | At the time the primary completion date is changed to "actual," the actual number of participants enrolled must be submitted. |
| Study Completion Date | 30 calendar days after the clinical trial reaches its actual study completion date. |
| Responsible Party, by Official Title | 30 calendar days after a change in the responsible party or the official title of the responsible party. |
| Responsible Party Contact Information | 30 calendar days after a change in the responsible party or the contact information for the responsible party. |
| Device Product Not Approved or Cleared by U.S. FDA | 15 calendar days after a change in approval or clearance status has occurred. |
| Record Verification Date | Any time the responsible party reviews the complete set of submitted clinical trial information for accuracy and not less than every 12 months, even if no other updated information is submitted at that time. |

**FIG. 8.18**

Table 3 data elements.

Table Source: https://prsinfo.clinicaltrials.gov/FinalRuleChanges-16Sept2016.pdf.[23]

Additionally, Responsible Parties are required to correct any errors, deficiencies, or inconsistencies within **15** days of submitting **registration** information, and within 25 days of submitting results information.

Please know that there are "potential legal consequences of non-compliance" per 42 CFR 11.66. Actions necessitating legal action include:

- Failing to submit clinical trial information
- Submitting false or misleading clinical trial information

Consequences may include:

- Civil monetary penalties
- Withholding of awarded grant money
- Withholding of future grant money for a new award

If you have questions, you can write to:
register@clinicaltrials.gov

In light of all of the changes explained in this chapter, research study teams and Research Administrators may wish to subscribe to e-mail notifications from the FDA and join research organizations in order to be provided with notifications when regulatory and GCP changes occur.

# ENDNOTES

[1] Federal Register Announcement, New Common Rule: https://www.federalregister.gov/documents/2018/02/21/2018-03244/human-subject-protection-acceptance-of-data-from-clinical-investigations-for-medical-devices?utm_campaign=FDA%20releases%20final%20rule%20on%20Acceptance%20of%20Data%20from%20Clinical%20Investigations%20for%20Medical%20Devices&utm_medium=email&utm_source=Eloqua&elqTrackId=A790E62E93937FE7627879A3C630AA39&elq=9e8a9f19bd4f400c81ef2d0d678cd829&elqaid=2484&elqat=1&elqCampaignId=1788.

[2] FAQs—New Common Rule https://www.fda.gov/downloads/MedicalDevices/DeviceRegulationandGuidance/GuidanceDocuments/UCM597273.pdf?utm_campaign=FDA%20releases%20final%20rule%20on%20Acceptance%20of%20Data%20from%20Clinical%20Investigations%20for%20Medical%20Devices&utm_medium=email&utm_source=Eloqua&elqTrackId=F4F5E63809CD6EC32B7CD25DAE698BDF&elq=9e8a9f19bd4f400c81ef2d0d678cd829&elqaid=2484&elqat=1&elqCampaignId=1788.

[3] New Definitions—Link here would be to NEW 45 CFR 46.

[4] Revised Definitions—Footnote and leave here (found in 45 CFR 46 .102).

[5] In 45 CFR 46.102.e.7.i, n 45 CFR 46.102.e.7.ii, n 45 CFR 46.110, the HHS Secretary.

[6] Reliance Agreement between IRBs (found in .103.e).

[7] Under Exempt Research .104(d)(7): Secondary research & broad consent.

[8] Cite for 17 items mentioned?

[9] https://www.fda.gov/RegulatoryInformation/Guidances/ucm126429.htm.

[10] Single I U.S. Department of Health and Human Services regulations for the Protection of Human Subjects at 45 CFR Part 46.

[11] https://grants.nih.gov/grants/guide/notice-files/NOT-OD-16-094.html.

[12] https://grants.nih.gov/grants/policy/faq_single_IRB_policy_research.htm#5167.

[13] https://osp.od.nih.gov/clinical-research/irb-review/.

[14] https://grants.nih.gov/grants/guide/notice-files/NOT-OD-17-109.html.

[15] https://grants.nih.gov/grants/guide/notice-files/NOT-OD-17-109.html.

[16] https://grants.nih.gov/grants/guide/notice-files/NOT-OD-17-109.html.

[17] https://humansubjects.nih.gov/coc/index.

[18] Source: https://grants.nih.gov/grants/guide/notice-files/NOT-OD-17-109.html.

[19] http://www.ich.org/fileadmin/Public_Web_Site/ICH_Products/Guidelines/Efficacy/E6/E6_R2__Step_4_2016_1109.pdf.

[20] http://www.fda.gov/ectd.

[21] https://prsinfo.clinicaltrials.gov/definitions.html.

[22] https://prsinfo.clinicaltrials.gov/FinalRuleChanges-16Sept2016.pdf.

[23] Ibid. https://prsinfo.clinicaltrials.gov/FinalRuleChanges-16Sept2016.pdf.

# AFTER THE STUDY HAS ENDED

# 9

*Purpose of chapter*:

- Provides information on study closeout procedures
- Provides Federal and ICH GCP regulatory guidance on Essential Document Retention following clinical trial conclusion
- Provides useful information on Publishing the Results of a Clinical Trial

## 9.1 STUDY CLOSEOUT

*Purpose of section*:

- Provides an overview of tasks leading to a successful study closeout
- Introduces the Study Closeout Checklist in Appendix 22
- Provides resource suggestions for developing the trial's final report

There are various tasks that need to be accomplished when closing out a trial. To help you, we have created a Study Closeout Checklist in Appendix 22. Use this checklist to identify what you need to do and to record the completion of each task.

Make sure your Regulatory Binder (see Appendix 14) and all Case Report Forms (whether paper or eCRF/EDC) are complete and correct.

Additionally, reference ICH GCP E6 R2 Section 8.4, essential documents that should be on file "After Completion or Termination of the Trial." The link is: http://www.ich.org/fileadmin/Public_Web_Site/ICH_Products/Guidelines/Efficacy/E6/E6_R2__Step_4_2016_1109.pdf.[1]

In a study performed for an Industry Sponsor, the Sponsor will have a CRO or Sponsor representative or/and a study monitor guide you through the closeout procedures and provide the necessary documents.

If you are conducting an Investigator-Initiated Study or a study with a Sponsor or funder that does not have an organized process for closure, following ICH GCP E6 R2 Section 8.4 and using the Study Closeout Checklist in Appendix 22 will help you to close out the study compliantly and without omitting any important documentation.

---

### AUTHOR'S CORNER

Make sure ALL Departments that manage a study process within your Institution are notified that the study is closed. Without this notification, what will ensue are the following possible missteps:

- The Finance Office will not know to close out a (bank) account for a study. Funds can be overspent in time if the account remains open.

The Sourcebook for Clinical Research. https://doi.org/10.1016/B978-0-12-816242-2.00009-6

- The Administration Office will not know that a Study ID (billing and registration system Study Identifier) has retired. It is possible that study activity from patient registration can be applied to the Study ID by mistake.
- The Research Pharmacy may not get the word on time and be late in performing a final account of the investigational agent and returning any remaining agent as expected. And,
- The Research Pharmacy may continue to charge maintenance and inventory fees without knowing the study has concluded.
- Other Departments may be scheduling staff to fulfill the needs of a study, not knowing the study has closed and that the extra staff are no longer needed.
- You get the idea. Your Institutional Departments and Operations Managers will appreciate timely notification of study closures.

### Final Report by PI

A final report must be written and submitted by the PI of a study. There are regulations and ICH Good Clinical Practice that mention it, but do not provide information on content. Therefore, we will explore this below.

Pursuant to ICH GCP E6 R2 Sections **4.13 Final Report(s) by Investigator and 6.9.6:**

Upon completion of the trial, the investigator, where applicable, should inform the institution; the investigator/institution should provide the IRB/IEC with a summary of the trial's outcome, and the regulatory authority(ies) with any reports required.

**6.9.6** Procedures for reporting any deviation(s) from the original statistical plan (any deviation(s) from the original statistical plan should be described and justified in protocol and/or in the final report, as appropriate).[2]

**Here are the Code of Federal Regulations references**:

**IND**

**Investigator**: 21 CFR 312.64(c) *Final report.* An investigator shall provide the sponsor with an adequate report shortly after completion of the investigator's participation in the investigation.

**IDE**

**Investigator**: 21 CFR 812.150(a)(6) *Final report.* An investigator shall, within **3 months** after termination or completion of the investigation or the investigator's part of the investigation, submit a final report to the sponsor and the reviewing IRB.

**Sponsor**: 21 CFR 812.150(b)(7) *Final report.* In the case of a significant risk device, the sponsor shall notify FDA within 30 working days of the completion or termination of the investigation and shall submit a final report to FDA and all reviewing IRBs and participating investigators within 6 months after completion or termination. In the case of a device that is not a significant risk device, the sponsor shall submit a final report to all reviewing IRBs within 6 months after termination or completion.[3]

### Contents of the Final Report

Following are three references and two suggestions for the content of a final report.

ↈICH

### 1. ICH Guideline

There is an ICH document available regarding the content of a final report (and other periodic clinical study reports), but it is old—from 1996. It is called the *Guideline for Industry: Structure and Content of Clinical Study Reports*, and can be found here: https://www.fda.gov/downloads/Drugs/GuidanceComplianceRegulatoryInformation/Guidances/UCM073113.pdf.[4]

It is from the International Council for Harmonisation (ICH) E3. The report structure is very long and comprehensive.

**2.** Guidance for Industry

A *Guidance for Industry* named *E3 Structure and Content of Clinical Study Reports*: *Questions and Answers (R1)* dated January 2013 by the U.S. Department of Health and Human Services, the Food and Drug Administration, the Center for Drug Evaluation and Research (CDER), and the Center for Biologics Evaluation and Research (CBER) builds upon the dated ICH Guideline noted above and answers questions regarding advances since 1996. The Guidance clarifies that "ICH E3 is a guidance, not a set of rigid requirements or a template, and flexibility is inherent in its use." The Guidance link is: https://www.fda.gov/downloads/Drugs/GuidanceComplianceRegulatoryInformation/Guidances/UCM336889.pdf.[5]

**IRB**

**3.** Your Institution's IRB resources

Your IRB may have a final report template. If not, your IRB should be able to communicate its expectations for final report content (which could be significantly shorter than the ICH E3 Guideline).

**4.** Use your Clinicaltrials.gov documentation

Another option is that if your study was listed on Clinicaltrials.gov, you can use your Clinicaltrials.gov results submission to help you formulate your final report. See https://clinicaltrials.gov/ct2/manage-recs/how-report.[6]

**5.** NIH grants

For studies funded by NIH grants, the NIH has a structured and required final report, called the "Final Research Performance Progress Report (RPPR)." It "is due within 120 calendar days of the end of the project period."

The specific Research Performance Progress Report (RPPR) website is: https://grants.nih.gov/grants/rppr/index.htm

You can open the NIH RPPR Instruction Guide from this website or go directly to it through: https://grants.nih.gov/sites/default/files/rppr_instruction_guide.pdf

eRA Commons has to be used to submit this report. eRA is the Electronic Research Administration web-based program from NIH. It is "an online interface where signing officials, principal investigators, trainees and post-docs at institutions/organizations can access and share administrative information relating to research grants." More information can be found at https://era.nih.gov.

eRA Commons has technical support available through its Service Desk. They can be reached directly through:

**Web:** http://grants.nih.gov/support (Preferred method of contact)
**Toll-free:** 1-866-504-9552;**Phone:** 301-402-7469
**Email**: s2ssupport@mail.nih.gov (for System-to-System support)
**Hours:** Mon-Fri, 7:00 a.m. to 8:00 p.m. Eastern Time, except for Federal Holidays

Please note: "NIH continues development of the RPPR for the final progress report and for administrative extensions (Type 4s; e.g., SBIR/STTR Fast-Track Phase II applications). NIH will continue to update the community as progress is made." Section 1.1 RPPR Instruction Guide.[7]

## 9.2 ESSENTIAL DOCUMENTS AND REGULATIONS FOR DOCUMENT RETENTION IN CLINICAL RESEARCH

*Purpose of section*:

- Provides information on trial document retention
- Reviews Federal regulations and ICH GCP for document retention

Retaining study documents is required for a period of time after the study is over. Reference the "Essential Documents" in Section 8.4 of ICH GCP E6 R2 to know what documents need to be retained, as mentioned in the study closeout, Section 9.2 of this chapter.

Below is a document retention table for quick reference and all of the regulatory and ethical sources that support it.

Of note, the Sponsor for a study may require a longer document retention period. The Authors have seen contracts that require document retention from 7 to 15 years after the trial has terminated. Check your contract at your study closeout meeting with the Sponsor to confirm the retention period, and make sure your budget has archival fees in it to cover all the years required.

| Clinical Research Timetable for Document Retention With Regulations and Good Clinical Practice References | | | |
|---|---|---|---|
| Item | By IRB | By PI | By Sponsor |
| Retention of essential documents | | 2 years* [Note 2, 4 and 6] | 2 years* [Note 1, 4, 7 and 7A] |
| Retention of IRB records for clinical research | 3 years* [Note 3 and 5] | | |

### FDA Regulations

21 CFR 312.57 Recordkeeping and record retention

**Note 1: (c)** A sponsor shall retain the records and reports required by this part for 2 years after a marketing application is approved for the drug; or, if an application is not approved for the drug, until 2 years after shipment and delivery of the drug for investigational use is discontinued and FDA has been so notified.

21 CFR 312.62 Investigator recordkeeping and record retention

**Note 2: (c)** *Record retention.* An investigator shall retain records required to be maintained under this part for a period of 2 years following the date a marketing application is approved for the drug for the indication for which it is being investigated; or, if no application is to be filed or if the application is not approved for such indication, until 2 years after the investigation is discontinued and FDA is notified.

45 CFR 46.115 IRB records Common Rule

**Note 3: (b)** The records required by this policy shall be retained for at least 3 years, and records relating to research which is conducted shall be retained for at least 3 years after completion of the research. All records shall be accessible for inspection and copying by authorized representatives of the department or agency at reasonable times and in a reasonable manner.

---

**45 CFR 46.115 (b) New Common Rule**
    **(b) The records required by this policy shall be retained for at least 3 years, and records relating to research that is conducted shall be retained for at least 3 years after completion of the research. The institution or IRB may maintain the records in printed form, or electronically. All records shall be accessible for inspection and copying by authorized representatives of the Federal department or agency at reasonable times and in a reasonable manner.**

---

### 21 CFR 812.140 (IDE) Records

**Note 4: (d)** Retention period. An investigator or sponsor shall maintain the records required by this subpart during the investigation and for a period of 2 years after the latter of the following two dates: The date on which the investigation is terminated or completed, or the date that the records are no longer required for purposes of supporting a premarket approval application or a notice of completion of a product development protocol.[8]

### ICH GCP E6 R2 references:

**Note 5: 3.4 Records**

The IRB/IEC should retain all relevant records (e.g., written procedures, membership lists, lists of occupations/affiliations of members, submitted documents, minutes of meetings, and correspondence) for a period of at least 3-years after completion of the trial and make them available upon request from the regulatory authority(ies).

The IRB/IEC may be asked by investigators, sponsors, or regulatory authorities to provide its written procedures and membership lists.

### 4.9 Records and Reports

### ADDENDUM

**4.9.0** The investigator/institution should maintain adequate and accurate source documents and trial records that include all pertinent observations on each of the site's trial subjects. Source data should be attributable, legible, contemporaneous, original, accurate, and complete. Changes to source data should be traceable, should not obscure the original entry, and should be explained if necessary (e.g., *via* an audit trail).

**4.9.4** The investigator/institution should maintain the trial documents as specified in essential documents for the Conduct of a Clinical Trial…and as required by the applicable regulatory requirement(s). The investigator/institution should take measures to prevent accidental or premature destruction of these documents.

**Note 6: 4.9.5** Essential documents should be retained until at least 2 years after the last approval of a marketing application in an ICH region and until there are no pending or contemplated marketing applications in an ICH region or at least 2 years have elapsed since the formal discontinuation of clinical development of the investigational product. These documents should be retained for a longer period however if required by the applicable regulatory requirements or by an agreement with the sponsor. It is the responsibility of the sponsor to inform the investigator/institution as to when these documents no longer need to be retained (see 5.5.12).

**Note 7: 5.5.8** If the sponsor discontinues the clinical development of an investigational product (i.e., for any or all indications, routes of administration, or dosage forms), the sponsor should maintain all sponsor-specific essential documents for at least 2 years after formal discontinuation or in conformance with the applicable regulatory requirement(s).

**Note 7A: 5.5.11** The sponsor-specific essential documents should be retained until at least 2 years after the last approval of a marketing application in an ICH region and until there are no pending or contemplated marketing applications in an ICH region or at least 2 years have elapsed since the formal discontinuation of clinical development of the investigational product. These documents should be retained for a longer period however if required by the applicable regulatory requirement(s) or if needed by the sponsor.

**5.5.12** The sponsor should inform the investigator(s)/institution(s) in writing of the need for record retention and should notify the investigator(s)/institution(s) in writing when the trial related records are no longer needed.[9]

## 9.3 PUBLISHING THE RESULTS OF A CLINICAL RESEARCH STUDY

*Purpose of section*:

- Provides Authorship Guidelines from the International Committee of Medical Journal Editors (ICMJE)
- Provides Author best practices on planning for authorship

The International Committee of Medical Journal Editors (ICMJE) is the definitive source for publishing. Organization literature recommends that authorship be based on *all four (4)* of the following four (4) criteria:

- Substantial contributions to the conception or design of the work; or the acquisition, analysis, or interpretation of data for the work; AND
- Drafting the work or revising it critically for important intellectual content; AND
- Final approval of the version to be published; AND
- Agreement to be accountable for all aspects of the work in ensuring that questions related to the accuracy or integrity of any part of the work are appropriately investigated and resolved.

For Contributors:

Individuals who were part of trial conduct, but do not meet all four (4) of the criteria for authorship cited above should be acknowledged as Contributors. Examples of activities that alone—(without other contributions)—*do not* qualify a contributor for authorship are acquisition of funding; general supervision of a research group or general administrative support; and writing assistance, technical editing, language editing, and proofreading.[10]

---

### 🕮 AUTHOR'S CORNER

One of the Authors was a member of a Publishing Committee. That experience confirmed that the PI and the study team need to decide *before the trial begins* the criteria for who will qualify as an author. This will avoid later disagreements, and hard feelings among your team, not to mention delays in publishing. Therefore, it is highly recommended that you **make authorship criteria a part of your study startup activities.**

---

Specifically, decide:

1. What percentage of time spent on the study qualifies an individual to be an author and how you are going to track that time throughout the study; *or*

2. What minimum number of hours (be specific) qualifies as a "substantial contribution" to be an author and how is this time going to be tracked throughout the study; *or*
3. What tasks, when added together, qualify as a "substantial contribution" and thus, earns the right to authorship for an individual. For example, if ALL of the following are done by an individual throughout the trial:
   **a.** Attends the Site Initiation Visit with a Sponsor (if applicable);
   **b.** Audits data entry into Case Report Forms against source documentation for accuracy at a __% sampling throughout the study;
   **c.** Reviews and edits documentation going to the IRB (or central IRB or Single IRB) prepared by a study team member prior to submission;
   **d.** Reviews and signs off on all Investigator Brochures or Instructions For Use (if applicable); and,
   **e.** Examines X% of subjects coming in for visits.
   The team might add further criteria based on the protocol design.

Ensure all team members weigh in and reach a consensus on the authorship criteria. Then, at the end of the study, there can be no disagreement, because everyone involved was a part of the decision-making process and aware of what was required for authorship. And, you will have an objective, quantifiable measure that can be tallied.

Authorship Guidelines

Sponsors will be looking for sites to comply with the authorship guidelines in the *Recommendations for the Conduct, Reporting, Editing, and Publication of Scholarly Work in Medical Journals* by the International Committee of Medical Journal Editors (ICMJE). The manuscript preparation and submission link can be found here: http://www.icmje.org/recommendations/browse/manuscript-preparation/.[11]

The Sponsor and the Publication of Study Results

For the purposes of good project management, take note:

- Sponsors will expect a **prepublication review**. This is typically written into your Clinical Trial Agreement (contract with the sponsor). The wording usually appears something like this:
  *Principal Investigator will provide (sponsor name) an opportunity to review any proposed publication of the Study results at least 30 days before it is submitted. (Sponsor name) will review for unprotected Inventions and may also provide comments on content (Some will read that a Sponsor will provide edits.) If any patent action is required to protect intellectual property rights, Principal Investigator agrees to delay the publication submission for a period not to exceed an additional 60 days.*

  As noted above, the timeline for publication may change due to the intellectual property rights of the Sponsor, so plan ahead.

  Tips for Manuscript Preparation:

- Make sure you redact any undisclosed confidential information of the Sponsor's. (The Sponsor will typically let you know what information they are uncomfortable with in your manuscript.) However, if you review and revise your manuscript for confidential information before sending it to the Sponsor for prepublication review, you will earn brownie points with the Sponsor.
- If you are participating in a multisite study, a joint publication representing all Study sites is usually expected before Investigators at individual sites can send their manuscripts to the Sponsor for prepublication review (or even think of publishing).

- 👍 ONLY SUBMIT TO ONE (1) JOURNAL AT A TIME. Yes, this makes it a lengthy process, but you will lose favor with publishers if you submit simultaneously. Keep your long-term goals in mind (for more publishing over time). Here's why:

  The rationale for this standard is the potential for disagreement when two (or more) journals claim the right to publish a manuscript that has been submitted simultaneously to more than one journal, and the possibility that two or more journals will unknowingly and unnecessarily undertake the work of peer review, edit the same manuscript, and publish the same article.[12]

- Once you are approved for a Journal Article through a Publisher, make sure to perform a HIGHLY DETAILED, sentence-by-sentence review of the proof the publisher will send you. (The proof is the draft before publication.) Catch any content errors, table, formatting or graph shifting, so that the final published article will be correct. You do not want to find errors after it has been published and distributed!

ꚍICH ICH GCP has the following to say regarding publishing:

4.8.10 (o) …If the results of the trial are published, the subject's identity will remain confidential.[13]

The completion of a trial is satisfying but it is important, both for the integrity of the trial and your reputation, along with the desire to obtain further Sponsor trials, to finish strong. The necessary administrative and project management diligence following the trial conclusion may seem anticlimactic, but it is critical.

## ENDNOTES

[1] http://www.ich.org/fileadmin/Public_Web_Site/ICH_Products/Guidelines/Efficacy/E6/E6_R2__Step_4_2016_1109.pdf [accessed 28.03.18].

[2] https://www.ich.org/fileadmin/Public_Web_Site/ICH_Products/Guidelines/Efficacy/E6/E6_R2__Addendum_Step2.pdf [accessed 28.03.18].

[3] https://www.accessdata.fda.gov/scripts/cdrh/cfdocs/cfcfr/CFRSearch.cfm?fr=312.64[accessed 28.03.18].

[4] https://www.fda.gov/downloads/Drugs/GuidanceComplianceRegulatoryInformation/Guidances/UCM073113.pdf [accessed 28.03.18].

[5] https://www.fda.gov/downloads/Drugs/GuidanceComplianceRegulatoryInformation/Guidances/UCM336889.pdf [accessed 28.03.18].

[6] See https://clinicaltrials.gov/ct2/manage-recs/how-report [accessed 28.03.18].

[7] NIH RPPR Instruction Guide https://grants.nih.gov/sites/default/files/rppr_instruction_guide.pdf.

[8] https://www.accessdata.fda.gov/scripts/cdrh/cfdocs/cfcfr/CFRSearch.cfm?fr=312.57[accessed 28.30.18].

[9] https://www.ich.org/fileadmin/Public_Web_Site/ICH_Products/Guidelines/Efficacy/E6/E6_R2__Addendum_Step2.pdf [accessed 28.03.18].

[10] http://www.icmje.org/recommendations/browse/roles-and-responsibilities/defining-the-role-of-authors-and-contributors.html [accessed 28.03.18].

[11] http://www.icmje.org/recommendations/browse/manuscript-preparation/ [accessed 28.03.19].

[12] http://www.icmje.org/recommendations/browse/publishing-and-editorial-issues/overlapping-publications.html [accessed 28.03.18].

[13] https://www.ich.org/fileadmin/Public_Web_Site/ICH_Products/Guidelines/Efficacy/E6/E6_R2__Addendum_Step2.pdf [accessed 28.03.18].

# Clinical Trials Glossary

**Adverse event** Any untoward medical occurrence associated with the use of a drug in humans, whether or not considered drug related. 21 CFR 312.32 (a)

**Amendment** A written description of a change(s) to, or formal clarification of, a protocol. Clinical Data Interchange Standards Consotirum (CDISC)

**Anonymized** Personal data, which have been processed to make it impossible to know the person with whom the data are associated. Applicable particularly for secondary use of health data. CDISC

**Assent** A child's affirmative agreement to participate in a clinical investigation. Mere failure to object should not, absent affirmative agreement, be construed as assent. 21 CFR 50.3 (n)

**Bias** Situation or condition that causes a result to depart from the true value in a consistent direction. Bias refers to defects in study design or measurement. CDISC

**Biomarker** A characteristic that is objectively measured and evaluated as an indicator of normal biological processes, pathogenic processes, or pharmacologic responses to a therapeutic intervention. CDISC

**Blinded study** A study in which the subject, the investigator, or anyone assessing the outcome is unaware of the treatment assignment(s). NOTE: Blinding is used to reduce the potential for bias. CDISC

**Blinding** A procedure to limit bias by preventing subjects and/or study personnel from identifying which treatments or procedures are administered, or from learning the results of tests and measures undertaken as part of a clinical investigation. NOTE: Masking, while often used synonymously with blinding, usually denotes concealing the specific study intervention used. [from ICH E9] The term masking is often preferred to blinding in the field of ophthalmology. [from AMA Manual of Style]. CDISC

With single blinding, the patient is unaware which treatment he is receiving, while with double blinding, neither the patient nor the investigator knows which treatment is planned. https://www.ncbi.nlm.nih.gov/pmc/articles/PMC2689572/

**Business associate** A person or entity who, on behalf of a covered entity, performs or assists in performance of a function or activity involving the use or disclosure of individually identifiable health information, such as data analysis, claims processing or administration, utilization review, and quality assurance reviews, or any other function or activity regulated by the HIPAA Administrative Simplification Rules, including the Privacy Rule. Business associates are also persons or entities performing legal, actuarial, accounting, consulting, data aggregation, management, administrative, accreditation, or financial services to or for a covered entity where performing those services involves disclosure of individually identifiable health information by the covered entity or another business associate of the covered entity to that person or entity. https://privacyruleandresearch.nih.gov/pr_06.asp

**Cadaver research** Research performed on the organs or body (cadaver) of a deceased person (through organ donation or whole body donation).

**Carry-over effect** Effects of treatment that persist after treatment has been stopped, sometimes beyond the time of a medication's known biological activity. CDISC

**Case history** An adequate and accurate record prepared and maintained by an investigator that records all observations and other data pertinent to the investigation on each individual administered the investigational drug (device or other therapy) or employed as a control in the investigation. NOTE: Case histories include the case report forms and supporting data including, for example, signed and dated consent forms and medical records including, for example, progress notes of the physician, the individual's hospital chart(s), and the nurses' notes. The case history for each individual shall document that informed consent was obtained prior to participation in the study. [21 CFR 312.62b] CDISC

**Case report form (CRF)** 1. A printed, optical, or electronic document designed to record all of the protocol-required information to be reported to the sponsor for each trial subject. 2. A record of clinical study observations and other information that a study protocol designates must be completed for each subject. NOTE: In common usage, CRF can refer to either a CRF page, which denotes a group of one or more data items linked together for collection and display, or a casebook, which includes the entire group of CRF pages on which a set of clinical study observations and other information can be or have been collected, or the information actually collected by completion of such CRF pages for a subject in a clinical study. CDISC

**Causality assessment** An evaluation performed by a medical professional concerning the likelihood that a therapy or product under study caused or contributed to an adverse event. CDISC

**CDISC SHARE** A global, accessible, electronic library, which, through advanced technology, enables precise and standardized data element definitions that can be used within applications and across studies to improve biomedical research and its link with healthcare. In the first iteration, CDISC SHARE will contain the existing CDISC standards, such as CDASH and SDTM, providing machine-readable elements (variables) within those standards. This will allow a range of applications used within organizations to automatically access those definitions. CDISC

**CDISC standard** (The) CDISC term for a proposed uniform CDISC standard intended to address the full life cycle of a clinical trial including protocol representation, capture of source data, submission, and archiving using a set of fully integrated and consistent models, terms, and controlled vocabularies derived from the current set of CDISC standards. CDISC

**Certified copy** A copy of original information that has been verified as indicated by a dated signature, as an exact copy having all of the same attributes and information as the original. CDISC

**Clinical pharmacology** Science that deals with the characteristics, effects, properties, reactions, and uses of drugs, particularly their therapeutic value in humans, including their toxicology, safety, pharmacodynamics, and pharmacokinetics (ADME). CDISC

**Clinical research** Clinical research is medical research that involves people to test new treatments and therapies. NIH

**Clinical research associate (CRA)** Person employed by a sponsor or by a contract research organization acting on a sponsor's behalf, who monitors the progress of investigator sites participating in a clinical study. CDISC

**Clinical research coordinator (CRC)** Person who handles most of the administrative responsibilities of a clinical trial on behalf of a site investigator, acts as liaison between investigative site and sponsor, and reviews all data and records before a monitor's visit. Synonyms: trial coordinator, study coordinator, research coordinator, clinical coordinator, research nurse, protocol nurse. CDISC

**Clinical significance** Change in a subject's clinical condition regarded as important whether or not due to the test intervention. NOTE: Some statistically significant changes (in blood tests, for example) have no clinical significance. The criterion or criteria for clinical significance should be stated in the protocol. CDISC

**Clinical trial** A research study in which one or more human subjects are prospectively assigned to one or more interventions (which may include placebo or other control) to evaluate the effects of those interventions on health-related biomedical or behavioral outcomes. NIH

**Cohort** 1. A group of individuals who share a common exposure, experience, or characteristic. 2. A group of individuals followed up or traced over time in a cohort study. CDISC

**Cohort study** Study of a group of individuals, some of whom are exposed to a variable of interest, in which subjects are followed over time. Cohort studies can be prospective or retrospective. CDISC

**Comparative study** One in which the investigative drug is compared against another product, either active drug or placebo. CDISC

**Compliance (in relation to trials)** Adherence to trial-related requirements, good clinical practice (GCP) requirements, and the applicable regulatory requirements. CDISC

**Confidence interval** A measure of the precision of an estimated value. The interval represents the range of values, consistent with the data that is believed to encompass the "true" value with high probability (usually 95%). The confidence interval is expressed in the same units as the estimate. Wider intervals indicate lower precision; narrow intervals, greater precision. CDISC

**Confidentiality** Prevention of disclosure to other than authorized individuals of a sponsor's proprietary information or of a subject's identity. CDISC

**Consent form** Document used during the informed consent process that is the basis for explaining to potential subjects the risks and potential benefits of a study and the rights and responsibilities of the parties involved. NOTE: The informed consent document provides a summary of a clinical trial (including its purpose, the treatment procedures and schedule, potential risks and benefits, alternatives to participation, etc.) and explains an individual's rights as a subject. It is designed to begin the informed consent process, which consists of conversations between the subject and the research team. If the individual then decides to enter the trial, s/he gives her/his official consent by signing the document. Synonym: informed consent form. CDISC

**Contract research organization (CRO)** A person or an organization (commercial, academic, or other) contracted by the sponsor to perform one or more of a sponsor's trial-related duties and functions. CDISC

**Control group** The group of subjects in a controlled study that receives no treatment, a standard treatment, or a placebo. [21 CFR 314.126] See also controls. CDISC

**Control(s)** 1. Comparator against which the study treatment is evaluated [e.g., concurrent (placebo, no treatment, dose-response, active), and external (historical, published literature)] 2. Computer: processes or operations intended to ensure authenticity, integrity, and confidentiality of electronic records. CDISC

**Controlled study** A study in which a test article is compared with a treatment that has known effects. The control group may receive no treatment, active treatment, placebo, or dose comparison concurrent control. CDISC

**Coordinating committee** A committee that a sponsor may organize to coordinate the conduct of a multicenter trial. [ICH E6] CDISC

**Coordinating investigator** An investigator assigned the responsibility for the coordination of investigators at different centers participating in a multicenter trial. [ICH E6] CDISC

**Covered entities** A designation in the HIPAA Privacy rules for (1) health plans, (2) health care clearing houses, and (3) health care providers who electronically transmit any health information in connection with transactions for which HHS has adopted standards. Covered entities can be institutions, organizations, or persons. https://privacyruleandresearch.nih.gov/pr_06.asp

**Crossover trial** A trial design for which subjects function as their own control and are assigned to receive investigational product and controls in an order determined by randomizations, typically with a washout period between the two products. [Center for the Advancement of Clinical Research; ADAM] CDISC

**Curriculum vitae (CV)** Document that outlines a person's educational and professional history. Representations of facts, concepts, or instructions in a manner suitable for communication, interpretation, or processing by humans or by automated means. CDISC

**Data coordinating center** One site within a multisite trial that collects data from all other sites in order to manage and analyze that data. Martien

**Data entry** Human input of data into a structured, computerized format using an interface such as a keyboard, pen-based tablet, or voice recognition. CDISC

**Data integrity** A dimension of data contributing to trustworthiness and pertaining to the systems and processes for data capture, correction, maintenance, transmission, and retention. Key elements of data integrity include security, privacy, access controls, a continuous pedigree from capture to archive, stability (of values, of attribution), protection against loss or destruction, ease of review by users responsible for data quality, proper operation and validation of systems, training of users. NOTE: In clinical research, the FDA requires that data relied on to determine safety and efficacy of therapeutic interventions be trustworthy and establishes guidance and regulations concerning practices and system requirements needed to promote an acceptable level of data integrity. CDISC

**Data management** Tasks associated with the entry, transfer, and/or preparation of source data and derived items for entry into a clinical trial database. NOTE: Data management could include database creation, data entry, review, coding, data editing, data QC, locking, or archiving; it typically does not include source data capture. CDISC

**Data monitoring** Process by which clinical data are examined for completeness, consistency, and accuracy. Data monitoring committee (DMc). Group of individuals with pertinent expertise that reviews on a regular basis accumulating data from an ongoing clinical trial. The DMC advises the sponsor regarding the continuing safety of current participants and those yet to be recruited, as well as the continuing validity and scientific merit of the trial. NOTE: A DMC can stop a trial if it finds toxicities or if treatment is proved beneficial. CDISC

**Data transfer agreement (DTA)** A contract that defines the terms under which data will be moved from one place of business to another. The terms include legal and regulatory obligations, HIPAA law requirements, how data will be stored and secured, the purposes for the data, intellectual property rights, and other contractual terms. Martien

**Database** A collection of data or information, typically organized for ease and speed of search and retrieval. CDISC

**Database lock** Action taken to prevent further changes to a clinical trial database. NOTE: Locking of a database is done after review, query resolution, and a determination has been made that the database is ready for analysis. CDISC

**Dataset** A collection of structured data in a single file. CDISC

**Decedent research** Medical research conducted with the use of deceased persons' protected health information.

**Decision rule** Succinct statement of how a decision will be reached, based upon the expected foreseen clinical benefits in terms of outcomes of the primary endpoint. CDISC

**Declaration of Helsinki** A set of recommendations or basic principles that guide medical doctors in the conduct of biomedical research involving human subjects. It was originally adopted by the 18th World Medical Assembly (Helsinki, Finland, 1964) and recently revised (52nd WMA General Assembly, Edinburgh, Scotland, October 2000). CDISC

**Deidentified** Removal of elements connected with data which might aid in associating those data with an individual. Examples include name, birth date, social security number, home address, telephone number, e-mail address, medical record numbers, health plan beneficiary numbers, full-face photographic images. CDISC

**Dependent variable** Outcomes that are measured in an experiment and that are expected to change as a result of an experimental manipulation of the independent variable(s). CDISC

**Digital signature** An electronic signature, based on cryptographic methods of originator authentication, computed by using a set of rules and a set of parameters, such that the identity of the signer and the integrity of the data can be verified. [21 CFR 11] CDISC

**Disease** Any deviation from or interruption of the normal structure or function of a part, organ, or system of the body as manifested by characteristic symptoms and signs. [Dorland's Medical Dictionary] CDISC

**Dosage** The amount of drug administered to a patient or test subject over the course of the clinical study; a regulated administration of individual doses. CDISC

**Dosage form** Physical characteristics of a drug product (e.g., tablet, capsule, or solution) that contains a drug substance, generally—but not necessarily—in association with one or more other ingredients. [21 CFR §314.3] CDISC

**Dosage regimen** The number of doses per given time period; the elapsed time between doses (e.g., every six hours) or the time that the doses are to be given (e.g., at 8 a.m. and 4 p.m. daily); and/or the amount of a medicine (the number of capsules, for example) to be given at each specific dosing time. CDISC

**Dosage strength** 1. Proportion of active substance to excipient, measured in units of volume or concentration. 2. The strength of a drug product tells how much of the active ingredient is present in each dosage. CDISC

**Dose** The amount of drug administered to a patient or test subject at one time or the total quantity administered. CDISC

**Double-blind study** A study in which neither the subject nor the investigator nor the research team interacting with the subject or data during the trial knows what treatment a subject is receiving. CDISC

**Dropout** A subject in a clinical trial who for any reason fails to continue in the trial until the last visit or observation required of him/her by the study protocol. [from ICH E9] CDISC

**Drug** 1. Article other than food intended for use in the diagnosis, cure, mitigation, treatment, or prevention of disease; or intended to affect the structure or any function of the body. Not a device or a component, part, or accessory of a device. 2. Substance recognized by an official pharmacopia or formulary. CDISC

**eClinical trial**  Clinical trial in which primarily electronic processes are used to plan, collect (acquire), access, exchange, and archive data required for conduct, management, analysis, and reporting of the trial. NOTE: FDA has recently drawn a distinction between studies and trials. Both words refer to systematic efforts to obtain evidence relevant to regulatory authorities, but, depending on regulatory context and particularly in the case of post-marketing commitments, a study might not be the appropriate word for a clinical trial (prospective, controlled, randomized), but should be reserved instead for surveillance, structured gathering of information, epidemiological studies, or even animal studies. CDISC

**eCRF**  1. Auditable electronic record designed to capture information required by the clinical trial protocol to be reported to the sponsor on each trial subject. 2. A CRF in which related data items and their associated comments, notes, and signatures are linked electronically. NOTE: eCRFs may include special display elements, electronic edit checks, and other special properties or functions and are used for both capture and display of the linked data. CDISC

**Efficacy**  The capacity of a drug or treatment to produce beneficial effects on the course or duration of a disease at the dose tested and against the illness (and patient population) for which it is designed. CDISC

**Electronic data capture (eDC)**  The process of collecting clinical trial data into a permanent electronic form. NOTE: Permanent in the context of these definitions implies that any changes made to the electronic data are recorded with an audit trail. EDC usually denotes manual entry of CRF data by transcription from source documents. The transcription is typically done by personnel at investigative sites. CDISC

**Electronic health record (eHR)**  An electronic record for healthcare providers to create, import, store, and use clinical information for patient care, according to nationally recognized interoperability standards. NOTE: The EHR has the following distinguishing features: able to be obtained from multiple sources; shareable; interoperable; accessible to authorized parties. CDISC

**Electronic medical record (eMR)**  An electronic record for healthcare providers within one healthcare organization to create, store, and use clinical information for patient care. An electronic record derived from a computerized system used primarily for delivering patient care in a clinical setting. NOTE: EMRs may serve as source documents, and such data could serve also as source data for clinical trials provided that the controls on the EMR system and the transfer of such data to the eClinical trial system were to fulfill regulatory requirements (e.g., 21 CFR 11). CDISC

**Electronic record**  Any combination of text, graphics, data, audio, pictorial, or other information representation in digital form that is created, modified, maintained, archived, retrieved, or distributed by a computer system. [21 CFR 11.3(b) (6)] CDISC

**Electronic signature**  A computer data compilation of any symbol or series of symbols, executed, adopted, or authorized by an individual to be the legally binding equivalent of the individual's handwritten signature. [CSUCT Glossary; 21 CFR 11.3(7)] CDISC

**Endpoint**  Variable that pertains to the efficacy or safety evaluations of a trial. CDISC

**Enroll**  To register or enter a subject into a clinical trial. NOTE: Once a subject has been enrolled, the clinical trial protocol applies to that subject. CDISC

**Epoch**  Interval of time in the planned conduct of a study. An epoch is associated with a purpose (e.g., screening, randomization, treatment, follow-up), which applies across all arms of a study. NOTE: Epoch is intended as a standardized term to replace: period, cycle, phase, stage. CDISC

**Equipoise**  A state in which an investigator is uncertain about which arm of a clinical trial would be therapeutically superior for a patient. NOTE: An investigator who has a treatment preference or finds out that one arm of a comparative trial offers a clinically therapeutic advantage should disclose this information to subjects participating in the trial. CDISC

**eRA Commons**  The eRA Commons is an online interface where signing officials, principal investigators, trainees, and postdocs at institutions/organizations can access and share administrative information relating to research grants. https://era.nih.gov

**Established name** The official name of a drug substance. [Food, Drug, and Cosmetic Act]. CDISC

**Ex vivo/in vitro** Outside of the living body or in an artificial environment outside of a living organism, such as a test tube.

**Exclusion criteria** List of characteristics in a protocol, any one of which may exclude a potential subject from participation in a study. CDISC

**Exploratory IND study** A clinical study that is conducted early in Phase 1; involves very limited human exposure and has no therapeutic or diagnostic intent (e.g., screening studies, microdose studies) [FDA Guidance for Industry, Investigators, and Reviewers: Exploratory IND Studies, January 2006] *See also Phase 0*. CDISC

**Exploratory study** Phase 1 or 2 study during which the actions of a therapeutic intervention are assessed and measured extraction transformation load (ETL). A class of software applications for data extraction, transformation, and loading that are used to implement data interfaces between disparate database systems, often to populate data warehouses. CDISC

**Field** Locus on a data collection instrument (usually a CRF) for recording or displaying a data element. *See data item*. CDISC

**File transfer protocol (FTP)** A standard protocol for exchanging files between computers on the Internet. *See also TCP/IP*. CDISC

**Final report** A written description of a trial/study of any therapeutic, prophylactic, or diagnostic agent conducted in human subjects, in which the clinical and statistical description, presentations, and analyses are fully integrated into a single report. [ICH E3] CDISC

**Finding** A meaningful interpretation of data or observations resulting from planned evaluations. *Compare to conclusion, hypothesis*. CDISC

**First subject in (FSI, FPI)** The date and time the first subject is enrolled and randomized into a study. The subject will have met the inclusion/exclusion criteria to participate in the trial and will have signed an informed consent form. *Synonym: first patient in*. CDISC

**First subject screened** First subject who signs the informed consent form and is screened for potential enrollment and randomization into a study but has not yet been determined to meet the inclusion/exclusion criteria for the trial. CDISC

**First subject treated** First subject who receives the test article or placebo in a clinical investigation. CDISC

**First-in-humans study** The first Phase 1 study in which the test product is administered to human beings. CDISC

**Frequentist methods** Statistical methods, such as significance tests and confidence intervals, which can be interpreted in terms of the frequency of certain outcomes occurring in hypothetical repeated realizations of the same experimental situation. [ICH E9] CDISC

**Generalizability** The extent to which the findings of a clinical trial can be reliably extrapolated from the subjects who participated in the trial to a broader patient population and a broader range of clinical settings. [ICH E9] CDISC

**Generic name** The drug identifying name to which all branded (proprietary) names for that indication are associated. CDISC

**Global assessment variable** A single variable, usually a scale of ordered categorical ratings, which integrates objective variables and the investigator's overall impression about the state or change in state of a subject. [ICH E9] CDISC

**Good clinical practice (GCP)** A standard for the design, conduct, performance, monitoring, auditing, recording, analyses, and reporting of clinical trials that provide assurance that the data and reported results are credible and accurate and that the rights, integrity, and confidentiality of trial subjects are protected. CDISC

**Granularity** Refers to the size of an information unit in relation to a whole. NOTE: Structuring "privileges" in electronic systems is said to be highly granular when each of many roles can differ in their capacity to act on electronic records. CDISC

**Health level 7 (HL7)** An ANSI-accredited Standards Developing Organization (SDO) operating in the healthcare arena. NOTE: Level 7 refers to the highest level of the International Standards Organization's (ISO) communications model for Open Systems Interconnection (OSI), the application level. The application level addresses definition of the data to be exchanged, the timing of the interchange, and the communication of certain errors to the application.

Level 7 supports such functions as security checks, participant identification, availability checks, exchange mechanism negotiations, and, most importantly, data exchange structuring. CDISC

**Healthy volunteer** A healthy volunteer is a person with no known significant health problems who participates in clinical research to test a new drug, device, or intervention. NIH

**HIPAA privacy rule, alteration of authorization** When An IRB or Privacy Board approves a request that removes some PHI, but not all, or alters the requirements for an Authorization (to use and disclose PHI). https://privacyruleandresearch.nih.gov

**HIPAA privacy rule, complete waiver of authorization** A complete waiver occurs when the IRB or Privacy Board determines that no Authorization will be required for a covered entity to use and disclose PHI for a particular research project. https://privacyruleandresearch.nih.gov

**HIPAA privacy rule, partial waiver of authorization** A partial waiver of Authorization occurs when an IRB or Privacy Board determines that a covered entity does not need Authorization for all PHI uses and disclosures for research purposes, such as disclosing PHI for research recruitment purposes. https://privacyruleandresearch.nih.gov

**Human subject** Individual who is or becomes a participant in research, either as a recipient of the test article or as a control. A subject may be either a healthy human or a patient. [21 CFR 50.3]. *Synonym: subject/trial subject.* CDISC

**Huriet law** France's regulations covering the initiation and conduct of clinical trials. CDISC

**IDE** (Investigational Device Exemption) An approved investigational device exemption (IDE) permits a device that otherwise would be required to comply with a performance standard or to have premarket approval to be shipped lawfully for the purpose of conducting investigations of that device. 21 CFR 812.1(a)

**In vivo** Occurring or carried out in the living organism. Collins English Dictionary–Complete & Unabridged 2012 Digital Edition

**Inclusion/Exclusion** Criteria     Inclusion/Exclusion Criteria are factors that allow someone to participate in a clinical trial are *inclusion criteria*. Those that exclude or not allow participation are *exclusion criteria*. NIH

**Inclusion criteria** The criteria in a protocol that prospective subjects must meet to be eligible for participation in a study. CDISC

**IND (Investigational New Drug)** Current Federal law requires that a drug be the subject of an approved marketing application before it is transported or distributed across state lines. Because a sponsor will probably want to ship the investigational drug to clinical investigators in many states, it must seek an exemption from that legal requirement. The IND is the means through which the sponsor technically obtains this exemption from the FDA. www.fda.gov, https://www.fda.gov/Drugs/DevelopmentApprovalProcess/HowDrugsareDevelopedandApproved/ApprovalApplications/InvestigationalNewDrugINDApplication

**Independent data monitoring committee (IDMC)** A committee established by the sponsor to assess at intervals the progress of a clinical trial, safety data, and critical efficacy variables and recommend to the sponsor whether to continue, modify, or terminate the trial. [ICH E9] *See also data monitoring committee.* CDISC

**Indication** A health problem or disease that is identified as likely to be benefited by a therapy being studied in clinical trials. NOTE: Where such a benefit has been established and approved by regulatory authorities, the therapy is said to be approved for such an indication. CDISC

**Informed consent** An ongoing process that provides the subject with explanations that will help in making educated decisions about whether to begin or continue participating in a trial. Informed consent is an ongoing, interactive process rather than a one-time information session. CDISC

**Informed consent form** This is the document that is presented to a subject for consideration of participation in a study and contains the eight basic elements found within 21 CFR 50.25(a), and one or more of the additional six elements found within 21 CFR 50.25(b) that are appropriate to the study. Martien

**Institutional review board (IRB)** Any board, committee, or other group formally designated by an institution to review, to approve the initiation of, and to conduct periodic review of, biomedical research involving human subjects. The primary purpose of such review is to assure the protection of the rights and welfare of the human subjects. 21 CFR 56.102 (g)

**Instrument** A means to capture data (e.g., questionnaire, diary) plus all the information and documentation that supports its use. CDISC

**Intention-to-treat** The principle that asserts that the effect of a treatment policy can be best assessed by evaluating the basis of the intention to treat a subject (i.e., the planned treatment regimen) rather than the actual treatment given. CDISC

**Interoperability** Ability of two or more systems or components to exchange information and to use the information that has been exchanged. CDISC

**Inter-rater reliability** The property of scales yielding equivalent results when used by different raters on different occasions. CDISC

**Intervention** The drug, device, therapy, or process under investigation in a clinical study that is believed to have an effect on outcomes of interest in a study (e.g., health-related quality of life, efficacy, safety, pharmacoeconomics). CDISC (Delete this one.)

**Intervention** A *manipulation* of the subject or subject's environment for the purpose of *modifying* one or more health-related biomedical or behavioral processes and/or endpoints Examples include drugs/small molecules/compounds; biologics; devices; procedures (e.g., surgical techniques); delivery systems (e.g., telemedicine, face-to-face interviews); strategies to change health-related behavior (e.g., diet, cognitive therapy, exercise, development of new habits); treatment strategies; prevention strategies; and, diagnostic strategies. NIH https://grants.nih.gov/grants/policy/faq_clinical_trial_definition.htm#5224

**Investigational product** A pharmaceutical form of an active ingredient or placebo being tested or used as a reference in a clinical trial, including a product with a marketing authorization when used or assembled (formulated or packaged) in a way different from the approved form, or when used for an unapproved indication, or when used to gain further information about an approved use. CDISC

**Investigator** An individual who actually conducts a clinical investigation (i.e., under whose immediate direction the test article is administered or dispensed to, or used involving a subject) or, in the event of an investigation conducted by a team of individuals, is the responsible leader of that team. [21 CFR 50.3 (d) and 21 CFR 56.102 (h)]

**Investigator's brochure (IB)** A document that compiles information on an investigational product such as the formula, pharmacological and toxicological effects, pharmacokinetics and biological disposition of the drug in animals, and, to the extent known, in humans, a description of possible risks and side effects to be anticipated, and more. Martien adapted from 21 CFR 312.23 (a) (5)

**Janus** 1. A logical design conceived by the FDA for a data warehouse intended to integrate submission data, protocol descriptions, and analysis plans from clinical and animal studies into as an FDA review environment that uses a set of validated, standards-based tools to allow reproducible cross-study, data mining, and retrospective comparative analysis. 2. The name assigned to a component of the NCI's caBIG Clinical Research Information Exchange (CRIX) initiative, representing a joint NCI/FDA project to develop a physical implementation of the Janus model. NOTE: Sometimes written as JANUS, the term is not an acronym, but harkens to the Roman god of gates and doors, beginnings and endings. CDISC

**Last subject out/complete (LSC/LPC or LSO/LPO)** 1. The date and time when the last subject has reached a planned or achieved milestone representing the completion of the trial. 2. The last subject to complete a trial. CDISC

**Last subject/patient in (LSI/LPI)** Date and time when the last subject to participate in a clinical trial is enrolled. CDISC

**Legal authentication** A completion status in which a document has been signed manually or electronically by the individual who is legally responsible for that document. CDISC

**Legally authorized representative** An individual or judicial or other body authorized under applicable law to consent on behalf of a prospective subject to the subject's participation in the procedure(s) involved in the research. 21 CFR 50.3 (l)

**Limited data set** Refers to PHI that excludes 16 categories of direct identifiers and may be used or disclosed, for purposes of research, public health, or health care operations, without obtaining either an individual's Authorization or a waiver or an alteration of Authorization for its use and disclosure, with a data use agreement. https://privacyrulean-dresearch.nih.gov/pr_08.asp#8c

**Longitudinal study** One in which participants are studied over time, with data being collected at multiple intervals. http://medical-dictionary.the-freedictionary.com

**Mapping** In the context of representing or exchanging data, connecting an item or symbol to a code or concept. CDISC

**Marketing support trials** Clinical studies that are designed to clarify therapeutic benefits of a marketed product or to show potential decision makers the rationale for preferring one therapy over another. CDISC

**Masking** See blinding. CDISC

**Matched-pair design** A type of parallel trial design in which investigators identify pairs of subjects who are "identical" with respect to relevant factors, then randomize them so that one receives Treatment A and the other Treatment B. See also pairing. CDISC

**Matching** See pairing. CDISC

**Material transfer agreement (MTA)** A document that defines the conditions under which research or other materials can be transferred and used among research laboratories Segen's Medical Dictionary. © 2012 Farlex, Inc.

**Mean** The sum of the values of all observations or data points divided by the number of observations; an arithmetical average. CDISC

**Median** The middle value in a data set; that is, just as many values are greater than the median and lower than the median value. CDISC

**Medical device** A medical device is "an instrument, apparatus, implement, machine, contrivance, implant, in vitro reagent, or other similar or related article, including a component part, or accessory which is:

• recognized in the official National Formulary, or the United States Pharmacopoeia, or any supplement to them,

• intended for use in the diagnosis of disease or other conditions, or in the cure, mitigation, treatment, or prevention of disease, in man or other animals, or

• intended to affect the structure or any function of the body of man or other animals, and which does not achieve any of its primary intended

purposes through chemical action within or on the body of man or other animals and which is not dependent upon being metabolized for the achievement of any of its primary intended purposes." https://www.fda.gov/AboutFDA/Transparency/Basics/ucm211822.htm

**Medical monitor** A sponsor representative who has medical authority for the evaluation of the safety aspects of a clinical trial. CDISC

**Medicines and healthcare products regulatory agency (MHRA)** The UK government agency responsible for ensuring that medicines and medical devices work, and are acceptably safe. [MHRA] CDISC

**Megatrials** Massive trials that test the advantages of therapeutic interventions by enrolling 10,000 or more subjects. Synonym: large sample trials. CDISC

**Memorandum of understanding (MOU)** A formal agreement between the Food and Drug Administration (FDA) and federal, state, or local government agencies; academic institutions; and other entities. NOTE: The MOU constitutes an understanding between the parties but is a non-binding agreement. It is FDA's policy to enter into MOUs with other entities whenever there is a need to define lines of authority or responsibility, or to clarify cooperative procedures. CDISC

**Message (Hl7)** The atomic unit of data transferred between systems. It comprises a group of segments in a defined sequence. Each message has a message type that defines its purpose. NOTE: For example, the Admission, Discharge and Transfer (ADT) Message type is used to transmit portions of a patient's ADT data from one system to another. In HL7, a three-character code contained within each message identifies its type. [HL7] CDISC

**Meta-analysis** The formal evaluation of the quantitative evidence from two or more trials bearing on the same question. NOTE: This most commonly involves the statistical combination of summary statistics from the various trials, but the term is sometimes also used to refer to the combination of the raw data. [from ICH E9 Glossary] CDISC

**Metabolism** The biochemical alteration of substances introduced into the body. metadata. Data that describe other data, particularly XML tags characterizing attributes of values in clinical data fields migration. The act of moving a system or software product (including data) from an old to new operational environment in accordance with a software quality system. [ISO/IEC/IEEE12207:1995 §5.5.5] CDISC

**Missing data** 1. Data not completed or corrupted in reports and case report forms. 2. Particularly the data not captured when a subject withdraws from a trial. NOTE: Reviewers are concerned about missing data (meaning 2) since patients who are not improved or who believe they have experienced side effects may be particularly prone to leave a trial, thus skewing the analysis of results if such analysis were to be done only on the subjects who had continued with the trial. Trial designs therefore specify plans for how such missing data will be treated in analysis. CDISC

**Mode** The most frequently occurring value in a data set. CDISC

**Model** A formal structure for representing and analyzing a process such as a clinical trial or the information pertaining to a restricted context (e.g., clinical trial data). CDISC

**Monitor** Person employed by the sponsor or CRO who is responsible for determining that a trial is being conducted in accordance with the protocol and GCP guidance. NOTE: A monitor's duties may include but are not limited to helping to plan and initiate a trial, assessing the conduct of trials, and assisting in data analysis, interpretation, and extrapolation. Monitors work with the clinical research coordinator to check all data and documentation from the trial. [from ICH E6, 5.18] See also clinical research associate. CDISC

**Monitoring** The act of overseeing the progress of a clinical trial and of ensuring that it is conducted, recorded, and reported in accordance with the protocol, standard operating procedures (SOPs), good clinical practice (GCP), and the applicable regulatory requirement(s). [ICH E6 Glossary] CDISC

**Monitoring report** A written report from the monitor to the sponsor after each site visit and/or other trial-related communication according to the sponsor's SOPs. [ICH] CDISC

**Monitoring visit** A visit to a study site to review the progress of a clinical study and to ensure

protocol adherence, accuracy of data, safety of subjects, and compliance with regulatory requirements and good clinical practice guidelines. [from ICH E6, 5.18] multicenter study. See multicenter trial. CDISC

**Multicenter trial** Clinical trial conducted according to a single protocol but at more than one site and, therefore, carried out by more than one investigator. [ICH E9 Glossary] Synonym: multicenter study. CDISC

**NCI enterprise vocabulary services (EVS)** Provides resources and services to meet NCI needs for controlled terminology, and to facilitate the standardization of terminology and information systems across the Institute and the larger biomedical community. CDISC

**New drug application (NDA)** An application to FDA for a license to market a new drug in the United States.

**New safety information** With respect to a drug, information derived from a clinical trial, an adverse event report, a postapproval study, or peer-reviewed biomedical literature; data derived from the postmarket risk identification and analysis system (REMS); or other scientific data regarding: (a) a serious risk or unexpected serious risk associated with use of the drug since the drug was approved, since the REMS was required or last assessed (b) the effectiveness of the approved REMS for the drug obtained since the last assessment of such strategy. [After 21 CFR, Part 505-1(b)] CDISC

**n-of-1 study** A trial in which an individual subject is administered a treatment repeatedly over a number of episodes to establish the treatment's effect in that person, often with the order of experimental and control treatments randomized. CDISC

**Nonclinical study** Biomedical studies not performed on human subjects. [ICH E6 Glossary] CDISC

**Not approvable letter** An official communication from FDA to inform a sponsor of a marketing application that the important deficiencies described in the letter preclude approval unless corrected. CDISC

**Null hypothesis** The assertion that no true association or difference in the study outcome or comparison of interest between comparison groups exists in the larger population from which the study samples are obtained. NOTE: A null hypothesis (e.g., "subjects will experience no change in blood pressure as a result of administration of the test product") is used to rule out every possibility except the one the researcher is trying to prove, and is used because most statistical methods are less able to prove something true than to provide strong evidence that it is false. The assertion that no true association or difference in the study outcome or comparison of interest between comparison groups exists in the larger population from which the study samples are obtained. See also research hypothesis [from AMA Manual of Style]. CDISC

**Nuremberg code** Code of ethics, set forth in 1947, for conducting human medical research. CDISC

**Objective** The reason for performing a trial in terms of the scientific questions to be answered by the analysis of data collected during the trial. NOTE: The primary objective is the main question to be answered and drives any statistical planning for the trial (e.g., calculation of the sample size to provide the appropriate power for statistical testing). Secondary objectives are goals of a trial that will provide further information on the use of the treatment. CDISC

**Objective measurement** A measurement of a physiological or medical variable such as blood glucose level that is obtained by a measuring device rather than a human judgment or assessment. CDISC

**Observational studies, also called "uncontrolled studies"** A type of study in which subjects are observed without interference (There is no control of any variables.) and data are recorded, based on what is seen and heard.

**Observer assessment** An assessment of patient condition made by an observer (investigator, nurse, clinician, family member, etc.). NOTE: Distinguished from self-assessment. The observer relies on his or her judgment to assess the subject. An interviewer simply capturing subject self assessments is not making an observer assessment. CDISC

**Open-label study** A trial in which subjects and investigators know which product each subject is receiving; opposite of a blinded or double-blind study. CDISC

**Open to enrollment** The status of a study such that a subject can be enrolled into that study. NOTE:

Registry terminology in common use is "open to recruitment"; however, recruitment can begin upon IRB approval of the site; whereas enrollment requires availability of study supplies, subject informed consent, etc., to allow participation of eligible subjects. CDISC

**Operational model** The set of CDISC data standards (including ODM and LAB) used to capture and archive data from clinical trials.

**Opinion** (in relation to independent ethics committee). The judgment and/or the advice provided by an independent ethics committee. [ICH E6 Glossary] CDISC

**Origin** 1. Source of information collected in the course of a clinical trial. Specifically used to differentiate between data collected at point of patient contact and data that are derived or calculated. 2. (SDTM) A metadata attribute defined for each dataset variable in the "Define" document of an SDTM submission that refers to the source of a variable (e.g., CRF, derived, sponsor defined, PRO, etc.). [1. CONSORT Statement. 2. from SDTM for descriptions of the Define document] CDISC

**Original data** The first recorded study data values. NOTE: FDA is allowing original documents and the original data recorded on those documents to be replaced by copies provided that the copies have been verified as identical in content and meaning. (See FDA Compliance Policy Guide 7150.13). CDISC

**Outcome (of adverse event)** Refers to the resolution of an adverse event. NOTE: Often denoted using a pick list from a controlled terminology such as Recovered/resolved, recovering/resolving, not recovered/not resolved, recovered/resolved with sequelae, fatal, or unknown. [SDTM Events class of observation] CDISC

**Outcome** 1. Events or experiences that clinicians or investigators examining the impact of an intervention or exposure measure because they believe such events or experiences may be influenced by the intervention or exposure. CDISC

**Outliers** Values outside of an expected range. CDISC

**Packaging** The material, both physical and informational, that contains or accompanies a marketed or investigational therapeutic agent once it is fully prepared for release to patients and/or subjects in clinical trials. CDISC

**Pairing** A method by which subjects are selected so that two subjects with similar characteristics (e.g., weight, smoking habits) are assigned to a set, but one receives Treatment A and the other receives Treatment B. See also matched-pair design. CDISC

**Parallel trial** Subjects are randomized to one of two or more differing treatment groups (usually investigational product and placebo) and usually receive the assigned treatment during the entire trial. Synonyms: parallel group trial, parallel design trial. CDISC

**Parameter** A variable in a model, or a variable that wholly or partially characterizes a probability distribution (mathematics and statistics). CDISC

**Participant** A live human being who enrolls in a clinical trial. Also known as a subject or patient.

**Password aging** A practice applying to multiuser computer systems where the validity of a password expires after a certain preset period. NOTE: FDA requires that passwords that are part of electronic signatures be "periodically checked, recalled or revised," but does not mandate password aging. [After NIST, 21 CFR 11] CDISC

**Patient** Person under a physician's care for a particular disease or condition. NOTE: A subject in a clinical trial is not necessarily a patient, but a patient in a clinical trial is a subject. See also subject, trial subject, healthy volunteer. Although often used interchangeably as a synonym for subject, a healthy volunteer is not a patient. CDISC

**Patient-reported outcome (PRO)** Information coming directly from patients or subjects through interviews or self-completed questionnaires or other data capture tools such as diaries about their life, health condition(s), and treatment. CDISC

**Performed activity** Clinical trial events as they actually occurred (as compared with events planned in the protocol). CDISC

**Per-protocol analysis set** The set of data generated by the subset of subjects who complied with the protocol sufficiently to ensure that these data would be likely to exhibit the effects of treatment according to the underlying scientific model. [ICH E9] CDISC

**Permanent data** Data that become or are intended to become part of an electronic record in relation to a regulatory submission. NOTE: Any changes made to such permanent data are recorded via an audit trail so that prior values are not obscured. CDISC

**Pharmacodynamics** Branch of pharmacology that studies reactions between drugs and living structures, including the physiological responses to pharmacological, biochemical, physiological, and therapeutic agents. CDISC

**Pharmacoeconomics** Branch of economics that applies cost-benefit, cost-utility, cost-minimization, and cost-effectiveness analyses to assess the utility of different pharmaceutical products or to compare drug therapy to other treatments. CDISC

**Pharmacogenetics** Study of the way drugs interact with genetic makeup or the study of genetic response to a drug. CDISC

**Pharmacogenetic test** An assay intended to study interindividual variations in DNA sequence related to drug absorption and disposition or drug action. Compare to pharmacogenomic test CDISC

**Pharmacogenomic test** An assay intended to study interindividual variations in whole genome or candidate gene maps, biomarkers, and alterations in gene expression or inactivation that may be correlated with pharmacological function and therapeutic response. Compare to pharmacogenetic test. CDISC

**Pharmacogenomics** Science that examines inherited variations in genes that dictate drug response and explores the ways such variations can be used to predict whether a person will respond favorably, adversely, or not at all to an investigational product. CDISC

**Pharmacokinetics** Study of the processes of bodily absorption, distribution, metabolism, and excretion (ADME) of medicinal products. CDISC

**Pharmacology** Science that deals with the characteristics, effects, and uses of drugs and their interactions with living organisms. CDISC

**Pharmacovigilance** Term used for adverse event monitoring and reporting. CDISC

**Phase** One in a set of successive stages in a progression or sequence such as 1. a step in the progression of a therapy from initial experimental use in humans to postmarket evaluation. 2. a stage in the conduct of a clinical trial. NOTE: Clinical trials are generally categorized into four (sometimes five) phases. A therapeutic intervention may be evaluated in two or more phases simultaneously in different trials, and some trials may overlap two different phases. For meaning 1, see Phase 0–5. For meaning 2, see epoch. CDISC

**Phase 0 study** First-in-human trials, in a small number of subjects, that are conducted before Phase 1 trials and are intended to assess new candidate therapeutic and imaging agents. The study agent is administered at a low dose for a limited time, and there is no therapeutic or diagnostic intent. NOTE: FDA Guidance for Industry, Investigators, and Reviewers: Exploratory IND Studies, January 2006 classifies such studies as (early in) Phase 1. NOTE: A Phase 0 study might not include any drug delivery but may be an exploration of human material from a study (e.g., tissue samples or biomarker determinations). [Improving the Quality of Cancer Clinical Trials: Workshop Summary—Proceedings of the National Cancer Policy Forum Workshop, Improving the Quality of Cancer Clinical Trials (Washington, DC, Oct 2007)] CDISC

**Phases of clinical trials** Clinical trials are conducted in "phases." The trials at each phase have a different purpose and help researchers answer different questions. NIH

- *Phase I trials*—An experimental drug or treatment in a small group of people (20–80) for the first time. The purpose is to evaluate its safety and identify side effects. NIH Phase 1 trials can run for several months. FDA
- *Phase II trials*—The experimental drug or treatment is administered to a larger group of people (100–300) to determine its effectiveness and to further evaluate its safety. NIH Phase 2 trials can run for several months to 2 years. FDA
- *Phase III trials*—The experimental drug or treatment is administered to large groups of people (1,000–3,000) to confirm its effectiveness, monitor side effects, compare it with standard or equivalent treatments. NIH Phase 3 trials can run for 1 to 4 years. FDA
- *Phase IV trials*—After a drug is licensed and approved by the FDA researchers track its safety, seeking more information about its risks, benefits, and optimal use. NIH There is no time constraint on Phase 4 trials from the FDA.

**Pilot study, pilot project, or pilot experiment** A small-scale preliminary study conducted in order to evaluate feasibility, time, cost, adverse events, and effect size (statistical variability) in an attempt to predict an appropriate sample size and improve upon the study design prior to performance of a full-scale research project. Wikipedia (not considered a great source, but it offers the best definition found.) Pilot studies can be run before different types of studies.

**Placebo** A pharmaceutical preparation that does not contain the investigational agent. In blinded studies, it is generally prepared to be physically indistinguishable from the preparation containing the investigational product. CDISC

**Postmarketing commitment (PMC)** Studies and clinical trials that applicants have agreed to conduct, but that will generally not be considered as meeting statutory purposes (see postmarketing requirement) and so will not be required. CDISC

**Postmarketing requirement (PMR)** FDA-required postmarketing studies or clinical trials. [FDAAA; 21 CFR Part 314, Subpart H; 21 CFR Part 601, Subpart E] CDISC

**Postmarketing surveillance** Ongoing safety monitoring of marketed drugs. CDISC

**Pragmatic trial** Term used to describe a clinical study designed to examine the benefits of a product under real world conditions. CDISC

**Preclinical studies** Animal studies that support Phase 1 safety and tolerance studies and must comply with good laboratory practice (GLP). NOTE: Data about a drug's activities and effects in animals help establish boundaries for safe use of the drug in subsequent human testing (clinical studies or trials). CDISC

**Pre-Market approval application (PMA)** An application to FDA for a license to market a new device in the United States. CDISC

**Prepublication review** A Sponsor's assessment of an Investigator's Study results' manuscript or abstract (at a specified timeframe) prior to submission for publication. Martien

**Primary completion date** The date that the last participant in a clinical study was examined or received an intervention and that data for the primary outcome measure were collected. Whether the clinical study ended according to the protocol or was terminated does not affect this date. National Institutes of Health Clinical Trial Glossary

**Primary objective** The primary objective(s) is the main question to be answered and drives any statistical planning for the trial (e.g., calculation of the sample size to provide the appropriate power for statistical testing). [ICH E6 6.3] CDISC

**Primary variable** An outcome variable specified in the protocol to be of greatest importance to the primary objective of the trial, usually the one used in the sample size calculation. CDISC

**Principal investigator** A Principal Investigator is a doctor who leads the clinical research team and, along with the other members of the research team, regularly monitors study participants' health to determine the study's safety and effectiveness. NIH

**PROMIS** NIH-sponsored project for the development and evaluation of PRO item banks and computer adaptive testing for pain, fatigue, physical function, social function, and emotional well-being. [NIH]

**Proprietary name** A commercial name granted by a naming authority for use in marketing a drug/device product. [SPL] Synonyms: trade name, brand name.

**Prospective study** Investigation in which a group of subjects is recruited and monitored in accordance with criteria described in a protocol.

**Protocol** A document that describes the objective(s), design, methodology, statistical considerations, and organization of a trial. The protocol usually also gives the background and rationale for the trial, but these could be provided in other protocol referenced documents. Throughout the ICH GCP Guideline, the term protocol refers to protocol and protocol amendments. NOTE: Present usage can refer to any of three distinct entities: 1) the plan (i.e., content) of a protocol, 2) the protocol document, and 3) a series of tests or treatments (as in oncology). [ICH E6 Glossary] CDISC

**Protocol amendment(s)** A written description of a change(s) to or formal clarification of a protocol. [ICH E3] CDISC

**Protocol approval (sponsor)** Sponsor action at the completion of protocol development that is marked when the signature of the last reviewer on the protocol approval form has been obtained, signifying that all reviewer changes to the protocol have been incorporated. NOTE: Approval by the sponsor usually initiates secondary approvals by IRBs, regulatory authorities, and sites. Protocol amendments usually also require a cycle of approval by sponsor and study staff prior to taking effect. CDISC

**Protocol deviation** A variation from processes or procedures defined in a protocol. Deviations usually do not preclude the overall evaluability of subject data for either efficacy or safety, and are often acknowledged and accepted in advance by the sponsor. NOTE: Good clinical practice recommends that deviations be summarized by site and by category as part of the report of study results so that the possible importance of the deviations to the findings of the study can be assessed. Compare to protocol violation. [See ICH E3] CDISC For example, a subject has a visit outside of a time window

**Protocol identifying number** Any of one or more unique codes that refers to a specific protocol. NOTE: There may be multiple numbers (Nat'l number, coop group number). [PR Project; eudraCT] CDISC

**Protocol violation** A significant departure from processes or procedures that were required by the protocol. Violations often result in data that are not deemed evaluable for a per-protocol analysis, and may require that the subject(s) who violate the protocol be discontinued from the study. Compare to protocol deviation CDISC for example, use of an unapproved medication, or the inclusion or exclusion criteria are determined to not have been met.

**Psychometrics** The science of assessing the measurement characteristics of scales that assess human psychological characteristics. CDISC

**Psychometric validation** The specialized process of validating questionnaires used in outcomes research to show that they measure what they purport to measure. CDISC

**p-value** Study findings can also be assessed in terms of their statistical significance. The p-value represents the probability that the observed data (or a more extreme result) could have arisen by chance when the interventions did not differ. CDISC

**Quality assurance (QA)** All those planned and systematic actions that are established to ensure that the trial is performed and the data are generated, documented (recorded), and reported in compliance with good clinical practice (GCP) and the applicable regulatory requirement(s). [ICH] CDISC

**Quality control (QC)** The operational techniques and activities undertaken within the quality assurance system to verify that the requirements for quality of the trial related activities have been fulfilled. [ICH] CDISC

**Quality of life** A broad-ranging concept that incorporates an individual's physical health, psychological state, level of independence, social relationships, personal beliefs, and their relationships to salient features of the environment. CDISC

**Query** A request for clarification on a data item collected for a clinical trial; specifically, a request from a sponsor or sponsor's representative to an investigator to resolve an error or inconsistency discovered during data review. CDISC

**Query management** Ongoing process of data review, discrepancy generation, and resolving errors and inconsistencies that arise in the entry and transcription of clinical trial data. CDISC

**Query resolution** The closure of a query usually based on information contained in a data clarification. CDISC

**Random number table** Table of numbers with no apparent pattern used in the selection of random samples for clinical trials. CDISC

**Random sample** Members of a population selected by a method designed to ensure that each person in the target group has an equal chance of selection. CDISC

**Randomization** The process of assigning trial subjects to treatment or control groups using an element of chance to determine the assignments in order to reduce bias. CDISC

**Raw data** Data as originally collected. Distinct from derived. Raw data includes records of original observations, measurements, and activities (such as laboratory notes, evaluations, data recorded by automated instruments) without conclusions or interpretations. Researcher's records of subjects/patients, such as patient medical charts, hospital records, X-rays, and attending physician's notes. CDISC

**Recruitment (investigators)** Process used by sponsors to identify, select, and arrange for investigators to serve in a clinical study. CDISC

**Recruitment (subjects)** Process used by investigators to find and enroll appropriate subjects (those selected on the basis of the protocol's inclusion and exclusion criteria) into a clinical study. CDISC

**Recruitment target** Number of subjects that must be recruited as candidates for enrollment into a study to meet the requirements of the protocol. In multicenter studies, each investigator has a recruitment target. CDISC

**Registry** A data bank of information on clinical trials for drugs for serious or life-threatening diseases and conditions. NOTE: The registry should contain basic information about each trial sufficient to inform interested subjects (and their healthcare practitioners) how to enroll in the trial. [FDAMA 113]

**Registry study** A data collection study.

**Reliability, psychometric** The degree to which a psychometric "instrument" is free from random error either by testing the homogeneity of content on multi-item tests with internal consistency evaluation or testing the degree to which the instrument yields stable scores over time. NOTE: Reliability pertains to questions concerning whether an instrument is accurate, repeatable, sensitive. CDISC

**Research hypothesis** The proposition that a study sets out to support (or disprove); for example, "blood pressure will be lowered by [specific endpoint] in subjects who receive the test product." CDISC

**Result synopsis** The brief report prepared by biostatisticians summarizing primary (and secondary) efficacy results and key demographic information. CDISC

**Retrospective** Looking back on or dealing with past events or situations.

**Retrospective data collection** Data that are gathered from medical charts from past visits.

**Risk** In clinical trials, the probability of harm or discomfort for subjects. CDISC

**Role** 1. The function or responsibility assumed by a person in the context of a clinical study. Examples include data manager, investigator. 2. Classifier for variables that describe "observations" in the SDTM. Role is a metadata attribute that determines the type of information conveyed by an observation-describing variable and standardizes rules for using the describing variable. [1. HL7. 2. SDTM] See also functional role. CDISC

**Routine costs (of a clinical trial)** All items and services that are otherwise generally available to Medicare beneficiaries. CMS

**Safety** Relative freedom from harm. In clinical trials, this refers to an absence of harmful side effects resulting from use of the product and may be assessed by laboratory testing of biological samples, special tests and procedures, psychiatric evaluation, and/or physical examination of subjects. CDISC

**Safety and tolerability** The safety of a medical product concerns the medical risk to the subject, usually assessed in a clinical trial by laboratory tests (including clinical chemistry and hematology), vital signs, clinical adverse events (diseases, signs, and symptoms), and other special safety tests (e.g., ECGs, ophthalmology). The tolerability of the medical product represents the degree to which overt adverse effects can be tolerated by the subject. [ICH E9] CDISC

**Sample size** 1. A subset of a larger population, selected for investigation to draw conclusions or make estimates about the larger population. 2. The number of subjects in a clinical trial. 3. Number of subjects required for primary analysis. CDISC

**Sample size adjustment** An interim check conducted on blinded data to validate the sample size calculations or reevaluate the sample size. CDISC

**Schedule of activities** A standardized representation of planned clinical trial activities including interventions (e.g., administering drug, surgery) and study administrative activities (e.g., obtaining informed consent, distributing clinical trial material and diaries, randomization) as well as assessments. CDISC

**Screen failure** A consented subject for a trial who does not pass one or more tests in the screening visit. Martien

**Screening (of sites)** Determining the suitability of an investigative site and personnel to participate in a clinical trial. CDISC

**Screening (of subjects)** A process of active consideration of potential subjects for enrollment in a trial. CDISC

**Screening trials** Trials conducted to detect persons with early, mild, and asymptomatic disease. CDISC

**Secondary variable** The primary outcome is the outcome of greatest importance. Data on secondary outcomes are used to evaluate additional effects of the intervention. [CONSORT Statement] See also outcome, endpoint. CDISC

**Sequential analysis** In statistics, sequential analysis or sequential hypothesis testing is statistical analysis where the sample size is not fixed in advance. Instead data are evaluated as they are collected, and further sampling is stopped in accordance with a predefined stopping rule as soon as significant results are observed. Thus, a conclusion may sometimes be reached at a much earlier stage than would be possible with more classical hypothesis testing or estimation, at consequently lower financial and/or human cost. www.wikipedia.org

**Serious adverse event (SAE)** An adverse event or suspected adverse reaction is considered "serious" if, in the view of either the investigator or sponsor, it results in any of the following outcomes: Death, a life-threatening adverse event, inpatient hospitalization or prolongation of existing hospitalization, a persistent or significant incapacity or substantial disruption of the ability to conduct normal life functions, or a congenital anomaly/birth defect. 21 CFR 312.32 (a) See Chapter 4 Section 4 for more information.

**Side effect** Any effect of a drug, chemical, or other medicine that is in addition to its intended effect, especially an effect that is harmful or unpleasant. www.dictionary.com

**Single-blind study** A study in which one party, either the investigator or the subject, does not know which medication or placebo is administered to the subject; also called single-masked study. CDISC

**Site investigator** A person responsible for the conduct of the clinical trial at a trial site. If a trial is conducted by a team of individuals at a trial site, the investigator is the responsible leader of the team and may be called the principal investigator. [ICH E6 1.35. 2.] CDISC

**Source** 1. The specific permanent record(s) upon which a user will rely for the reconstruction and evaluation of a clinical investigation. 2. Sometimes used as shorthand for source documents and/or source data… records… that provide the information underlying the analyses and findings of a clinical investigation. CDISC

**Source data** All information in original records and certified copies of original records of clinical findings, observations, or other activities in a clinical trial necessary for the reconstruction and evaluation of the trial. Source data are contained in source documents (original records or certified copies). [ICH E6; CSUCT] CDISC

**Source data verification** The process of ensuring that data that have been derived from source data accurately represent the source data. CDISC

**Source document verification** The process by which the information reported by an investigator is compared with the source records or original records to ensure that it is complete, accurate, and valid. CDISC

**Source documents** Original documents, data, and records (e.g., hospital records, clinical and office charts, laboratory notes, memoranda, subjects' diaries or evaluation checklists, pharmacy dispensing records, recorded data from automated instruments, copies or transcriptions certified after verification as being accurate copies, microfiches, photographic negatives, microfilm or magnetic media, x-rays, subject files, and records kept at the pharmacy, at the laboratories, and at medicotechnical departments involved in the clinical trial). See also eSource document, source, original data, certified copy. [ICH; CSUICI] CDISC

**Sponsor** 1. An individual, company, institution or organization responsible for initiating and managing a clinical trial; it may or may not be the main funding body Segen's Medical Dictionary 2012 2. An individual or an organization providing the financial backing for a clinic, hospital, medical mission, professorship, or research study. Medical Dictionary 2009 Farlex and Partners

**Sponsor investigator** An individual who both initiates and conducts, alone or with others, a clinical trial and under whose immediate direction the investigational product is administered to, dispensed to, or used by a subject. NOTE: The term does not include any person other than an individual (i.e., it does not include a corporation or an agency). The obligations of a sponsor-investigator include both those of a sponsor and those of an investigator. [21 CFR 50.3f] [ICH] CDISC

**Standard** Criterion or specification established by authority or consensus for 1. measuring performance or quality; 2. specifying conventions that support interchange of common materials and information. CDISC

**Standard deviation** Indicator of the relative variability of a variable around its mean; the square root of the variance. CDISC

**Standard of care** In legal terms, the level at which the average, prudent provider in a given community would practice. It is how similarly qualified practitioners would have managed the patient's *care* under the same or similar circumstances. www.medicinenet.com

**Statistical analysis plan** A document that contains a more technical and detailed elaboration of the principal features of the analysis described in the protocol, and includes detailed procedures for executing the statistical analysis of the primary and secondary variables and other data. [ICH E9] statistical method. The particular mathematical tests and techniques that are to be used to evaluate the clinical data in a trial. [ICH E9; from the Center for Advancement of Clinical Research] CDISC

**Statistical significance** An interpretation of statistical data that indicate that an occurrence was probably the result of a causative factor and not simply a chance result. Statistical significance at the 1% level indicates a 1 in 100 probability that a result can be ascribed to chance. Mosby's Medical Dictionary, 9th edition

**Stopping rules** A statistical criterion that, when met by the accumulating data, indicates that the trial can or should be stopped early to avoid putting participants at risk unnecessarily or because the intervention effect is so great that further data collection is unnecessary. CDISC

**Study completion date** The date that the final data for a clinical study were collected because the last study participant has made the final visit to the study location (i.e., "last subject, last visit") National Institutes of Health Clinical Trial Glossary.

**Study coordinator** See clinical research coordinator. CDISC

**Study data tabulation model (SDTM)** SDTM provides a standard for organizing and formatting data to streamline processes in collection, management, analysis, and reporting. CDISC

**Study design** A plan that delineates the precise procedures to be followed in a clinical trial, including planned and actual timing of events, choice of control group, method of allocating treatments and blinding methods. The study design assigns a subject/patient to one or more epochs during the trial. Segen's Medical Dictionary 2012

**Subinvestigator** Any member of a clinical trial team—for example, associate, resident, research fellow—who is supervised by the investigator at a trial site and allowed to perform critical trial-related procedures and/or to make key trial-related decisions. Segen's Medical Dictionary 2012

**Subject identification code** A unique identifier assigned by the investigator to each trial subject to protect the subject's identity and used in lieu of the subject's name when the investigator reports adverse events and/or other trial-related data. [ICH] CDISC

**Subject/trial subject** An individual who participates in a clinical trial, either as recipient of the investigational product(s) or as a control. [ICH] CDISC

**Subject-reported outcome (SRO)** An outcome reported directly by a subject in a clinical trial. CDISC

**Surrogate marker** A measurement of a drug's biological activity that substitutes for a clinical endpoint such as death or pain relief. CDISC

**Survey** Any means (e.g., questionnaire, diary, interview script, group of items) that is used to collect PRO data. NOTE: Survey refers to the content of the group of items and does not necessarily include the training and scoring documents generally not seen by respondents. CDISC

**Syntactic** The order, format, content of clinical trial data and/or documents as distinct from their meaning. CDISC

**Termination (of trial)** Premature discontinuation of a trial prior to plan. CDISC

**Treatment trials** Test new treatments, new combinations of drugs, or new approaches to surgery or radiation therapy. NIH

**Trial monitoring** Oversight of quality of study conduct and statistical interim analysis. [ICH E9] trial site. Synonym for investigative site, investigator site, site, site of the trial, study site. [ICH E6] CDISC

**Triple-blind study** A study in which knowledge of the treatment assignment(s) is concealed from the people who organize and analyze the data of a study as well as from subjects and investigators. CDISC

**Type 1 (or type i) error** Error made when a null hypothesis is rejected but is actually true. Synonym: false positive. CDISC

**Type 2 (or type ii) error** Error made when an alternative hypothesis is rejected when it is actually true. Synonym: false negative. CDISC

**Type 3 (or type iii) error** Some statisticians use this designation for an error made when calling the less effective treatment the more effective one. CDISC

**Types of clinical research**
- *Diagnostic trials*—Determine better tests or procedures for diagnosing a particular disease or condition. NIH
- *Natural history studies*—Provide valuable information about how disease and health progress. NIH
- *Prevention trials*—Look for better ways to prevent a disease in people who have never had the disease or to prevent the disease from returning. NIH
- *Quality-of-life trials*—(or supportive care trials) Explore and measure ways to improve the comfort and quality of life of people with a chronic illness. NIH
- *Screening trials*—Test the best way to detect certain diseases or health conditions. NIH

**Variance** A measure of the variability in a sample or population. It is calculated as the mean squared deviation (MSD) of the individual values from their common mean. In calculating the MSD, the divisor n is commonly used for a population variance and the divisor n-1 for a sample variance. CDISC

**Verification** 1. The act of reviewing, inspecting, testing, checking, auditing, or otherwise establishing and documenting whether items, processes, services, or documents conform to specified requirements. 2. (of software). Provides objective evidence that the design outputs of a particular phase of the software development life cycle meet all of the specified requirements for that phase. CDISC

**(Study) Visit** An appointment for specified tests, tasks or/and procedures to be performed within a specific time range for a study as specified in the protocol. Martien

**Vulnerable subjects** Individuals whose willingness to volunteer in a clinical trial may be unduly influenced by the expectation, whether justified or not, of benefits associated with participation, or of a retaliatory response from senior members of a hierarchy in case of refusal to participate. Examples are members of a group with a hierarchical structure, such as medical, pharmacy, dental, and nursing students, subordinate hospital and laboratory personnel, employees of the pharmaceutical industry, members of the armed forces, and persons kept in detention. Other vulnerable subjects include patients with incurable diseases, persons in nursing homes, unemployed, or impoverished persons, patients in emergency situations, ethnic minority groups, homeless persons, nomads, refugees, minors, and those incapable of giving consent. ICH GCP E6

**Witness or impartial** Witness a person, who is independent of the trial, who cannot be unfairly influenced by people involved with the trial, who attends the informed consent process if the subject or the subject's legally acceptable representative cannot read, and who reads the informed consent form and any other written information supplied to the subject. ICH GCP E6 R2

# Index

Note: Page numbers followed by "*f*" indicate figures, and "*t*" indicate tables.

Printed in the United States
By Bookmasters